Drama, Psychotherapy and Psychosis

Drama, Psychotherapy and Psychosis explores the use of drama and theatre with people who hear voices, focusing especially on survivors of abuse and those diagnosed as suffering from schizophrenia. In examining the often baffling and frightening world of psychosis the book offers alternative models of madness and the self, which form the basis for therapeutic interventions.

Illustrated by case histories and practical examples, the book includes chapters covering:

- Historical perspectives on psychosis and hearing voices
- Individual psychodrama
- Dramatherapy with groups

Drama, Psychotherapy and Psychosis demonstrates how creative action methods can be helpful to those who hear voices. It provides guidelines for good practice, essential to all those interested in promoting the safe use of these methods in therapy.

John Casson is a psychotherapist and supervisor in private practice, and is a senior trainer in the Northern School of Psychodrama. He works part-time as a psychodrama psychotherapist and dramatherapist at the Bowness High Dependency Unit (NHS), Prestwich Hospital, Manchester, UK. He has also written a full length play, 'Voices and Visions', based on his research with people who hear voices.

Drama, Psychotherapy and Psychosis

Dramatherapy and psychodrama
with people who hear voices

John Casson

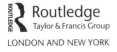 Routledge
Taylor & Francis Group

LONDON AND NEW YORK

First published 2004
by Routledge
27 Church Road, Hove, East Sussex BN3 2FA

Simultaneously published in the USA and Canada
by Routledge
711 Third Avenue, New York NY 10017

Routledge is an imprint of the Taylor & Francis Group, an Informa business

Typeset in Times by Keystroke, Jacaranda Lodge, Wolverhampton
Paperback cover design by Jim Wilkie

British Library Cataloguing in Publication Data
A catalogue record for this book is available from the British Library

Library of Congress Cataloging in Publication Data
Casson, John Witham.
  Drama, psychotherapy and psychosis / John Casson.
     p. cm.
Includes bibliographical references and index.
  ISBN 1-58391-804-3 (hbk. : alk. paper) — ISBN 1-58391-805-1 (pbk. :
alk. paper)
  1. Psychodrama. 2. Psychoses—Treatment. 3. Auditory
hallucinations—Treatment. I. Title.

  RC489.P7C37 2004
  616.89'1523—dc22

                            2003019633

ISBN 978-1-58391-805-0 (pbk)

This book is dedicated
with love, gratitude and admiration to my sister,
Mrs Lesley Austin SRN

Contents

Illustrations and figures

Foreword

With this book John Casson has undertaken an ambitious task: to cover the field of mental illness, especially as expressed in the phenomenon of hearing voices. He has produced a first-class exhaustive volume on a topic which has been largely neglected in psychiatric literature when compared to that dealing with other symptoms. He also reminds us that hearing voices does not by itself indicate mental illness and that many creative beings, Socrates among them, as well as psychiatrists have themselves admitted to such experiences. In many instances these voices have been a source of inspiration. But there are others, not so productive, and these are what the author has dedicated himself to treat.

Dr Casson brings to our attention that the treatment of insanity and hearing voices goes far back, that it has a history in shamanism, poetry, literature, philosophy, theology, music and art. It is fairly safe to surmise that the history is actually a good deal older than we know since there are no records that point us to even more distant origins. Regrettably, in our time, with the advent of biological psychiatry, psychotherapy has largely been relegated to non-psychiatrists. It is among the ranks of those that the most daring practitioners have recently been active, psychiatrists now being in the minority. But it was they originally who first undertook the direct approach to the mentally ill. Now John Casson has undertaken the detailed task of researching all the pioneers who brought their energy and inventiveness to this area of their concern. His special focus is on the ways in which patients who hear voices can be treated and what have been the results of these interventions, including those of his own.

From J. L. Moreno, I learned that we can think of the role player as having three component parts: the director, the one that tells us what to do as 'Get up, it's time to get started'; the actor is the second part, it gets up and does what it has to do; the third part is the observer, which can be a positive or a negative force, as 'You're dawdling and you're going to be late', or 'Well done.' It is my observation that in the psychotic experience the director and observer temporarily drop away and the actor takes over. I believe the other two are burnt up in 'the white heat of action'. It is part of the therapeutic function to restore these two parts within the patient. They are essential to the wholeness of the person but they have to be reorganised into positive structures. The voices may be an autonomous attempt by patients to reconstruct themselves. Regrettably, they appear largely as critics and add to the confusion.

Having assisted J. L. Moreno in his work with patients in psychodrama, I will always be grateful for the learning obtained in this practice; it has been the basis for understanding what suffering human beings experience while struggling to find their way back into the world at large and to feel humble when some of them are successful. Being in the function of doubling with them and expressing some of these voices has opened up an entirely new series of vistas of being. I particularly recall two different approaches to patients for whom Moreno appointed me as their auxiliary ego. One was a young schizophrenic who in psychodrama introduced us to his family. According to his presentation, his wife and twelve children were always with him in bed. When surrounded by this loving family, he heard the voice of God. Showing us the role of God in role reversal he whispered benign, soothing messages. I then took over that whispering voice and the patient listened with his eyes closed and a smile of heavenly bliss on his face. As this was a demonstration session in a mental hospital abroad, Moreno could do no more than recommend a further treatment programme for him, but this had been the first time the patient had so opened up. We were not kept informed as to the follow-up treatment but I went away with a question in my heart: 'Why would he want to get well if in his current state he had such a blissful relationship with his maker? Could in such a case treatment only disturb his equilibrium further?' That strikes me as a very pertinent question in therapy. Either therapy must give the patient something of equal value as what they are giving up, or else it leads to great disillusionment.

The second example involved the case of a young woman who fell severely ill immediately after her child's birth. She was mute, catatonic and obviously boiling with rage within. Her hands were balled into tight fists and the nurses had to massage them open daily as well as keep them open with large bandages so she would not lose their function. We found out later that the rage was directed at her husband for not being the mate she had expected him to be, but that discovery came after she had again found speech and faced him with his failure in psychodrama. Because of her profound muteness, Moreno appointed several of his staff members to be the voices the patient could not utter, by only making sounds, no words were to be spoken. I chose to scream and did so from my guts for as long and hard as I could, while others produced different sounds. The patient listened and her face became more mobile, losing some of its formerly frozen mask. I had the best endorsement for my sound from a student who had been called to the telephone outside of our theatre, as Moreno started the session. The student entered the theatre and was coming down the backstairs where he could not see the proceedings. But he reported to us that as he heard my voice he told himself: 'Ah, Judy is screaming, how wonderful.' He regretted to see it was only an auxiliary ego, but the session bore fruit anyway. A few days later Moreno conducted a session in which Judy was watching a nurse carrying 'her baby' (actually a pillow) to hell to be taken care of by the devil, because according to Moreno's dictum out loud: 'A child without a mother is in hell anyway.' This psychodramatic shock therapy hit its mark. Judy started to scream as I had done, this time stop-watched by Moreno, who told us not to interfere, and for almost ten minutes. Judy's body relaxed for the very first time and she began to speak a day or two later.

John Casson's book is a most valuable and inspiring resource and he is to be congratulated for having made his work available to us. He also hopes it will encourage others to venture into this field which is filled with question marks and challenges.

Zerka T. Moreno, Charlottesville, VA, USA

Introduction

This book is the result of six years' doctoral research into dramatherapy and psychodrama as psychotherapeutic interventions with people who hear voices and eighteen years' experience as a therapist. It is based on my PhD thesis (Casson, 2002). That research, while building on the work of previous therapists and researchers, was ground-breaking because there had not been previous focused research into what people who heard voices found helpful or not helpful in dramatherapy and psychodrama. I present some of the research findings, though I do not present all the material in the thesis to ensure this book is not overly academic: readers who wish to know more can apply to the university for the thesis or to me for a copy on CDRom (email: joncassun@beeb.net). I see this book then as a starter, hoping that it will inspire other therapists and researchers to follow up the insights I have gathered, to the eventual benefit of voice hearers and the development of creative action methods in psychotherapy.

The research in brief

The research was carried out between 1996 and 2000 in two adjacent National Health Service (NHS) psychiatric services: over the years I gradually received a total of forty-two referrals. Just half of those referred, twenty-one people – nine women (aged 24–44) and twelve men (aged 20–50) – completed an assessment of six sessions and chose to enter the study, taking up offers of individual or group therapy. Six (four women and two men) were offered forty-four sessions of individual therapy. Another woman was offered forty sessions of individual therapy. Three men who were waiting for a group were given seventeen sessions of individual therapy. (All individual therapy was in weekly one-hour sessions.) There were three groups (twenty weekly sessions of up to two hours' duration) offered sequentially: a men's group and two mixed gender groups. Two men chose to attend two groups (of these, one man dropped out of the second group) and one woman chose to join a group after her individual therapy had ended. The low dropout rate (one woman and three men) suggests that the long and careful assessment had built up a sufficient therapeutic alliance to sustain the person through the therapy. Not counting assessment sessions, the research comprised 349 individual therapy sessions and 60 group sessions (340 client sessions).

In the first period of the research the participants met periodically in a group to discuss the work and express their opinions. In the second period of the research participants were interviewed by research assistants before, during and at the end of therapy to ascertain their opinions as to what was helpful or not helpful in dramatherapy and psychodrama. A questionnaire was also devised and completed in final follow-up interviews. For the study I was not able to gather the opinions of those who dropped out, except in one case, so the results of the study are based on the opinions of eighteen people.

The following description of the characteristics of the participants reveals the diversity of the study.

Age and ethnic diversity

Age (at time of entry into the research) ranged from 20 to 50: six in their twenties, ten in their thirties, four in their forties and one aged 50.

The participants included one African, one south-east Asian, one Asian, one half-Jewish, one descendant of Second World War Ukrainian immigrants, one half-Spanish adopted at birth by British couple: all of these had experienced the impact of racism. Three experienced the dislocation of being refugees from violent political upheaval; they had survived terrorism and genocide.

Diagnoses

- Schizophrenia: five women, two men (including two survivors of rape, three of sexual abuse, one of physical abuse)
- Paranoid schizophrenia: five men, two women (including two survivors of sexual abuse, two of physical abuse)
- Depression: two women, one man (one survivor of rape, two of physical abuse, one of sexual abuse)
- Paranoid psychosis: two men (one survivor of physical abuse, one of bullying)
- Drug induced psychosis: one man, one woman (both survivors of physical abuse)
- Organic psychotic illness: one man (survivor of physical abuse)
- Personality disorder: two women (both survivors of rape, one of sexual abuse)
- 'Neurotic with voices' (originally diagnosed schizophrenic when 21): one man (bullied).

Several had more than one diagnosis. Two people did not have any diagnosis of a mental illness: both were survivors of abuse. Once diagnosed with a mental illness, other elements of a person's experience, such as experiences of childhood physical or sexual abuse, may not be attended to; however, there is evidence to suggest that hearing voices is a response to traumatic experiences (Romme and Escher, 2000: see Chapter 2). It is therefore relevant to consider the incidence of trauma in the participants' lives.

Experiences of trauma

- Survivor of sexual abuse as a child: seven women
- Survivor of rape as an adult: two women, two men
- Survivor of physical abuse as a child: five men, two women
- Survivor of bullying as a child or young person: three men.

There were many other traumas: the death of siblings, assaults, head injuries, near-death experiences, witnessing murder, other losses and the traumas of mental illness. There were also traumas in the parents' and grandparents' lives.

It is possible, even likely, that there were some traumas that were not disclosed: in the case of two men I had some evidence that they had been sexually abused, but they did not disclose. Abuse may be disguised in psychotic/dissociative experiences, for example one woman said she had a three-way split in her personality:

- the white side of treacle (she mentioned an overpowering teacher)
- her bad self 'Twat'
- herself now.

She said she felt 6 years old: she didn't want to be, she wanted to be grown up, but she could not or would not remember nor let me know her secret. I did not insist that she tell me: the symbolism of a sticky white substance and the words she used seem thinly veiled references to sexual abuse. Her sexualised behaviour as a child may also be relevant evidence. She said that she carried a secret, which her father also carried, which was unspeakable, which she would keep forever. One of her voices told her not to speak: 'he' made her words disappear. The issue of not being able to speak will be further explored in Chapter 6.

The presentation of material in this book

Verbatim quotations from clients are used throughout. These are taken from taped research interviews, journals and clinical notes. I have obtained permission for the use of these quotations. Whenever I have used a transcription of the actual words of a participant I have put their words in a different font. When there are words in ordinary type or in parentheses these are not their actual words but my paraphrase. When there are three dots (. . .) it means that there is a break in the record or change to another interview: I have omitted hesitations, repetitions, deviations or statements by the interviewer. I have also edited quotations, cutting out phrases that do not address the point I am illustrating. I have punctuated the speech as I saw fit. I have not corrected grammar or spelling in entries from people's journals. When I have wanted to emphasise words I have *italicised* them, or in the transcripts, printed them in bold.

Confidentiality

To protect the confidentiality of those who took part in the research I have changed names and possible identifying details. All names are fictitious. Those names in **bold** were participants in my research, other names not in bold were clients in my private or NHS practice: all have given permission for me to refer to their work. When I have needed to further ensure someone's anonymity I have written, 'One man/woman said . . . '. I have also used other appropriate ways to conceal the identity of clients. I have not altered any of the verbatim statements of people's opinions except for names that might identify someone. I have used details about their lives only in order to illustrate the points I am making and where possible I have disguised these, without, I hope, losing the essence of the person's experience.

An outline of the book

In Chapter 1, 'Psychosis and hearing voices 1: a historical perspective', I look back over the history of hearing voices, psychosis and psychotherapy beginning with shamanism. I explore whether psychotic experience has meaning or not and provide a brief survey of some relevant literature on psychotherapy with people diagnosed as schizophrenic.

In Chapter 2, 'Psychosis and hearing voices 2: making sense of voices', I introduce the Hearing Voices Network and the work of Professor Marius Romme. I provide a description of the voices that people hear based on an analysis of my research findings.

In Chapter 3, 'Psychosis and hearing voices 3: models of madness', I consider the medical, biopsychosocial, dimensional, psychodramatic models of madness, definitions of psychosis, and explore different realities. I present a new environmental model of the development and process of psychosis.

In Chapter 4, 'Theatre, madness and healing', I review the phenomenon of hearing voices in theatre from shamanism, via Shakespeare and Goethe, to twentieth-century texts. I examine the history of healing through theatre, introduce J. C. Reil and sketch the development of theatre therapy at the dawn of psychotherapy.

In Chapter 5, 'The twentieth century: theatrotherapy, psychodrama and dramatherapy', I provide a history of the development of these creative action methods and a survey of relevant literature on their use with people who hear voices or have a diagnosis of schizophrenia. I provide definitions of dramatherapy and psychodrama; note the research recently carried out into the value of the creative arts for people with mental distress and other methods that use action in psychotherapy. I introduce the issues of distance and safe practice.

Chapter 6, 'Dramatherapy with individuals: finding a voice and telling stories', explores the difficulty of being able to speak and how in dramatherapy people can be empowered through voice work. I describe methods of assessment and ways of ensuring that practice is safe for vulnerable clients. I describe projected play, especially the use of miniature objects including toy theatre. I introduce the Five Story Self Structure. I explore the empowerment of clients through enactment and role play.

In Chapter 7, 'The wave and the whelm: distance and empowerment', I tell the story of the emergence of significant theory underpinning safe practice of dramatherapy and psychodrama in the value of distancing techniques. I apply distance theory to psychosis.

In Chapter 8, 'Individual dramatherapy: Cheryll', I describe the therapy of one woman using many dramatherapy methods in 156 sessions over three and a half years.

In Chapter 9, 'The theatre model of the self', I offer a theory of the self that can inform clinical practice, offering the therapist a template metaphor to contain the many possible aspect of self.

In Chapter 10, 'Group dramatherapy', I describe my practice of dramatherapy in groups of people who hear voices and have psychotic experiences, in both out-patient and in-patient settings. I explore embodiment, projected and role play including voice work, work with text and video. I reflect on the value of structure.

In Chapter 11, 'Individual psychodrama: Harry', I offer a description of the therapy of one man using psychodrama over 44 sessions.

In Chapter 12, 'Group psychodrama', I describe group sociodramas and psychodramas exploring voices, dreams and one case of an obsessional rumination. I consider the core psychodrama methods of warm-up, doubling, mirroring, role reversal, concretising, future projection (behavioural rehearsals), auxiliary work and the use of coloured lights. I also give examples of catharsis. I consider the value of spontaneity and creativity.

In Chapter 13, 'What is helpful and not helpful in dramatherapy and psychodrama', I reveal the research results, the participants' opinions of these creative action methods, which are the evidence base from which I am then able to offer the following chapter's guidelines.

Finally in Chapter 14, 'Guidelines for good practice', I offer a summary of theoretical and practical approaches to safe, effective dramatherapy and psychodrama with people who hear voice and struggle with psychotic experiences.

The case for dramatherapy and psychodrama

My aim in this book is not to claim that dramatherapy and psychodrama are superior to other therapies. I do make a case for them to be regarded as effective methods and to be offered alongside other ways of working such as cognitive behavioural therapy (CBT: see Chadwick et al., 1996; Haddock and Slade, 1996) and art therapy (Killick and Schaverien, 1997) so that the client has a choice. As Hogman and Sandamas (2000: 7) conclude: 'Positive outcomes are increased if people are informed about their choices, allowed to choose and given their choice.'

It is clear to me from the findings of my research that voice hearing is multifactoral and therefore needs a flexible multidimensional response. While some voice hearers continue to point to spiritual explanations of voice hearing it is hardly surprising that in the rational culture of university-based research and NHS psychiatry and psychology, CBT has gained such pre-eminence. Dramatherapy and psychodrama incorporate many ways of working and offer different perspectives, including the spiritual dimension (see Grainger, 1995; Lindqvist, 1994): these creative action methods have an important contribution to make to services.

Acknowledgements

I am grateful to the following who have helped me write this book: Ms Di Adderley, Dr Anne Bannister, Mr Francis Batten, Dr Elspeth Campbell, Dr Chris Farmer, Mr John Harris, Ms Cynthia Lees (Oldham Libraries), Ms Hazel McKay, Dr Alan Tait, Ms. Janet Tolan, Mr Nick Totton, Ms Barbara Tregear, Ms Morag Williams (Crichton Museum), Dr Guy Undrill.

Photographs by Stonehouse Graphic Design and Photography

Figure 1 computerised by Mr Ben Pitman

Figure 2 drawn by Mr Andy Smith

I am grateful to Faber and Faber Ltd for permission to quote from Alan Ayckbourn's play *Woman in Mind* (in Chapter 4).

I also thank the people who hear voices who worked with me during the research. I am grateful to my university tutors, Dr Bill Campbell and Dr Paul Wilkins; my psychotherapy supervisor Ms Jan Costa; Dr Alistair Stewart, consultant psychiatrist; the North West Regional Health Authority for funding the clinical work; the Manchester Metropolitan University's Centre for Human Communication for funding the academic work; and the many colleagues who have supported me through the years of the research.

Chapter 1

Psychosis and hearing voices 1

A historical perspective

Prehistory

Hearing voices is an ancient and widespread human experience. From time immemorial shamans and mediums have heard the voices of spirits and relayed their messages to audiences. Voices thus became a source of culture. The gods spoke to humankind, giving guidance (Watkins, 1998: 35). Jaynes (1990) in a study of the *Iliad* and the *Odyssey* analysed the nature of the voices of the gods and suggested that in the ancient world, voice hearing was a normal way that people made important decisions. Voice hearers have found his book helpful.

Creative action methods of healing have been used in individual therapy and community ceremonies for thousands of years by the shamans, who enacted dramatic encounters with 'demons' and rescued the lost soul of the patient (Casson, 1979, 1984; Eliade, 1989). In the early 1990s,

> a range of shamanic techniques have been successfully employed in treating people in a community mental health centre. Interestingly, approximately two-thirds of the clients with long histories of troublesome auditory hallucinations have reported experiencing immediate relief as a result.
>
> (Watkins, 1998: 58, referring to Eshowski, 1993)

The historical context

In the west, over the past 2,000 years, hearing voices became a sign of divine or demonic visitation. Many saints and religious leaders, including Jesus, Mary his mother, John the Baptist, Muhammad, St Francis, Joan of Arc, John Bunyan, St Teresa of Avila and Meister Eckhart, heard voices (Watkins, 1998: 30). These people drew inspiration from their voices which they regarded as profoundly meaningful. The voices were, for them, a calling: 'what Jung called vocation' (Romme and Escher, 1993: 59). As the dominance of the church in matters of the soul (psyche) gave way to the rise of psychiatry, hearing voices came to be seen as a symptom of mental illness. Nevertheless religious, creative and political leaders including Schumann, Swedenborg, Mahatma Gandhi, Martin Luther King and Simone de Beauvoir continued to hear voices and draw inspiration from them. The founders of psychoanalysis (Freud), analytic psychology (Jung) and group psychotherapy and psychodrama (Moreno, see Chapter 5) all heard voices (Nettle, 2001: 93; Watkins, 1998: 27, 30–31; Fox, 1987: 212). These examples of the inspirational guidance of voice hearing show there are positive aspects to the experience that need not be reduced to pathology. However, until recently the experience of hearing voices was regarded as probably pathological, indeed as a 'first rank symptom' of schizophrenia.

A short history of schizophrenia and therapy

Reil (1759–1813, see Chapter 4), Heinroth (1773–1843), Ideler (1795–1860) and Newmann (1814–1884) emphasised the psychogenesis of mental illness, the symbolic meaning of certain symptoms, and the possibility of the psychotherapy of psychosis (Ellenberger, 1994: 729). Dr Eugen Bleuler (1857–1939) introduced the term 'schizophrenia' in 1908.

> The word schizophrenia – splitting of the mind – stresses the dissociation of psychic functions (associations), which to Bleuler was the feature common to a group of heterogeneous psychoses.
>
> (Ellwood, 1995: 24)

Bleuler was a humane man who treated his patients as people and witnessed their struggles and recoveries. His son Manfred (1903–1994), who also became a psychiatrist, considered

> his father's main contribution to the problem of schizophrenia was to favour the study of what was going on psychodynamically in a schizophrenic patient, and so to create a basis for a psychotherapeutic and psychosocial approach.
>
> (Ellwood, 1995: 25)

Interestingly, Eugen Bleuler encouraged his children 'to take part in theatricals' with patients (Ellwood, 1995: 24). Manfred observed that

> Some of the patients who hardly ever uttered coherent sentences started to speak or behave as if they were healthy on certain occasions, for instance, when on leave, at hospital festivities.
>
> (Bleuler, 1978: 633)

After a lifetime of study of schizophrenia Manfred stated that there was insufficient evidence for either the dopamine hypothesis or any somatic, metabolic or genetic causation. He suggested that many life experiences, particularly those connected with members of the patient's family, played a role in the development of schizophrenia (Shepherd, 1982). A psychosis developed when the conflict between the patient and his/her social environment became *overwhelming*: the patient then denied realistic experience and logical thinking to inhabit a world of phantasy. In Manfred Bleuler's view effective treatment of schizophrenics included clear and steady personal relations, activity, interests, responsibility, appropriate risk taking and relaxation. He considered that the same influences which developed the healthy ego were the main therapy for the split ego. From this therapeutic experience he argued in favour of the assumption that schizophrenia developed in the same spheres as the normal human personality.

However, such was the criticism directed against Eugen Bleuler's first psychological theory of psychosis by the German psychiatric establishment that as a consequence, from 1913 onwards, Bleuler began to move away from Freud and closer to organic psychiatry (Ellwood, 1995).

Road blocks

While some theories of psychology and therapy enable us to move forward, other theories can become road blocks. Freud and Ferenczi both considered the possibility of the pathogenesis of psychosis in sexual abuse (Masson, 1992). Freud wrote that childhood sexual trauma was symbolised in the symptoms of psychosis: that what appeared unintelligible was meaningful and pointed back to the original reality (see Masson, 1992: 117). Freud subsequently abandoned this 'seduction' theory. He also came to the conclusion that psychosis could not be treated by psychoanalysis (a view proved correct by later researchers, as we shall see). Freud's abandonment of the 'seduction' theory in favour of his idea of infantile sexual fantasy led to a generation of therapists not believing what their clients told them. It is necessary therefore to go back to the people who are actually hearing voices and, bracketing our preconceived ideas, listen to what they have to tell us (see Chapter 2). There are, however, the road blocks to be negotiated. The massive structure of ideas about schizophrenia has actually obscured the real experiences of people (Read, 1997). The hearing of voices has become stigmatised as a symptom of mental illness to such an extent that people keep such experiences secret for fear of being labelled mad, hospitalised and their medication increased.

Psychosis: meaning or meaninglessness?

Perry outlined the orthodox view:

> A valuation of the symbolic imagery of psychotic individuals is often denied under the prevailing 'medical model' which views such imagery as 'either meaningless primary process atavism or, if not meaningless, at least without therapeutic import'.
>
> (Perry 1974: 15)

The Bleulers' views, however, were confirmed by Mollon:

> The fundamental dissociation in schizophrenic states often does seem to correspond to the process of 'decathexis' originally described by Freud (1911). This is the fateful break with reality, the withdrawal of psychic interest from the world, and the subsequent creation of an alternative delusional world . . . The 'decathexis' of reality then places part of the mind in a state akin to the withdrawal from the external world during sleep, resulting in dreams, which display thought processes that carry no respect of reality. Whilst dreaming the schizophrenic person is still awake – hence the interweaving of rational and dreamlike thought in this state of mind.
>
> (Mollon 1996: 10)

This suggests that just as therapists work with dream material as meaningful it may be possible to work with such dreamlike psychotic material (Casson, 1999b; see also Chapters 9 and 12 in this volume). Many psychotherapists have regarded psychotic experience as meaningful (see Eigen, 1993: 15; Young, 1995: 40). Jung worked alongside Eugen Bleuler with people struggling with psychotic experiences and developed many of his ideas concerning the collective unconscious and archetypes from what they told him. Jung believed that auditory hallucinations were an exaggerated form of the dialogue, necessary for healthy living, between different voices in the psyche. Jung developed active imagination to facilitate a dialogue between different personified aspects of the psyche (the complexes and archetypes). He used creative methods including painting, dance and play-writing, where different personalities, each one representing a different voice from the author's psyche, argued for what they want (Newham, 1993: 66). This is just what Snow (1996: 229), a dramatherapist, did with a psychotic client (see Chapter 5).

A polarity then developed between biological psychiatry that regarded psychosis as the result of biochemical processes in the brain (and so not meaningful) and psychotherapists who believe it is possible to work psychologically with psychotic experience. Nevertheless, some psychiatrists do take a wider view, for example:

> An alternative approach to primary process material is taken by such psychiatrists as Grof (1986, 3–4) who articulates: 'the new understanding of psychosis as a potentially healing and transforming process' in which the mythic imagery is of great potential value in therapy.
>
> (Snow, 1996: 216; see also Perry, 1974; Eigen, 1993: 134; Thomas, 1997: 170, 181)

Following in the footsteps of Jung, Snow went on to show how psychotic material is mythic, dramatic, and follows archetypal, ancient ritual processes. Perry (1974:

145) described how the arts can help guide the patient towards reintegration: creative expression giving form to the phases in the self's transformation.

Johnson, a dramatherapist, further stated:

> The nature of the drama, with its tolerance of the unreal and the imaginative, entices the inner self of the schizophrenic, which is occupied in fantasy, to reveal some part of itself. The patient finds he can explore with some freedom, the various fragments of himself while, at the same time, actualising them for others. In this way, the inner self makes contact with the world, and the individual's fantasies become part of objective existence.
>
> (Johnson 1981: 60)

This is exactly Moreno's original discovery in the 1930s (see Chapter 5): that enacting the psychotic material enabled the protagonist to move gradually from pathological fantasy to social reality. It is however contrary to orthodox psychiatric practice which attempts to suppress voices with medication, denies that psychotic material has any meaning and would regard such practice as potentially dangerous.

Psychotherapy with people diagnosed as schizophrenic

Roth and Fonagy's (1996) review of the research literature on the effectiveness of psychotherapy goes some way to explain why therapy is *not* usually offered to people struggling with psychotic experiences. In their chapter on schizophrenia they report on studies which show some benefits from social skills training groups and cognitive behavioural therapy. Furthermore, CBT research has shown positive benefit for voice hearers (Haddock and Slade, 1996; Chadwick *et al.*, 1996). Martindale *et al.* (2000: 39) reported on CBT studies that did reduce or eliminate delusions and hallucinations in people with schizophrenia (Bouchard *et al.*, 1996). On the other hand Roth and Fonagy (1996) point to studies which show positive harm or no benefit from psychodynamic – expressive psychotherapy, though they report some benefit from supportive therapy. They do not, however, mention hearing voices, auditory hallucinations or dramatherapy. Of particular significance is their report on the value of social skills training which included modelling, rehearsal and role play. However, although some studies demonstrated benefit there is 'rather limited evidence of positive impacts [and] only a modest degree of generalisation of skills' (Roth and Fonagy, 1996: 191). They concluded that the benefit of social skills training remained to be demonstrated.

In contrast Wallace and Liberman (1985) did indicate a modest advantage for the social skills training. Furthermore Hogarty *et al.* (1986) reported that social skills training was effective in reducing the relapse rate below that found in patients who received only maintenance pharmacotherapy. It was seen as just as effective as family therapy and most effective when combined with the latter. However, the effects of social skills training alone faded in the subsequent follow-up year. Bellack's (1984) controlled clinical trial of social skills showed that at the end of a twelve-week treatment programme there were

> few differences in clinical state or social skills, but at 6 month follow-up, participants in the social skills training group were rated as significantly more improved clinically in their retention of the social skills. However, very disappointing was the finding that 50% of the patients in each group relapsed subsequently and had to be rehospitalised, indicating that social skills training had little impact on this very negative outcome.
>
> (Goldstein, 1991: 121)

However, Goldstein did not state what factors had led to relapse. Breggin (1993) reported on studies that confirm the efficacy of psychotherapy for individuals diagnosed as schizophrenic.

> Patients who received psychotherapy as compared to those receiving medication showed less thought disorder . . . spent less time in hospital . . . these effects became more marked the longer the patients were followed, and psychotherapy proved to be less costly in the long run.
>
> (Karon and VandenBos, 1981: 371)

Later Karon and VandenBos (cited in Fisher and Greenberg, 1989; Breggin, 1993: 482) stated that the optimal treatment for a schizophrenic is psychotherapy and that the conclusion that schizophrenic patients must be treated with medication, whatever else is done, is based on poorly designed studies. Goldstein (1991) however advised that effective psychotherapy with schizophrenic patients must operate within a problem solving model to assist the patient to deal with day-to-day problems of living. Furthermore Chadwick warned:

> psychosis is a lot to do with excessively seeing meanings and significance in things, even in such trivialities as a man dropping his newspaper . . . talk about 'the profound significance of things' was extremely counter-therapeutic and mentally loosening. I do not think that many psychodynamically oriented professionals realise this.
>
> (Chadwick, 1997: 147–148)

These views seem to be borne out by further research. Drake and Sederer (1986) reported that intensive treatment of chronic schizophrenia through exploratory, insight-oriented psychotherapy (at least three times a week) conducted by experienced analysts had negative outcomes: 50 per cent dropped out, spent more time in hospital, were less likely to return to function in the community, and within two years, five people committed suicide. In contrast those receiving supportive psychotherapy once a week did improve. Fairweather et al. (1960) found that hospitalised chronic psychotic patients deteriorated when given intensive psychoanalytic psychotherapy several times a week. Controls, who were given support and rehabilitation, improved (cited in Drake and Sederer, 1986). Truax (1963) found that schizophrenic patients who were given empathy, positive regard and a relationship with a therapist who presented himself as real, tended to improve, whereas those who got low levels of support and more interpretative work tended to get worse (cited in Drake and Sederer, 1986).

After these and other studies cast doubt on the value of psychoanalytic and psychodynamic psychotherapy for people diagnosed as schizophrenic (Grinspoon *et al.*, 1972), a major two-year randomised controlled trial contrasted expressive insight oriented psychotherapy (EIO) with reality adaptive psychotherapy (RAS) (Stanton *et al.*, 1984). This was a complex and thorough study. The insight oriented therapy was psychoanalytic, expressive, looking at present and past, at relationships, feelings and meanings. The reality adaptive therapy was less intense, focused on present and future, encouraged more positive experiences, ego strengthening activities and coping strategies. RAS was found to be more effective than EIO (Stanton *et al.*, 1984). There are many things that can be learned from this study including the difference in therapist styles of relating: RAS therapists were more active, self-revealing, problem solving. Therapist style may well be as important as technique:

> The therapist . . . should . . . make contact with the frightened patient, to reassure him, and to provide for basic needs such as safety and sustenance. This relationship needs to be respectful and, in particular, to respect the patient's **need for distance and need to regain some sense of mastery**.
> (Drake and Sederer, 1986: 316 added emphasis)

A therapeutic environment, they suggest, should provide a moderate amount of stimulation and take into account the person's need for structure and clarity. They advised therapists to be active, offer support and focus on problem solving and develop social skills. **'Above all self-esteem must be protected'** (Drake and Sederer, 1986: 317 added emphasis).

None of these studies, into individual, group or social skills interventions, mentions any effect of the treatment on voice hearing. These studies seem to indicate that a treatment that combined structured, supportive psychotherapy with social skills training can be more effective for people with a diagnosis of schizophrenia. Dramatherapy seems then to fit the bill.

In order to offer therapy to people who hear voices and/or struggle with psychotic experiences, therapists need to have some understanding of those experiences and by carefully listening to clients, learn from them. In the next chapter we do just that: hearing their voices as we seek a way forward.

Chapter 2

Psychosis and hearing voices 2

Making sense of voices

The Hearing Voices Network

New thinking about auditory hallucinations was prompted by a patient (Patsy Hage) who was able to voice her distress and challenge her psychiatrist (Dr Marius Romme), who *listened* and *heard* what she said (James, 2001: 31). She changed his life and the lives of countless others: the result was the Hearing Voices Network, established from 1987, by Dutch and British voice hearers and mental health workers (Romme and Escher, 1993). This self-help organisation has encouraged new thinking about the experience of hearing voices, resulting in research and the discovery of self-help and coping strategies. Patsy has since recovered and no longer hears voices (Voices, 2002; Hage, 2003: 3). Romme and his team in the Netherlands and Ivan Leudar at Manchester University (Leudar and Thomas, 2000) have discovered that two-thirds of people who hear voices cope well and do not need psychiatric care (Romme, 2001: 7). While Slade and Bentall (1988), Tien (1991), Eaton *et al.* (1991), Romme and Escher (1993), Watkins (1998) and Leudar and Thomas (2000) have shown that hearing voices is a human experience shared by many 'normal' people – about 2–3 per cent of the population according to Romme (2001) and 4–5 per cent according to Tien (1991) – only about 1 per cent are in receipt of psychiatric services. Thus hearing voices *per se* cannot now be regarded as necessarily a symptom of mental illness but a variety of human experience. People who hear voices are *not* all the same, indeed they are as heterogeneous as the general population. They are individuals and just as it is not very meaningful to suggest that all people who are gay are the same, so it is not helpful to think of people who hear voices as one class (Romme, 1998: 54). As already stated in Chapter 1, some people who hear voices have been great religious leaders and artists. Others are healers, actors, workers, children, deaf people, psychiatric patients and professionals. Hearing voices and other hallucinatory experiences are found across diagnostic categories and in the 'normal' population. *Not all people who hear voices are psychotic.* For some, voices are not problematic: voices can be helpful advisers as well as unhelpful persecutors.

> The difference between patients hearing voices and non-patients hearing voices, is their relationship with the voices. Those who never became patients

accepted their voices and use them as advisers. In patients however voices are not accepted and seen as evil messengers.

(Romme, 2001: 7)

Many voice hearing experiences have been found to start after a traumatic or stressful experience. It is the negative, persecutory voices that are the problem and the attitude the person takes to their voices. One man heard friendly voices but was terrified that they were evil witches trying to drive him mad (Haddock, 1995: 6). The person's attitude to the voices may be as important as the voices themselves (Romme, 1998: 53). There's a world of difference between believing your voices are a gift that can help you and believing they are the symptoms of an incurable illness. Romme's research found the following differences between those who coped with their voices and those who did not cope:

Copers	Non-copers
Feel stronger than voices;	Feel weaker . . .
Can ignore voices;	Less able to ignore . . .
More likely to listen selectively to voices;	Less likely to listen selectively . . .
Set more limits to voices;	Afraid/unable to set limits . . .
Experience more positive/helpful voices;	Experience voices as negative . . .
Feel supported by others;	Feel alone, unsupported . . .
Communicate re voices;	Communicate with others less . . .

(Romme and Escher, 1993: 15)

The copers are interacting with the voices and others: they are in relationship to *self and other*. The non-copers are less able to relate, more isolated and tend to be *overwhelmed*. Furthermore Watkins (1998: 109) suggested that some people found the most fruitful and effective coping strategy involved selecting the positive voices and paying close attention to them while at the same time trying to ignore the negative voices. Therapy might aim therefore to enable someone to move from the non-coping to the coping column: out of powerless isolation, through therapeutic relationship, to empowerment.

Romme and Escher (1993) provided a comprehensive survey of different explanations of the phenomenon and many accounts of how people cope. They noted that certain themes are repeated in the different accounts:

1   It is unhelpful to deny the experience: indeed acceptance (of voices and self) is essential to developing a coping strategy. (20, 70, 79, 87, 105, 140, 143, 180)
2   Voices have meaning: discovering the meaning can help someone cope. (25, 155, 162, 180–1, 190)
3   Limits and boundaries must be set. Structure is helpful. (21, 135)

4   People benefit from talking to others, including to the voices. (26, 50–51, 208)
5   Voice hearers must take responsibility and say 'No' to unacceptable suggestions by the voices. (21, 58, 81, 114)
6   Methods that empower, putting the person more in control, are helpful. Conversely powerlessness is unhelpful. (53, 132, 142–3, 176, 187, 199–243)
7   Negotiate with or refuse the negative; listen to the positive. (161)

(Romme and Escher, 1993)

Romme and Escher (1996) wondered if hearing voices is a survival strategy instead of a symptom of illness. In my research **Diane** said her voices were *a coping mechanism*. People often begin to hear voices at a moment of extreme emotional pain, a time when reality may have seemed almost too difficult to bear (Watkins, 1998; Leudar and Thomas, 2000). Romme and Escher's (1996: 144) research identified certain categories of life influences related to the onset of voices:

- intolerable or unsatisfying living situations
- recent traumas
- aspirations or ideals
- childhood trauma
- emotional intolerance and control.

They assert that discovering these meanings behind the voices can help resolve them:

> Curiosity about the meaning of the voices, and getting more control over them, both help to diminish voice hearing's disabling effects. Children's voices disappear, just as they do for adults, when underlying problems are resolved or integrated. Some voices are triggered by developmental crises, like having to learn to cope with grief, or to make choices in life, or to forge a separate identity . . . normalisation of the voice hearing experience does help. Voices might be a problem, but not every problem is an illness.
>
> (Escher *et al*., 1998: 14)

This has been confirmed in Romme's (2001) study of children in the Netherlands:

> 64% of children's voices disappeared . . . [as they learned] to cope with emotions and became less stressed. In children with whom the voices were psychiatrised and made part of an illness and not given proper attention, voices did not vanish, but became worse, the development of those children was delayed.
>
> (Romme, 2001: 8)

It is useful at this point to reflect on the nature of voices: to consider 'who they are'. From what voice hearers have told me, I am able to offer the following description of different types of voice hearing experiences. This is useful because therapists need to know something of the nature of this experience to enable them to work with people who hear voices (see Slade and Bentall, 1988). I illustrate the description with actual examples of what people have said to me during the research.

The voices

It appears that voices fall into positive, negative and neutral categories; however even apparently benign sounds such as 'whiffs' (**Leah**'s descriptive word for the whispered sounds she heard) can scare and disturb people. I suggest that voices fall into the following categories.

Voices of known people

Voices of known people in the person's past and present environment including parents, relatives, friends, enemies, abusers, neighbours, professionals. For example:

Diane: I know that I can hear my dad in my head . . .

Gloria: I am plagued with my sister-in-law's image and sulky expression; disapproving of my thoughts on any subject about her. I've started hearing her criticism as badly as she used to criticise me in real life. She liked to blame me of something or other, real or unreal. I hate it! Seeing her image before my eyes annoys me and shows me how powerless I am about these voices and hallucinations . . .

Three women heard the voice of their abuser or rapist.

Internal commentators

Internal commentators can be experienced as critics, persecutors, controllers, sometimes commanding self-harm, suicide or violence to others. These are often in relation to the person's self-esteem. For example, **Pat** heard a conversation in my head . . . I'm criticised right, left and centre, that's the voices. The female voice that criticised her behaviour as a mother voiced her guilt about past behaviour, communicated a super-ego standard of 'perfect' parenting from Victorian times and seemed veiled criticism of her own mentally ill mother. **Pat**'s grandfather was a high court judge who criticised her mother as a stupid woman.

Tina: I have asthma and they (the voices) told me to stop taking my steroids so I had an asthma attack. They put me in intensive care on a ventilator.

Anton's voices told him to kill, to cut off his genitals.

This category overlaps with the next; indeed voices seem, like iron filings, to gravitate towards positive or negative poles.

Simon: *One voice was a piss take, take the mickey. The other chap was trying to be helpful . . .*

Jimmy: *Some voices are friendly, some are aggressive. Friendly ones younger, the more antagonistic ones are older.*

Supportive voices

Supportive voices include advisers or reminders, voices which may call the person's name. For example:

Diane: *The voices are real today . . . I like listening to the good people they make me feel secure and wanted and that I have a purpose in life. They say that they love me and that they care about me and I really like them being around, like for example last night . . . the good voices – stopped me from feeling paranoid while I was on the train and up until I met my friend . . . I could ask them all night if they was still there for security . . . Today I felt anxious about going out . . . so the good voices Sue, George, Jeannie and Annie kept me smiling as I was hearing bad voices through the wind and in my ears. So Sandra and Tara told them to fucking shut their mouths so I felt alright but Annie kept making me laugh so I felt like a nutter!! . . . The voices were nice to me last night because they told me beautiful fantasies and they made me relaxed and comfortable . . .*

Gloria: Voices give *a commentary on what I'm doing. Feels intrusive but also sometimes helpful and also controlling . . . sometimes feel a guidance.* This was helpful when she could choose whether to follow the guidance, sometimes exercising choice was a struggle.

Voices of spiritual forces

Voices of 'spiritual forces' include deities, demons, archetypes, characters: real or imaginary figures of power (and therefore possibly linked back to the category of voices of known people). For example:

Dillon identified his voices as British politicians, inter-galactic power figures, Buddhist deities; one voice called 'Cotcrap' was made up of people's excrement and controlled paranoid schizophrenics.

Simon: *Three voices: one female, helpful male, unhelpful male* (of the latter voice:) *he's changed over the years, less difficult now . . . He's dominant . . . military style . . . a prisoner one time was very aggressive.*

Unknown voices

Unknown voices form a distinctive group and are characterised by unidentified whisperers, babblers, gossips, jokers, indistinct noises and music.

Leah didn't want to think of where the voices came from because it frightened her. I used to hear noises from my wee. A noise: dur, dur, dur (like a telephone ringing). Whiffs: an airvent talking to her when there's a strong wind. Nonsense: like another language – can't understand it.

Diane: I was hearing bad voices due to sleep deprivation, through traffic, the shower . . . when I'm stressed up I hear them through water running . . . TV, kettle, microwave, fridge freezer . . .

Gloria heard music before she heard voices.

Overlapping categories

These categories overlap in that a voice might first be identified as a demon and then emerge as a known other such as an abuser or, in **Tina**'s case, her husband.

Tina: I thought they were demons . . . a spiritual thing, but now I know it's not . . . I'm sure it's my mind, my subconscious, doing it . . . I'm learning to understand why (I hear voices). They just kept saying to me at the hospital, 'Are you under a lot of stress?' which I have been, under a bit of stress. But my husband's always said, 'It's me, I'm doing it to you.' I've found out through John that it is him. He's a nagger, he picks and he's gone on at me that much he's done my head in. He's nagged me out of my mind. He's picked and picked and picked. He's lovely and I love him but he's a nuisance. (laughs) . . . I've been with him for 20 years. People have seen the way he is. I knew I couldn't stand being nagged at. My mother nagged at me when I was a kid and I can't stand being nagged at. John asked me something that no one has ever asked me: why do you think these voices are so angry? And all of a sudden I thought, 'Well my husband's angry all the time, he's angry,' so I said, 'That's what my husband's like: he's angry all the time. I do this wrong, I do that wrong, I don't do this and I don't do that and he's always flaring up because there's something not right and that's how the voices are. They're angry at me and critical of me,' so the two went together. They (the voices) tell me I've got to leave him because he's the devil. Every time I hear voices I leave him, because he's the devil.

A critical voice, as in **Gloria**'s case, may be identified as a sister. Such a critic may become supportive, as when **Pat**'s critical voice told her it was stupid to abuse medication (tablets she had bought) so she flushed them down the toilet. Some of the voices are characters, with names, histories and changing natures, others just odd words or noises. Voices can thus be seen as roles, having function and meaning. Nayani and David (1996: 185, 181) discovered that: 'Men and women were more likely to hear male voices. With respect to the reported age, middle-aged voices were more common . . . The next most common being a young adult man' (over twice as common as a young adult female).

As many of the voices are of power figures this seems to reflect the patriarchal structure of our society where, despite women's progress in the past hundred years, men are still dominant. Oppression keeps people suppressed by lowering their self-esteem. Those who do not cope experience voices which were stronger than self and negative (Romme and Escher, 1996: 142).

To further elucidate the voice hearing experience I will now identify certain themes that recur.

Voices and self-esteem

Watkins (1998: 219) pointed out that 'Disturbing voices sometimes begin to disappear spontaneously as a person's self-esteem improves.' Indeed negative voices indicate low self-esteem: as one man said, his voices were related to how I feel bad about myself: the voices of my paranoia. The voices reinforced his low self-esteem by reminding him of things of which he was ashamed. This is confirmed by **Sheila**: I used to hear voices all week, every week, because I had such a low opinion of myself. It has changed . . . I think because I'm feeling a bit better about myself I'm having more positive thoughts than negative thoughts . . . (See p. 21 for a section on voices and thought.)

Voices and stress

Watkins (1998: 16) observed that 'stress of sufficient severity can act as a trigger which will instigate the experience of hearing voices in certain individuals.' There is a relationship between voices, mood and stress levels: the greater the stress, the lower the mood, the more voices a person hears. For example:

Pat: When I'm stressed that's when it's bad.

Diane: I feel either high for five minutes then low for three hours. It's like the voices are tuned in to you . . . They are my worst fears, hopes and even dreams.

In particular many statements people made about their voices concerned the impact of high levels of negative emotion expressed in families. This is in line with previous research (Romme and Escher, 1993; Martindale *et al.*, 2000).

Furthermore, as if in a feedback loop, the voices apparently add to stress levels:

Jimmy: *Voices . . . make me feel aggressive, I get so fed up with the constant bombardment . . .*

There also appears to be a relationship between stress, mood, loneliness and voices as, for example:

Cheryll (speaking of her voices): *depends on the level of depression – when I'm down or stressed, hurt or something goes wrong or alone for a long period . . . When crowded/down they (voices) make things worse.*

It is important to note that stimulating activity alleviates voices, conversely lack of stimulus and isolation seem to exacerbate voices. This has implications in relation to the potential value of creative therapy:

Cheryll: *When I'm stimulated or active I can go through them (voices) without them bothering me.*

Tom: *One funny thing about the voices is why they always come at night time: I'm fine in the day time. I think that might be because I'm with people and I'm keeping active. When you're on your own and quiet anything can happen.*

Anton: *When I'm sat around doing nothing, **if I'm not thinking/concentrating the voices creep in**.*

Voices and thought

Bentall (1990, cited in Romme and Escher, 1993: 171) proposed a cognitive theory, namely that people who hear voices mistake inner thoughts for external stimuli: he and others have developed cognitive models and therapy (Chadwick *et al.*, 1996; Haddock and Slade, 1996). For some in my research, there was a link between thoughts and voices. One man said: *I'm paranoid and the voices express that, they're like **thoughts** . . . critical and referring to past experiences.*

Tina said that after her second marriage to a man who was domineering, *I stopped having my own thoughts and kept my thoughts to myself. I've lost part of my personality.* After therapy she wondered if her voices were her 'evil' thoughts: *what I've noticed . . . sometimes when I'm in bed I'll get **a thought**: and I think, 'Eeee that sounds like my voices: something that my voice would say: **a condemnative thought** about myself.' Two or three times that's happened and I've thought, 'That's funny,' but it just makes it more obvious to me **they are my thoughts**.*

At the end of therapy **Anton** said he was feeling *a lot better actually, I've had a few bad voices but mainly they're just **intrusive thoughts** . . . Less than when we started: (they're) more like thoughts . . . There have been long periods tonight of feeling people are inside me and trying to put **awful thoughts** into my head. They seem to pass through me, these people. For so long I battle mentally with one **thought** from one person. Achieve success, then another one comes along!*

Voices, distraction and concentration

One treatment offered to voice hearers has been distraction: 'any kind of behaviour which serves to take the hearer's mind off the voices' (Romme and Escher, 1993: 211). While some have found this helpful, Haddock and Bentall (1993) were concerned that, although it may have short-term benefits as a coping mechanism, distraction does not address the underlying content of the voices and therefore is unlikely to offer any enduring resolution of the person's difficulties. Distraction may not help the already distracted person. Voices, like intrusive thoughts, are distracting, making concentration, communication and relating difficult: such distraction can create confusion (for voice hearer and therapist) and is an aspect of the controlling influence of voices. For example, **Dillon** said his voices challenged him to concentrate and then distracted him.

Simon: I really don't have much opportunity to mix . . . (Then in response to a question:) Sorry, I missed that: I was trying to concentrate on two things at once: I heard a voice saying something and I missed what you said. (What did the voice say?) Something like 'Maybe'. Also there **may be** people in libraries if I got to know them I might share some interest . . . (Did the dramatherapy we did help people communicate more?) It **may** have done but it's very difficult to assess when you're trying to concentrate on something else like there were people talking and I was occasionally hearing voices and there were lapses in concentration while I thought about things . . .

Jenny said, of her individual therapy, that it could be quite difficult having three (herself, her voice, 'Mr', and the therapist) in the room: Sometimes when I come out Mr goes on and on for hours. 'You've only been saying what I've been telling you, I've told you so; You shouldn't listen; listening to other people just makes you worse.' Here the voice, 'Mr', who was originally her abuser, was attempting to reinforce isolation: isolating the child is a tactic of abusers (Warner, 2000: 39). Abused children have difficulty concentrating.

Voices and boundaries

In order to have a coherent, separate sense of self, we must be able to separate from the other and establish clear boundaries. **Anton** sometimes had difficulty when he felt he was merging with others: Sometimes I'm in my father's body when I was conceived . . . I feel my father's heart attack in my own body . . . He heard voices when confronted with vulnerability or powerlessness and a lack of boundaries, as when his grandmother was ill and when he saw babies. Thomas presented a similar case of Peg, a woman who heard voices in the context of vulnerable children or elderly people who were ill (Leudar and Thomas, 2000: 134). In psychotic experience the boundary between self and other dissolves so the person may feel overwhelmed by the other. **Dillon** said he was not sure of his boundaries: where he began and ended. **Tom** said: There's no boundaries to your imagination. Hallucinations are waking nightmares. The boundaries between phantasy and reality, waking and dreaming are blurred. Unconscious material erupts, spilling over the boundary of consciousness to overwhelm the vulnerable ego.

Voices seem to cross boundaries between people. Bosga (1993) and Watkins (1998) give accounts of people who consider voices to be the result of clairvoyance and extra sensory perception (ESP). My study revealed similar views. For example:

Simon: I have a view it's got ESP connections and psychical . . . There does appear to be some telepathic involvement.

Dillon, **Leah** and **Diane** thought hearing voices was telepathic. **Diane** wondered if she was psychic: she thought this would explain the voices. In fact the voices suggested this to her (though it was originally her father's idea, as we shall see). Without commenting on the possibility of clairvoyance, I noted that this idea could express her need for contact at a safe *distance* and a wish that people could know, without her stating, her needs. Speaking of her isolation she said: it was painful because people couldn't read my thoughts. When, as a small child, she came home one day, with soiled underpants, after being anally raped, her mother did not guess what had happened: perhaps **Diane** had wished her parents could have read her thoughts, guessed her trauma, which was then unspeakable. Her father suggested they were in telepathic communication at the time of her grandfather's death when she had heard a rushing noise and a voice saying, 'Don't be afraid,' the day before, and her father (in another country) said he had heard her voice telling him grandfather had died. The idea of such communication at a *distance* may have comforted them at that time. **Diane**'s experience of abuse combined being catastrophically *underdistanced* from her abusers and *overdistanced* from her parents. I will further examine the issue of distance in Chapter 7.

Voices and abuse

Voices breach boundaries: abuse is also a breach of boundaries. The frequency with which voices are associated with the aftermath of abuse deserves special notice. I know two sisters, one of whom was sexually abused by her father, the other was not. The one who was abused hears voices, the other does not. Romme and Escher (2000) confirmed the prevalence of voice hearing in the aftermath of sexual abuse. Chu and Dill (1990) found that:

> 63 per cent of female inpatients had suffered child abuse and noted the common occurrence in these patients of psychotic symptoms, particularly auditory hallucinations.

> (cited in Read, 1997: 451)

Out of the twenty-one people in my study, fourteen (66.6 per cent) disclosed physical and/or sexual abuse and/or rape.

Diane: I hear (voices that say) that my brother-in-law is going to come up to the house and rape and strangle me. I wish he would then I could knife him in the stomach for abusing me . . . (voices reminded her of details of abuse). One, supposed to be my brother-in-law, said he'd rape me, 'bastard, fuck off, piss off, you're dirty, you smell' . . . I need therapy for the experience of abuse not so much for voices: though they are connected.

In Coleman's (1998) opinion voices are part of the scenario – they re-live the experience of the abuse through the voice.
Harry was physically abused by his father: his voices told him to physically harm himself and attack his son. One woman's voices started when she was raped at 15: she heard the voice of the rapist. Many participants in my study had experiences of being a victim or felt victimised by the voices: **Theo** was bullied as a child and attacked as a young man. He said: (I) sometimes fear people ganging up on me: it's in my mind. I feel victimised . . . The voices can be seen as a re-enactment, as **Tom** said: I'm a victim of the voices now really . . .

In contrast **Diane** saw her voices as helpful and protested in her journal: I DONT WANT TO BE A *VICTIM* ANYMORE I WANT TO BE A SURVIVOR with all the help of my little helpers in my head . . .

The link with abuse throws light on one particular aspect of the voice hearing experience: secrecy and isolation increase the *power* of the voices: disclosure reduces their impact.

Simon: They (voices) want it to be secret, they don't want me to discuss certain things.

Jenny: It's something I've never talked about . . . It was my secret . . . I suppose I was frightened of making it worse, which it did, still does sometimes . . . Yeah I'm not as scared anymore. I think before . . . nobody knew and I felt since I've talked to you about it and you know and P. (social work assistant) knows and K. (community psychiatric nurse – CPN) now knows and T. (husband) knows, doing that has taken away some of its power, well I think so: I'm not alone anymore with it. It were just me and Mr ('Mr' is the voice of her abuser). It was my secret and that were it: I didn't dare tell anybody. Since people do know about Mr the impact is not as (bad).

Warner (2000: 39) has described the tactics of abusers who ensure children keep abuse secret.

Voices, history and illness

Past events, traumatic experiences that have been kept secret, not talked about or sufficiently processed or metabolised by the person or previous generations, are then passed down the generations: it is Schutzenberger's view that it takes two generations of poor communication to create a schizophrenic: 'Analytic therapy of psychotic patients pinpoints that these patients unconsciously express what happened in their mother's life before expressing what has happened in their own' (Schutzenberger, 1998: 32).

Of the twenty-one participants in the study, ten had mothers with mental health problems; one person had both parents mentally ill, two had a mentally ill grandparent and one a mentally ill uncle.

From the above I suggest that participants' psychotic experiences referred to real events in the past. Many of the voices referred to past events: they were often 'out of date'.

Gloria (speaking about her voices): When we oppress ourselves the messages we draw on are often from the past and **out of date**: the here and now is what we must refer to for ourselves.

Grief and loss in a previous generation can be transmitted down a generation. For example, **Sheila** said: Before I was born mother lost two daughters . . . (one at three days, one at three months). Mum would never talk about it . . . Mum didn't express her feelings because of the way Dad treated her. **Sheila** felt 'presences' and used to talk to them. From 3 years old Sheila had an imaginary, invisible friend. This friend would talk to her, keep her company: it was not a problem but a comforting experience. Mum said it was from when I first started talking . . . It used to annoy me Mum: if I was naughty it was my friend: they told me to do it. (This is exactly what happens in Dowie's (1987) play *Adult Child/Dead Child*, see Chapter 4.)

Dillon was interested in history: in fascism, communism and revolution. Some members of his father's family had escaped the Holocaust, others had perished. His grandfather had 'hidden' in a English Protestant family and lost his Jewish identity. His grandfather did not talk about the Holocaust. **Dillon** became ill while at university where he was studying history: he likened his breakdown to the ice-axe murder of Trotsky (who was Jewish). **Dillon** believed the Germans were against him. (See Slade and Bentall (1988: 3) for another example of voice hearing in a man whose mother and girlfriend were from Germany and Holocaust survivors; see also Bloom (1997) about the intergenerational transmission of the effects of the Holocaust.)

In these two examples the theme of not being able to speak again occurs. I further explore this issue in Chapter 6.

Voices, power and control

As the above references to abuse, dysfunction and bullying suggest, in relationships between self and other a central issue is power/control. Slade and Bentall (1988: 24) argued that it was the inability of the person hallucinating to control, modify or stop their voices that is the single most important factor in contributing to fear and distress.

Tina: When the voices are there I have no control.

Ben: spoke of voices, physical – shocking, (I feel) thrown about . . . it causes problems for me/my body . . . I have panic attacks. **It's not up to me** . . . Who's **controlling** me? There are always obstacles: if **I can't help myself**, no one can help me.

I will further explore this issue in subsequent chapters.

The onset of voices

Escher *et al.* (1998) have shown that some children hear voices. If family history and child abuse are important we could expect voice hearing to emerge in childhood. As did **Sheila**, some participants began to hear voices when they were children or adolescent. **Dirk** heard voices from aged 5 or 6; **Anton** first heard voices when he was 12; **Diane** was 16 when, her general practitioner (GP) said, she suffered from an amphetamine psychosis but **Diane** said she'd been hearing voices before taking drugs. At 19 **Dave** tried 'magic mushrooms' and became paranoid. A relationship ended. He became obsessed with this girl and heard her voice. It seems that the emergence of voices here has connections with the isolation of the young person. However, for others voices emerged in adulthood (for example, following rape or a head injury) and here isolation also appears to have a deleterious effect.

Voices and isolation

Leah, after the diagnosis of her psychotic illness, couldn't go out for four months. Such isolation can lead to depression and may exacerbate the voices: indeed the voices may 'people' the loneliness and comfort by their presence. Sensory deprivation can trigger voices (Slade and Bentall, 1988: 30–31). Just as I might switch on the radio when alone, voice hearing may be a creative response to loneliness: the brain generating company! Speaking of his voices **Jimmy** said: sometimes they're quite entertaining . . . it's nice to have company instead of being alone.

This is confirmed by Watkins (1998):

The fact that hallucinations of various kinds may be elicited in many people under conditions of extreme social isolation raises the possibility that people with a psychotic disorder such as schizophrenia who have become largely cut off from the normal social world might experience hallucinatory voices as a result of their sensory isolation alone.

(Watkins, 1998: 19)

Diane said: I do feel lonely and isolated so I don't know whether it's my mind creating voices people . . . I feel so lonely and unwanted . . . I was self-reliant from 13 (mother was ill, father disengaged, **Diane** lonely at school). Her inner world was then populated by voices to offset the outer world of loneliness. During therapy this intrapsychic creativity resulted in the emergence of a new voice who said she was coming to take **Diane** away: in effect to rescue and love her. Thomas also describes the emergence of a new, positive voice during therapy (Leudar and Thomas, 2000: 136). **Diane** described the voices as a substitute family. She complained of not receiving enough support from the psychiatric service: history was repeating itself. Such chronic loneliness starts in childhood: **Cheryll** wrote in her journal: som-how birthdays for me never were parties, deep inside I felt a solitude, I hadn't relationships with children that could support a party . . . I went un-noticed much of the time.

Such feelings of loneliness may be expressed by the voices:

Anton: The voices are voices of loneliness and depression.

Theo heard the voices as soon as he put his key in the door of his flat: they seemed to express and exacerbate his loneliness.

'Eighty per cent said being alone worsened their hallucinations' (Nayani and David, 1996: 180). Many had had experiences of abandonment and rejection, deprivation and neglect. Professionals, including researchers, also repeat this pattern: when asked whether she would take part in the research if invited to do so again **Cheryll** replied: Yes, not sure, I heard of someone who took part in research and then was abandoned (she connected this with Jed, her ex-boyfriend, 'dumping her in the gutter').

Dr R. Marton, psychiatrist, addressing a conference concerned with the well-being of Mordecai Vanunu (a political prisoner in Israel) who has been held in solitary confinement for over ten years, said:

The most common feeling people in solitary confinement have is that of extreme and profound anxiety. Gradually fear and despair take over and the person's mental and physical strength are shattered. The feelings of total abandonment and deep anxiety coupled with the factors of thought disorder and hallucination rapidly put a person into a state of doubt and uncertainty in which they lose their self-confidence, self-esteem and finally lose their identity.

(Marton, reported in *Guardian*, 3 January 1998, p. 2)

Isolation might not just be in a room, but in a culture:

> Pronounced effects have been reported when individuals have been separated by one means or another from their usual social or physical environments, with resulting reports of 'culture shock', the psychoses of language-isolated refugees.
>
> (Haggard, 1964: 443)

A number of people in my research were refugees or from refugee families. **Ben**, who had lost father, mother, grandparents, relatives, his country, language and culture, said, I feel I've lost myself.

In *Isolation and Personality*, Haggard (1964) stated that normal subjects experiencing temporary isolation reported perceptual disturbances such as

> the spontaneous appearance of partial or full-blown visual, auditory, and somatic hallucinations or delusions, color anomalies and distortions of tactual experience, body image and the time sense. Affective disturbances, including spontaneous bursts of such affects as fear, anxiety, and anger, or reactions involving restlessness, boredom, agitation, and a sense of depersonalisation were frequently reported. As for cognitive processes, some subjects reported a rapid disintegration of their ability to attend, concentrate, or think in a directed and sustained manner, to solve abstract problems or even to carry out such simple tasks as serial counting. Instead, they reported that their minds went blank or, if active, were involuntarily filled with emotionally toned and highly personalised images . . . the subjects in these experiments may show any or virtually all of the 'symptoms' which characterise mentally ill patients such as schizophrenics.
>
> (Haggard, 1964: 435)

In these experiments the subjects knew they were being observed and could terminate the experiment whenever they wanted: they had some control. Their symptoms mostly dissipated within half an hour. However, some reported that certain reactions persisted a good deal longer, such as feelings of fatigue, dizziness, drowsiness, loss of motivation, feelings of being confused or disoriented; others reported continued preoccupation with various thoughts and feelings, such as fears and anxieties or suggestions which occurred during isolation. What if the person had withdrawn into isolation and knew that no one was there, that they were, or believed themselves to be abandoned. Some children are left alone for hours and recently some have been found abandoned by callous or disturbed parents for days. One person in my research remembered going hopelessly to his room as a child and hallucinating a figure coming through his bedroom wall to offer comfort. Such a hallucination would be a creative response to loneliness and distress; it could also however mean a child might begin to rely on such self-generated sources of nurture when the outer world offered none. Isolation might even be protective in an emotionally abusive environment: children might withdraw for self-preservation (although they might also be sent to their room in preparation for sexual or physical abuse so that aloneness would be mixed with dread). Self-imposed isolation may be a way of coping: a withdrawal to prevent the person being *overwhelmed*: she or he may be attempting to protect themselves or others from hostility, abuse, judgement and criticism. The isolation is thus a way of *distancing oneself from the other* (see Chapter 7).

Gloria: I thought I would harm my family (in response to voices) so I **distanced** myself.

This can result in a lack/loss of relationship: in extreme it becomes an *overdistance*.

Diane: I felt great comfort in being isolated but . . . People couldn't help me to get out of this cocoon . . .

This disassociation from others can also signal a dissociation from feelings and aspects of self, resulting in an experience of blankness and a lack of ability to relate to others.

Cheryll: I cut myself off from normal people . . . If I got back to normality I would have normal feelings but now I cut off from feelings and people . . . **I don't live in ordinary reality.**

The experience of sadness was particularly mentioned as encouraging hallucinations in 52% of the sample [of 100 people who had experienced auditory hallucinations], fear (16%) and anger (8%) . . . In eight out of nine (89%) psychotic depressive patients, sadness was described as a precipitant . . . Sadness was expressed not infrequently in association with being alone or lonely.

(Nayani and David, 1996: 180)

Martindale *et al.* (2000: 141) reported on the social isolation of people diagnosed as schizophrenic that resulted in them positively valuing their stay in hospital as a welcome respite from their loneliness in the community.

Voices, dissociation and denial of reality

Dissociation is a normal, even creative process which, when used excessively as a coping or survival strategy, can become problematic as the self/ego fragments. Dissociation and denial can be coping strategies when reality is intolerable: 'I don't feel anything.' 'This is not happening.' Denial and projection of unbearable thoughts and feelings out into the environment may protect the fragile ego from being flooded with 'previously distanced affects' (Drake and Sederer, 1986: 319).

Dissociation however can result in a loss of reality as it is our feelings that are a major source of our sense of what is real.

'The sense of reality depends on this role of feeling to create meaningful connections with the objective world, and these are cut across when feeling is withdrawn' (Perry, 1987: 73).

In 1932 Ferenczi accepted that child sexual abuse was pathogenic.

> As a defence the child sinks into a dream or trance state . . . the child's need to deny altogether what has happened loosens her hold on reality. The child may well become psychotic which is a defence not dissimilar to the original trance state, a protected but lonely hiding place.
>
> (Masson, 1992: 149)

Tina reported: When the voices are there . . . I go into trance.

Diane wrote in her journal: I keep spacing out for some unknown reason. I think it is because I'm starting to remember more abuse . . .

Voice hearers' reality may also have been denied by others: abusers deny or distort the reality of their victims' experience (some abusers threaten to kill if the victim discloses). Professionals may also deny the reality of voices or be unable to hear what people say:

Jenny: I never talked about it (hearing voices). I tried one time. I got smacked back and told I was living in a fantasy land. When I was about 13/14. I thought this psychiatrist was on my side and he wasn't . . .

Having attempted to speak of her reality and being rejected, **Jenny** withdrew. Years later she did not tell her psychologist that she was hearing voices through over a year of therapy.

Withdrawal from others and the world may be a withdrawal from hostile reality, turning instead to fantasy. Reality then comes to mean the *other* – outer, non-self, hostile – while fantasy is the realm of the inner *self*, a haven from disappointment. Fantasy may make up for something lacking in outer reality:

Dave (reflecting on inner city poverty, mental illness and emotional deprivation): My early memories are of a surreal life amongst dereliction (slum clearance) and fantasy . . . (I) remember sending psychic message at the age of 16 to a girl I fancied whilst masturbating.

Listening to voices, hallucinating, daydreaming may be a creative way of coping with social and psychological deprivation. In his journal **Dillon** stated that day after day he spent the rest of the day in solitary contemplation . . . A non descript day of shadows and silence . . . Alone he received communications and empowerments from deities, and conversed with academics and inter-planetary figures.

Voices may also soothe, comfort and support and when they diminish due to therapy they may be missed:

Diane: The voices are real today. They want me to tell them what I'm writing. I like listening to the good people they make me feel secure and wanted and that I have a purpose in life. They say that they love me and that they care about me and I really like them being around . . . I'm really pissed off because I am beginning to hear the voices less and less . . . I don't know what to do with myself, I mean it's good the voices are down to a minimum but I feel isolated and alone. I could always rely on the good voices to help me get whatever I was doing or going somewhere. Now I am frightened that I won't be able to go out . . .

The withdrawal from reality and consequent loss of reality also results in confusion as to what is real/not real.

Diane: Sometimes I'm very irrational . . . I don't understand the difference between reality and fantasy . . . I know that they're real but then Oh it's not real . . . cutting myself helps me forget about the abuse and keeps me in touch with reality whatever that is . . . I have created a world inside my head where they (voices) can help me all the time so what every body else says is wrong . . .

When one man was gang raped he was confused as to what was real due to the drugs that had been put in his drink.

On not remembering

Just as people can practise memory skills and therefore remember more, so I have come to believe people can practise not thinking, not feeling, not remembering. Sometimes people may prefer not to feel, think or remember. As **Leah** said: I try to forget about what I've suffered. I have memory problems.

Another woman said: He's (voice) wearing my brain down so I've got no recollection of what's going on. He makes me forget . . . he knows what I think and he stops my thinking process . . . The voice has blocked the past . . . when I was 17/18 I used to block things out, the rape.

Cheryll chose a button with holes in it to represent the holes in herself, left by gaps in her memory. She said that she liked this ability to blank out memories. Forgetting was a way of coping with her partner's violence: each time he assaulted her she forgot it. Such forgetting may be defensive and can be exacerbated by the effects of medication and electroconvulsive therapy (ECT). Prolonged stress can also damage the hippocampus which plays a critical role in memory. The resultant memory loss may mean a loss of self and identity as our memory is one of the ways that we construct our sense of self. Memory problems affect relationships:

Pat said she had a *problem with short-term memory*. This affected her ability to recall things her husband said and caused frustration in their relationship. In a drama when we reviewed a past scene **Pat** role reversed as one of her voices said: 'We won't let you forget this.' As herself she wanted to forget those things of which she was ashamed. As herself in the past she would deny it all. She had learned denial as a child and in this way coped with her own mother's mental illness.

Denial of reality, if habitual, can lead, through lies, to madness and/or evil: hence, possibly, the prevalence of the devil in psychotic imagery. Many of the voice hearers have had experiences of evil, of being overwhelmed by destructive power that threatens their survival, both in having been abused and in experiencing voices that command them to do evil acts:

Tina: I thought I was under spiritual attack . . . I tried to kill my mother when I was poorly. I thought that she was, that everybody, was against me. The voices tell me that as well. They got me down, the doctors, as being paranoid psychosis. I see demons on their faces. I hallucinate: and their faces change and they look evil. And I thought she was trying to hurt me. She lives in a flat on the top and she stood at the top of the stairs. I felt very very strong. And she's only little my mum and I just grabbed hold of her by the scruff of the neck, picked her up. I was going to throw her down the stairs. She shouted at me (called her name.) I came to my sense and put her down. She was very frightened . . . They (the voices) tell me I've got to leave him (husband) because he's the devil.

Harry heard an evil voice he named as Satan, a destructive part of him he did not want to own. **Jenny** wanted her therapist to be an ally . . . in the fight against the demons! In projective work she spoke of ghosts, identifying them as grandmother, father and other controlling figures in her childhood: they had stolen/possessed her child self. This statement is in harmony with shamanic ideas of illness: the loss of soul.

Shamanic healing involved travel, in altered states of consciousness, to different, spiritual levels of reality to rescue the lost soul of the patient from demons. The shamanic model of illness served humankind for thousands of years. Each culture develops models to explain madness and I now turn to an examination of some of the current western models and offer my own in Chapter 3.

Psychosis and hearing voices 3
Models of madness

Why do we need a model of madness? Such is the disturbing, overwhelming power of psychosis that therapists approaching work in this area can feel frightened and bewildered. Furthermore, the fact that most therapists have not heard voices nor experienced other psychotic disturbance and cannot hear the voices their clients hear, often means that they can quite simply be at a loss to empathise or understand the client's experience and so may feel out of their depth. Engel (1977: 130) defined a model as 'a belief system utilised to explain natural phenomena, to make sense out of what is puzzling or disturbing.' A map of the territory can clarify the journey to be undertaken. Shamans had a cosmology that gave them a sense of direction during their trance journeys in search of the lost soul of the patient (Eliade, 1989). The model a therapist chooses must empower him or her to travel through the landscape of madness and accompany their clients on their healing journey.

The medical model

The medical model is a sophisticated, continuously evolving system of diagnosis and treatment supported internationally by thousands of doctors, researchers and drug companies. Its effect in clinical practice has been to deny that there is meaning in psychotic experiences. The model states that the content of voices (what they say) is meaningless: it is the form of the voices (whether they are third person etc.) that indicates the diagnostic category of illness and is indicative of biological dysfunction which, if properly understood, would lead to the correct medication relieving this symptom of disease.

Diagnosis

Diagnosis is a process by which doctors attempt to orient themselves in the landscape of madness. A 'correct diagnosis' can result in the establishment of effective treatment: the medical, psychological and social management of 'illness'. In my view diagnosis is not the business of therapists who must accompany people, whatever the diagnosis, on their therapeutic journey. Therapists must be able to see the person first, not the diagnosis. Diagnosis, moreover, is problematic. Despite a century of diagnostic research during which entire generations of psychiatrists and patients have accepted there is an illness called schizophrenia, many have now come to the conclusion that schizophrenia does not exist as a discrete disease entity (see Slade and Bentall, 1988; Bentall, 1990; Boyle, 1990; Parker *et al.*, 1995; Marshall, 1995: 58–59, 62–63; Thomas, 1997: 102; Watkins, 1998: 275–278; Romme, 1998: 54). Schizophrenia may now more accurately be described as a group of symptoms, i.e. a syndrome. Being diagnosed as schizophrenic may mean that other experiences are discounted or not paid sufficient attention. The diagnosis can blind clinicians to the need for therapy of someone diagnosed as schizophrenic who is also a survivor of trauma. In psychiatry the definition of insight, in terms of psychotic illness, is that patients accept that they are ill, that they have the illness that the psychiatrist says they have, or at least accept that their voices are medically defined 'hallucinations' (and not, for example, the voices of spirits). This is problematic as some people have been misdiagnosed as schizophrenic when they are survivors of abuse and their voice hearing experiences are post-traumatic symptoms. Some feel 'haunted' by their abuser or by the 'presences' of deceased significant others. Psychosis can alternatively be seen as a spiritual emergency: when individuals are struggling with the meaning of their life experience and their very survival is at stake. Hallucinations should be labelled as pathological only when they are seen by the psychiatrist as being outside the person's cultural/ spiritual context. However, in normal practice people's spiritual experiences may be regarded as pathological symptoms and their meaning ignored.

Due to the social stigma of a diagnosis, a patient can experience discrimination, exclusion and oppression. A diagnosis may also bring secondary gains including incapacity benefit (in the United Kingdom) and so keep people in the sick role (recovery might result in poverty).

Some people want a diagnosis (as helping them get a handle on their experience), while others doubt their diagnosis. For example, we can compare **Diane** and **Gloria**.

Diane, who did *not* have a diagnosis of schizophrenia, is *white* and a survivor of sexual abuse and rape, said: I do think I'm partly schizophrenic, a little bit schizophrenic: 50 per cent schizophrenic, 50 per cent emotional. **Diane** would not accept that she was *not* schizophrenic, despite being told she was not: to be schizophrenic would have explained her desperation, her voices and her sense of 'illness', whereas the psychiatrist told her she had a personality disorder in the context of being a survivor of childhood sexual abuse.

Conversely **Gloria**, who *did* have a diagnosis of schizophrenia, is *black* and a survivor of sexual abuse and rape, said: I didn't know who I could trust. I'd fought to get out of hospital – I was being misdiagnosed. No one was willing to listen – people said this is in your best interest. Eventually **Gloria** was proved right: she was in fact suffering from hypothyroidism and had indeed been misdiagnosed. **Gloria**'s experience seems to be in line with much evidence that suggests black people are more likely to be diagnosed schizophrenic than white people (Littlewood and Lipsedge, 1982; Burke, 1984; Harrison *et al.*, 1999).

Medication

Tina recalled her diagnosis thus: *They (doctors) just said to me, 'You'll have to take these tablets for the rest of your life,' **and that was it**. 'You've got a chemical imbalance and you'll have to take these tablets for the rest of your life'* . . . **Tina** did find her medication very helpful: it silenced her voices. *I've been on haloperidol since then. It stops the voices altogether . . . At least mine (voices) are under control by the medication.*

From the mid-1950s the development of 'anti-psychotic' medication brought hope and benefit to many patients. While neuroleptic medication has been seen as 'the treatment of choice' for schizophrenia, there 'is evidence that despite appropriate levels of medication, many patients continue to experience residual psychotic symptoms which, though often less severe than those occurring in acute episodes, are unresponsive to further medication' (Roth and Fonagy, 1996: 185).

Leah: *Medication has helped; medication dampens the voices but doesn't stop them.*

Diane: *Medication: it helps calm them (the voices) down, they're not so loud but don't go away. The tablets numb them down a bit . . .*

Others doubted the value of their medication:

Dave: *Modecate has never stopped voices for me . . . largactil – not good for voices . . . One of the problems with medication is that it flattens your emotions; it induces a tranquillity of sorts but this is more like a numbness or hollow feeling. Consequently while using medication it's difficult to realise your emotional potential . . . Sometimes wondered if depressions are due to medication . . . on the nature of anti-psychotic medication, at first you control it then it controls you . . .*

Roger complained that *All the psychiatrist wants to do is change my medication, they don't want to listen to how I feel.*

While often helpful, medication is not, by itself, the solution.

Even **Tina**, who found her medication beneficial, felt the need for further help: *I think you need more than that. I think . . . when their minds are a little bit better and they've got the voices sorted out with medication I think they should meet in a group and discuss it so they know exactly what is wrong with them and they know that they're not on their own and that other people suffer from the same thing.* Group therapy (see Chapters 10, 12 and 13) can provide much needed support and therapeutic benefit, which the diagnosis and medication cannot. A combination of medication and therapy may offer the best outcome (combined with a holistic assessment of needs such as housing, diet, education, employment, hobbies, work, physical exercise, social, spiritual, cultural opportunities): the reliance on medication alone can result in people being dangerously over medicated. Since medication is not the whole answer, indeed it may become part of the problem as neuroleptics can cause irreversible brain damage (Breggin, 1993) and numerous distressing side-effects, even sudden death (Healy, 1993; Martensson, 1998) it seems logical further to explore the potential value of appropriately designed psychotherapy to this distressed group of people. Therapy can be regarded as expensive and some may argue that 'the National Health Service cannot afford such a luxury': in fact less than six days in hospital could pay for a whole year of individual therapy or three years of group therapy; some of the medications offered to such clients are substantially more expensive than therapy (for comparative costings see Appendix 4).

The danger of a diagnosis of schizophrenia or other major mental illness is that once so labelled people are offered medication and some supportive activities but no psychological therapy. This may be due to several factors:

- a belief that therapy is not helpful, is even dangerous, for people with psychotic illness
- a lack of skilled therapists
- a climate of fear around the person which makes the person withdraw from contact and others also draw back.

Rowe (Breggin, 1993: 483) pointed out that in the United Kingdom psychiatrists have, until recently, been taught that psychotherapy was 'contraindicated' for schizophrenia (research had shown that psychoanalytic psychotherapy was not helpful to people diagnosed as schizophrenic, see Chapter 1). Leudar and Thomas (2000: 119) stated that the dominant view in psychiatry 'is that the voices are not to be explored psychologically.' This situation is changing to some extent. Current guidelines from the National Institute for Clinical Excellence (NICE, 2003: 1.3.3.6) state that cognitive behavioural therapy and family interventions should be available but that

> Counselling and supportive psychotherapy are not recommended as discrete interventions in the routine care of people with schizophrenia where other psychological interventions of proven efficacy are indicated and available.
>
> (NICE, 2003)

In effect this means that CBT and family interventions may be the only therapy offered. Consequently people may be denied even the simple counselling they need to get their life back to normal after a period of psychosis. In practice many mental health workers have counselling training and do offer their clients such support but in a busy psychiatric service this is often not available in a regular way.

Even when the psychotic experiences are the result of physical processes in the brain, the person may still need psychological support to cope with voices and other psychotic and life experiences. These may also relate to traumatic experiences previously not recognised by psychiatrists searching for biological substrata.

Theo was variously diagnosed with 'definite organic pathology, early cortical atrophy, abnormal patch in left hemisphere', 'organic mood (hypomanic) syndrome'. He had suffered several head injuries. (However, CT and MRI brain scans showed very little atrophy and were virtually normal.) The psychiatrists had not paid attention to the facts that he had been physically abused as a child and as a young adult; that he was chronically lonely; his mother had been depressed; his father was abusive. No psychological treatment had been offered as he had been assessed as not suitable for cognitive therapy. Nevertheless within weeks of starting dramatherapy his persecutory voices were reduced.

A definition of psychosis

How then does the medical model define psychosis? The medical model proposes that psychoses are illnesses which result from physical, organic vulnerability, for some genetically determined, manifest in brain biochemical abnormalities (the 'chemical imbalance' mentioned above by **Tina**). Professor Alex Jenner defined psychoses as illnesses in which one has lost contact with reality (Romme and Escher 1993, 149). Psychiatrists are trained to take into account a client's cultural beliefs about reality yet in practice this can be problematic as **Dave** wrote in his journal:

> Anyway who is the arbiter of *reality*:- Dr E.? (psychiatrist) (are you fucking joking?) T. S. (CPN)? (No) C. M. (nurse) (No) Dr T. (psychiatrist) (No – and I think he would admit that ultimately) Dr D. (My GP, No) You John (I think you know ultimately that reality is relative and not a fixed article; No) Einstein (No, far too intelligent to not realise that he ultimately knew nothing in the greater scheme of the cosmos). We are as insignificant as a gnat to the solar system and in that relativity even less. Everything is ultimately true or false if you want to believe it.

The medical model as dogma

Engel (1977: 130) criticised the medical model as having become a dogma: 'In science, a model is revised or abandoned when it fails to account adequately for all the data. A dogma, on the other hand, requires that discrepant data be forced to fit the model or be excluded.' Furthermore Engel (1977: 135) recognised the obstacles in the way of developing alternatives: 'The power of vested interests, social, political, and economic, are formidable deterrents to any effective assault on biomedical dogmatism.' Coleman (1999: 32) pointed out the political pressures that enforce the views of the psychiatric establishment: 'that mental illness is a biological condition and that the way to treat it is to ensure compliance with medication.' This is not unrelated to gender as the positivist, materialist science behind biopsychiatry is male dominated and of a worldview that seeks to control nature.

A biopsychosocial model

Goldberg and Huxley (1992) revising the medical model, proposed a biosocial model and a stress vulnerability model, namely that those who are constitutionally vulnerable to stress are more likely to break down when stressed (see also Martindale *et al.* 2000: 32). The vulnerability may be due to genes, to neurodevelopmental problems in the womb, brain injury after birth or substance misuse. This biological vulnerability renders the person less able to cope with stress and so when they experience sufficient stress they become ill. The stress vulnerability model has led to the development of psychosocial interventions which aim to reduce stress, increase the person's coping ability, promote social skills, improve family and other relationships. Creative activities and therapy can be part of such a package of care.

Engel (1977: 132) proposed a biopsychosocial model. 'Psychological and social factors are also crucial in determining whether and when patients with the biochemical abnormality of schizophrenia come to view themselves or be viewed by others as sick.' Martindale *et al.* (2000) continue to work towards a synthesis: an integrated biopsychosocial model, to provide a multidisciplinary response to psychotic experiences that includes medication, supportive activities and psychotherapy.

A dimensional model

Rather than being the result of discrete diseases it is possible to view mental distress as occurring on a continuum; likewise hallucinations can be seen to be at one end of a continuum with vivid mental imagery at the other end (Slade and Bentall 1988: 19, 58). Voices may begin as thoughts, feelings, intuitions, fantasies or simply recollected echoes of what we have heard repeated like a tape loop. Dissociation is a normal, even creative process which, when used extensively as a coping or survival strategy, can become problematic as the self/ego fragments. Hallucinations are experienced by people who have many different diagnoses, and none. Instead of a split between 'them' as insane and 'us' as sane, I see a continuum of experience at one end of which are people who are diagnosed as schizophrenic: their experiences are similar to ours only taken to extremes (see Thomas, 1997: 100; Nettle, 2001: 33–35).

A dimensional model has been developed from the observation that many clients cross diagnostic boundaries and even those who have no diagnosed 'illness' may still be on a continuum of vulnerability. Tsuang and Faraone (2002) suggested a dimensional model which states that schizophrenia is the result of a genetic predisposition, 'schizotaxia' (Meehl, 1962), which in some family members is 'unexpressed' as the illness, but is evident in 'related conditions such as schizotypal personality disorder, negative symptoms, neuropsychological impairment or other neurobiological manifestations of the predisposition to schizophrenia.'

The psychodramatic model

Since the 1930s psychodramatists have had a model of 'madness' developed from the philosophy of the founder of psychodrama, Dr J. L. Moreno. This model is entirely consistent with the method. It states that 'madness' is the manifestation of inadequately channelled (or pathological) spontaneity and creativity derived

> from the split which occurs in the life of the infant during the first year and which results in the division between 'objective reality' and 'surplus reality', or fantasy. In the first few months after birth, the child experiences itself as the totality of the universe. It is not aware that there is a distinction between itself, a separateness from itself, and other beings and objects. When this separateness is first experienced, there is an undermining of the power which the earlier universe gave the child. From that moment on, the child must live in these two dimensions. The more impoverished, in every sense, is the experience in objective reality, the more the child will retreat into the subjective reality where once again it is all powerful, the only being in the world. When the breach between these two areas of experience becomes unbridgeable, this retreat into the first universe in which the child is unrestrained in its fantasy productions, madness may plant its seed.
>
> (Moreno and Moreno, 1984: 28–29)

The causes are interpersonal and the treatment is therefore interpersonal. The prognosis is good if the person can develop positive relationships (tele) with the therapist and others (auxiliaries) and eventually expand their social network (their social atom, see Chapter 9). The patient is given the right to explore his or her hallucinations and delusions through psychodrama: to act these out and be accepted as a creative human being. The aim of treatment is to enable the person to be more spontaneous and creative in multiple roles; to gain greater control; to achieve flexibility, both intrapsychically and interpersonally; to trust him/herself to try out new behaviours and reach out for new relationships.

Towards a model for dramatherapists

The definition of such a complex experience as psychosis may forever remain elusive, 'fuzzy' and debatable: nevertheless to be able to work in this field therapists must develop their thinking and engage in the debate. These different models then are beliefs which inform the way we behave towards people who have unusual experiences. We need to be aware of our beliefs and the effects they have on the way we construct people's suffering and how we, as therapists, respond. Dramatherapists need a model for their work and so I offer the following, which taken together with the theory of distance (Chapter 7) and the theatre model of the self (Chapter 9) can provide a theoretical framework and foundation for the safe practice of dramatherapy with people who hear voices and have psychotic experiences.

Two dramatherapists' definitions of psychosis

Jenner's definition of psychosis cited earlier raises the question: 'What is reality?' I propose that reality is socially and culturally constructed: multiple, diverse, complex. Ordinary reality is a containing culture we share with others: it is social. Each person's individual sense of reality is coloured by their perceptions, emotions, beliefs, history and yes, brain chemistry (as the effects of alcohol, drugs, hormones and head injury can affect our sense of reality). This suggests however that within the socially constructed 'consensus' reality there are different, even multiple, individual realities.

Jennings (1998: 119) describes people struggling with psychosis as 'trapped in dramatic reality'. By this, she means that they fail to distinguish the boundaries between the ordinary, everyday, social reality and the inner, symbolic reality of the imagination, which she calls 'dramatic reality' (Jennings, 1998: 117; see also Chapter 9.) Their inner world of fantasy, delusion, fear is projected out onto external reality and they are lost in the confusion between these worlds.

I will define psychosis as a process in which a person escapes from intolerable reality and creates another fantastic 'reality' (as **Leah** put it: I daydream a lot . . . of rescue and love. I create stories in my head. She said that these fantasies helped her cope: hearing voices . . . you . . . feel isolated in your own mind and thoughts about fantasies in life or dream fantasy or realities of life. When I have these it makes me afterwards think I'm ill cause then I day dreams regularly). Someone 'may seek this altered state of consciousness for its excitement value because in one's heart, one is depressed or feeling low about oneself' (Chadwick, 1997: 145). People dissociate from the unbearable in search of safety, nurture, power, survival when no other way of escape is possible (Watkins, 1998: 139–140, 156; Mollon, 1996: 9–10, 121; Bloom, 1997: 34). Levinson (1966) quoted a patient who said, 'The voices . . . were telling me what to do just **as if** a mother were talking to a child. I guess I wanted a mother so badly I just imagined one' (Watkins, 1998: 136).

The psychotic fantasies will then be symbolic of what was intolerable in the rejected/denied social reality: the characters/images/delusions/voices will contain, at one remove (at a safer distance), those feelings and experiences from which the person needed to escape. What cannot be expressed directly is then expressed through the psychotic imagery (just as in dreams). This new 'reality' may have its satisfactions and compensate for the deficits of the other, unbearable reality. Voices may be friends who fill the silence of loneliness. Spirituality may provide comfort, strength, meaning and a feeling of being special. Imagination may enable a powerless person to feel powerful. The psychotic person's 'pain-staking construction of his lonely world may be seen as an abortive attempt at creativity' (Miller, 1972: 60). For a time this alternative reality may be preferable to the social reality and help the person survive. Moreno saw that social reality can be deficient at times and that 'surplus' reality (in psychodrama) can provide opportunities that the social reality cannot: the chance to be special, powerful, have friends (auxiliary egos), express feelings and needs. Moreno provided an example of this psychotic creativity when a woman created a hallucinatory lover (Moreno, 1945a: 14). 'Surplus reality', like Jennings' (1998) 'dramatic reality', offers the opportunity to play out things we cannot have in life on the psychodrama stage and so satisfy such needs and 'act hungers'.

Thus psychosis can be seen as a creative act, but one in which the creative process can destroy social reality, destroying the psychotic person's ability to relate to or function in the social reality, resulting in withdrawal, isolation and dysfunction. This psychotic creativity is not wholly conscious nor in the control of the person: indeed unconscious processes may drive the creative process. The person is then overwhelmed by a combination of intrapsychic and interpersonal forces: historical, environmental, emotional, spiritual, psychological, biochemical. They may be overwhelmed by fear (paranoia), joy/excitement (mania), confusion (thought disorder), nightmares (hallucinations). They may experience voices and delusions that they are unable to comprehend or control, loss of self or parts of self and loss of a sense of (social) reality. Alternatively they may be empowered by psychotic strength, delusional conviction, grandiosity, manic energy that temporarily protects them from, or impels them towards, that other possible escape from intolerable reality – suicide.

An environmental model

Listening to people who hear voices has enabled me to construct an environmental model of psychosis: it is a contribution to the development of the biopsychosocial model and is multidimensional, taking into account the complexity of life. The simplistic search for a single cause, whether genetic or biochemical is doomed to failure and we must understand that psychosis is multifactoral with many interpersonal and intrapsychic elements interacting. This view is supported by Romme and Escher:

> the hearing of voices is not solely . . . a discrete individual psychological experience, but . . . an interactional phenomenon reflecting the nature of the individual's relationship to his or her environment, and indeed vice versa . . . it is not only a psychological but also a social phenomenon.
>
> (Romme and Escher, 1993: 16)

The environment surrounding the genesis of psychosis is complex and many layered: for clarity I divide it into sections but it must be remembered that these sections continuously interrelate and that what may appear discrete sections are in fact processes that influence each other. For example the historic, cultural message 'boys don't cry' has impacted directly on the ability of individual boys to process trauma.

This model can be seen as a wave slowly developing with gathering momentum. The wave begins its journey long before conception. The forces accumulate until they eventually overwhelm the person. In some cases other factors can protect and prevent the onset of psychosis. However, a specific crisis can result in the wave reaching the critical height and crashing over the person's head. Look in the background of someone with a drug induced psychosis or a post-puerperal psychosis and these other factors will be found adding to the stress that eventually precipitates the psychosis.

> Virchow argued that 'diseases have no independent or isolated existence . . . they are only the manifestations of life processes under altered conditions'. Psychiatrists like Adolf Meyer (1955) argued that mental disorders were reactions of the whole organism to its total environment, rather than being produced by some discrete inner lesion.
>
> (Goldberg and Huxley, 1992: 53–54)

Chadwick (1992: 131) insisted that 'external factors are critically important in the genesis and exacerbation of the psychotic state.'

All the questions and ideas in this model are drawn from research participants' actual experiences. The model is consistent with the stress vulnerability model (see p. 38). In considering the development of psychotic and voice hearing experiences, the following elements may be significant.

The external environment before birth

The historical environment

Wars and civil wars; oppression; murder; terrorism and torture; dislocation (emigration/immigration) and being a refugee; the impact of politics; of economics, social upheavals.

The cultural environment

Messages from religion, imperialism, racism, sexism, homophobia; scapegoating; the stigma of mental illness.

The psychological environment

Of mental illness or mental disability in previous generations; parents' psychological dysfunction, disability and deprivation, inability to process their own losses, hostility, traumas, emotions and achieve/maintain clear boundaries. The death of siblings before birth.

The pre-conception physical environment

Parents' diet; drugs and alcohol; housing.

The womb environment

From conception: is the baby wanted? Mother's diet (medication or drug misuse) and well-being (physical and psychological). The loss of a twin, dying in the womb. The foetus can hear sounds/voices from beyond the womb: what is their tone?

The interacting environment

The environment in infancy

At birth does the infant suffer trauma or brain injury? Is the baby premature? How is the baby received into the world? Can the baby take the mother's milk? Is basic attachment achieved between mother/carer and child? Is the mother in mourning for a previous lost child? Are there potential boundaries or is symbiosis maintained/denied? What is the interplay of baby and carers? The emergence of the vulnerable self/ego: does the environment offer nurture or abandonment/deprivation, stress, abuse? '[E]xposing [children] to overwhelming stress appears to cause actual impairments in normal brain development' (Bloom, 1997: 21).

Childhood environment

Is there lack of nurture, loss, hostility, criticism, poor emotional education, lack of boundaries, invasiveness, physical trauma (head injury), epilepsy, abuse (emotional, physical, sexual), denial of abuse (and therefore reality), oppression, dysfunction in relationships, abandonment, confusing messages? What is the effect of their place in the order of siblings or are they an only child? Are there siblings who die or are miscarried? Is there marital conflict or divorce? The impact of sexism: are boys preferred to girls? Is a parent mentally or physically ill, withdrawn, unavailable? Does the child have to look after a parent? Is the parent/carer unable or unwilling to hear what the child says and so unable to protect? Is the child put in care? Is the child shy, lonely, bullied at school? Does the child hear voices? And are they able to disclose this? Do they receive support or further rejection/criticism? Failure in education (due to difficulty concentrating, poor peer relations, dyslexia or other problems).

The environment in youth

Continuance of the above exacerbated by repeated moves of home, school and country; the crises of puberty, low self-esteem, further trauma, more bullying, homophobia (heterosexual boys can be victims of innuendo about their sexuality), overwhelming emotions, including violent feelings and behaviour, self-harm, alcohol/drugs, withdrawal from external reality to escape into inner fantasy/spirituality, offending behaviour, further criticism.

The young adult environment

Continuance of the above exacerbated by relationship dysfunction, loss of first love, isolation, sexual dysfunction; rape, torture, humiliation, self-criticism and social ostracism/scapegoating. Suicide of sibling or friend and other losses. Becoming a parent: post-natal depression and loss of a child or abortion. Stress and failure in work (due to lack of ability to concentrate and function) and consequent unemployment. 'I have known people suffer such "psychogenetic" stresses in offices, in the army, the police force, at school, etc.' (Chadwick, 1992: 63).

The current environment

Care in the community (nurture or abandonment?), social withdrawal, dysfunction, isolation, hostility from the community/family, outer and inner criticism, nightmares, lack of sleep, illness role, the effects of medication, death or suicide of significant others, voices oppressing the vulnerable ego.

In noticing the impact of past events on the developing person I would not wish to suggest that the present is simply determined by the past: a person's view of the future can also be an important influence on their present functioning as construct psychology (Kelly, 1955) suggests. Perry (1987), influenced by Jung, stated:

> we do not look for causes in the fortuitous circumstances of early infancy, as if the psyche were only an inert lump of raw material moulded solely by the hands of caprice, so much as for ends towards which the psyche as a living organism is striving – namely for its self-fulfilment in its several aspects and functions.
>
> (Perry, 1987: 6)

Romme and Escher (1996: 144) have suggested that the onset of voices may sometimes occur with the frustration of youthful ideals.

Dramatherapy and psychodrama pay attention to the past but are grounded in the here and now with a future orientation of what could be: whatever the past, healing is possible and change (positive or negative) inevitable. However, in the confusing maze of psychotic experience the therapist needs a map and I have constructed the following schema to help find a way through the labyrinth.

Elements in the psychotic process

Self/ego is my term for the whole psyche, body, mind, soul and spirit, acknowledging conscious and unconscious. Self/ego is a relationship between these two: the smaller, vulnerable ego (the conscious 'I' part) and the greater (the whole – conscious and unconscious) self.

The vulnerable self/ego

At first there is no clear sense of a separate self/ego and other: normally boundaries gradually develop but in some circumstances are weak, even non-existent due to overinvolvement, invasive disrespect and lack of empathy for the developing, vulnerable personhood of the infant; in other circumstances due to a lack of nurture, loss, abandonment, deprivation, the child reaches out into the world and meets an emptiness, without clear boundaries or emotional support. A vulnerable ego develops which may be overwhelmed by experiences and learn to dissociate, to withdraw into protective non-feeling oblivion (loss of sense of self). A split develops between the ego and the self, the former being conscious, small and vulnerable (and therefore anxious), the latter containing all other aspects of the whole being of the person including split-off experiences of overwhelming affect.

The vulnerable self/ego under attack

The child experiences not only lack of nurture and emotional deprivation but also active attacks threatening his/her survival: oppression, abuse, trauma, hostility, criticism, humiliation.

The vulnerable self/ego is unable to defend him/herself

Without clear boundaries or protection from carers, the child is powerless and overwhelmed, both externally and internally (indeed without clear boundaries it is difficult to tell what is internal and what is external). Overwhelming feelings threaten the vulnerable self/ego and so are split off/denied/lost to consciousness through dissociation, and/or the flooding of the stress hormone cortisol, destroying nerve cells in the hypocampus (and resulting in a loss of memory of the trauma), or through other self-administered methods such as drinking to unconsciousness or using opiates and other drugs. The vulnerable self/ego fragments (see Bloom, 1997: 34).

The person suffers a loss of sense of self, of identity

Oppressed by her/his environment and experience, unable to process this or cope, the person is unable to speak and 'loses her/his own voice': the trauma is literally unspeakable, or occurs in an environment where people do not speak of such things. This may be because it occurs in infancy before speech develops or may simply take her/his breath, and ability to speak, away. It may also be because no one is willing or available to hear: when parents are mentally ill or unable to process their own trauma they are not able to listen, respond to or hear the emotional needs of the child. There may be things in previous generations that the family do not speak about (Schutzenberger, 1998). The person may be threatened by an abuser not to speak, may be too ashamed to speak or be protecting others (see Chapter 6). Unable to process the indigestible trauma or metabolise feelings, the person is powerless and confused. Not being able to process feelings means that other losses, traumas and emotional difficulties are also not dealt with and not feeling becomes a survival strategy. A blank appears: a numb deadening of feeling, a not knowing resultant from not feeling and not remembering. The emptiness may be the only soothing available. This deadening of feeling can become a coping strategy of dissociation; a loss of consciousness through fainting or trance (see Mollon, 1996: 69). Dissociation may lead to the development of dissociative identity disorder in which the voices are those of different personalities. The blank also means no clear thinking, a loss of reality and a sense of not knowing what to do or say and consequent inability to make effective decisions and function in social reality. Without feeling or thought, without a sense of identity, there is a growing sense of being depersonalised, of not being human, feeling unreal, perhaps of being controlled by some unfeeling machine or technology (see Baars, 1997: 149–150). This loss of sense of self is sometimes described as having died (or the child inside being dead) or no longer being human. Some people report that they have survived near-death experiences.

The person withdraws or is lost

The withdrawal into silence and isolation from potentially dangerous contact with others means that the person cannot access nurture/support to process their experience. He/she withdraws from oppressive external reality into inner fantasy and spirituality – the haven of the self: but this is a dangerous haven where all denied and split off aspects of the person's experience lurk; a haven which is a heaven and a hell inhabited by ghosts, demons, fairies, angels, God, *voices*. The voices have power (the power of feelings and experiences lost to consciousness). The powerlessness of the vulnerable (conscious) ego is reinforced. Depression ensues. Isolation has psychological consequences and can result in hallucinations (Haggard, 1964: 433–470). Loneliness itself may stimulate the voices to occupy the void in relationships. The person may come to prefer the voices and rely on them for company. They may keep this secret, so not speaking is reinforced. Not speaking out loud may eventually result in voices developing or becoming louder. In isolation the person feels lost or that they have lost their identity (Coleman, 1999: 55).

Voices and delusions

The voices and delusions the person now experiences *encapsulate and encode feelings and traumatic experiences*: but being encoded they are not immediately comprehended. Voices 'metaphorically express the trouble people are having with their emotions reflecting confusing experiences, ideals or the lack of certain capacities like making decisions on one's own' (Romme, 1998: 54).

The encoding may also be an attempt to gain mastery through an explanation, such as: 'I am hearing the voice of God who has chosen me for a special mission and is testing me.' This grandiosity may be expressive of feelings of abandonment and a lack of meaning/purpose in life. Such spirituality is common and reflects the truth that people's souls, their whole being, is at stake. Spiritual explanations of their experience may also be regarded as attempts to comprehend and frame their experience in a personally meaningful way. However, they may also be metaphoric. The omnipotence of God is at the opposite polarity from experiences of powerlessness of the vulnerable ego. God may also be the self: that greater whole that encompasses the smaller, vulnerable ego. Spirituality may provide metaphors/symbols for what cannot be expressed on another level. Such symbols contain power, meaning and potential. We must not reduce spirituality to pathology: psychosis can be seen as a spiritual emergency, demanding that the person reassess their life.

The feelings encoded in voices and delusions are hidden: there is some protection for the vulnerable ego inherent in such denial/dissociation/avoidance. The feelings do not immediately overwhelm but threaten to overwhelm: survival is still at risk. An inner civil war between such split off aspects of the self has the person struggling with unseen psychic forces. These have escaped from the person's control and threaten to control him/her in a replay of the original abusive experience. Thus voices can be seen as encapsulating parts or fragments of the self that threaten the vulnerable ego. In Prouty's (1986) view a hallucination is a self-fragment that expresses an actual life experience. Delusions likewise may be seen to be act hungers in metaphorical dress. Feelings that cannot be expressed (or even felt) are translated into images/dreams and experienced by the psychotic person as real because feelings are what give us our sense of what is real. The images must therefore be processed to extract their meaning and thus the feelings be expressed (see Watkins, 1998: 186). However, as we have seen in Chapter 1, Chadwick (1997: 147–148) warned that therapists' interpretation of meaning can be unhelpful: the disturbing material of psychosis is held at a safe, metaphoric distance and to interpret the metaphor risks collapsing that distance prematurely. As Benedetti states:

> In the case of a psychotic ego that is being dissolved the primary therapeutic task does not lie in the interpretation of symptoms. What is primordial is to be with the client and with his symptom. In order to understand this, one should consider that the psychotic symptom hides a double aspect. It has two functions, two interpersonal aspects, namely communication on the one hand and defence on the other.
>
> (Benedetti, 1983: 189, cited in Tselikas and Burmeister, 1997: 169)

The delusions are fixed because they are a defensive adaptation to protect the vulnerable ego from being overwhelmed by feelings: they are the wall that holds back the sea, though storms (stress) may still whip up the waves and threaten to breach the wall. Stress and real life events can also reinforce and exacerbate the psychotic pattern/process.

In subsequent chapters I present theory (7, 9, 14) and practice (6, 8, 10, 11, 12, 13) of working through safe distancing methods in dramatherapy and psychodrama to ensure people are not overwhelmed.

Hostility/aggression

In their lives psychotic people have often been the victims of others' aggression and hostility. Many are victims of abuse, rape, criticism, insults. In turn they do not learn to handle their own aggression, anger, frustration, hostility and violent feelings in safe ways. Indeed they may split off their aggression and experience it as alien to themselves. The voices often then speak out their aggression, but against themselves, repeating and reinforcing their role as victim. This inner hostility may be reinforced by external, real hostility from others such as family members, neighbours or professionals. This repetition compulsion cries out for others' caring attention so that the psychotic person can gain the caring attention he/she so needed at earlier times. Is the environment now able to respond or is the pattern reinforced? Are they accused of being 'attention seeking' in a judgemental tone? There is a danger that 'Care in the Community' could become neglect/ abandonment in the community (Martindale *et al.*, 2000: 134). This may contribute to the high suicide rate of people in distress and despair.

Power/powerlessness: power and control

Many research participants had been powerless at times during their lives: they had experienced war, rape, abuse, being sectioned into hospital and being controlled by voices. A person overwhelmed by psychosis does not experience him/herself as being in control of the self/ego or life. The locus of control is not within the ego but in the voices or some other: whether in an abuser, a delusional identity or a professional intervention. This concern with control is the result of past and present experiences of powerlessness. Janet (1889) considered that traumatisation resulted from the inability to take effective action against a potential threat. Freud (1926) viewed the essence of trauma as the experience of helplessness, of being overwhelmed, in the face of an accumulation of tension or excitation which the ego could not master (Mollon, 1996: 17, 36). Dissociation may be the only escape or way of coping in such circumstances.

For some a delusion may offer a sense of control: **Dillon** wrote in his journal: I'm becoming more radioactive as an empowerment – spiritual power to control over things . . . I should be able to totally control myself. The voices are trying to challenge my control. Sometimes he was in control of his fears, sometimes they were in control of him.

This concern with control then is the result of past experiences of powerlessness. During the rape **Gloria** said she *was paralysed by fear and anger and couldn't fight back.* One man said his feeling of being controlled dated from when he was raped. **Jenny** was also a survivor of abuse, her voice 'Mr' being her abuser. Having been controlled by men in childhood, she had chosen controlling men as partners.

This experience can be continued in relation to professionals on occasions (such as when sectioned) and in relation to the voices. **Ben** was sectioned by a large force of police in riot gear (because of his fear and anger he was holding a knife to protect himself). He had experienced the power and control of the military during a civil war when his father was shot dead in front of him. He also experienced feelings of powerlessness in relation to his voices. **Ben** was very troubled and disabled by a delusion that a controlling technical, non-human, agency outside him was the source of his problems.

When the person feels powerless his or her disowned power becomes unconscious, returning in nightmares, delusions, voices or is projected outwards into the environment onto others, causing anxiety and fear. Paradoxically this has a powerful effect causing the mobilisation of large forces of personnel and resources to contain and treat: hospitals, teams of professionals, drug companies, researchers, anxious for their own reasons to contain and restrain the sick person. The services then can further disempower the person (see Coursey *et al.*, 1995: 298). Staff can also feel powerless in the face of the profound disturbance and chaos of psychosis. Nurses retreat into the office or 'assertively' take control. Psychiatrists and psychologists can retreat behind professional personas. Romme, a psychiatrist, 'felt quite powerless' in his attempts to assist people with auditory hallucinations and this motivated his research to find ways of helping people cope. It was voice hearers themselves who showed that it was possible to cope and since the establishment of the Hearing Voices Network they have worked increasingly in partnership with professionals to achieve change (Romme and Escher, 1996: 140).

Coleman (1999: 48) stated that: 'recovery has at its very heart the reclamation of personal power.' Professional services must not further disempower people, nor deny their experience. The processing of power and control are key issues. Coleman (1998: 36) doubted that professionals can empower people: 'power is never freely given, power is taken.' However, Coursey (*et al.* 1995: 298, added emphasis) found that psychotherapy could empower people and there was 'a strong relationship between *acting empowered* in the therapeutic relationship and clients' perception of therapist permission to act in such a way . . . acting empowered in therapy' correlated with better mental health. Dramatherapy and psychodrama involve people making choices and are permission giving: through creative drama people can take power. 'In dramatherapy . . . the client's potential to make choices within and at every single point in that process is central. His ability to act and have an effect in his world is a central issue in psychosis and in creative therapies' (Birdfield, 1998–1999: 26).

The uncontrollable psyche

As well as external interpersonal experiences of powerlessness the vulnerable ego finds there are intrapsychic forces that may be beyond ego control, such as dreams, emotions and voices.

Tom: The only time I start worrying is when I go to bed . . . You can have dreams nilly willy, **you can't control them** . . . they (voices) may be very harsh, it's like a very loud whisper. They've got more persistent. (Here he links dreams, voices, anxiety and loss of control.)

Tom was also alarmed by emotional expression: emotion is another psychological experience not easily controlled: We was enacting this woman's predicament, she got a bit upset. I thought I'd like it to stop but it wasn't that bad really. She was in tears. That was quite alarming.

Dreams, (unconscious) phantasy, (conscious) fantasy, thoughts, emotions (including sexual feelings), voices, relationships may be impossible or difficult to control. The vulnerable ego may attempt control. Professionals may attempt control. Over-control may result in tension and anxiety. Letting go of control however may be frightening or difficult. Letting go will involve some relaxation of tension and can thus be therapeutic. Dramatherapy and psychodrama can offer *a safe experience of letting go of control* (see Chapter 13). Control is often experienced in the body: a sense of someone/something having control of the body. Dramatherapy and psychodrama, in using physical activities, can provide physical release and foster a greater sense of physical self control. Dramatherapy and psychodrama also offer *a safe experience of being in control. Dramatherapy and psychodrama must, above all, empower people and return control into their own hands.*

In Chapters 4 and 5 we will look at the origin of these creative action methods in shamanism, theatre and psychotherapy, their historical development and the way previous therapists have worked.

Chapter 4

Theatre, madness and healing

Hearing voices in theatre

Theatre developed from shamanism, ritual, play and storytelling. From its beginnings drama was a healing art. Many of the tricks of theatre illusion were developed by the shamans: ventriloquism for example enabled the shamans to simulate the voices of spirits in dramatic seances; masks and puppets enabled them to present the spirits who spoke to the people of other levels of reality. During rituals in ecstatic religions, the ululations and speaking in tongues of ordinary members of the congregation or the possession of mediums (such as in Voodoo or western spiritualism) enable the members of the cult to hear the spirits' voices. In many myths and stories the voice of a god, spirit or magical object has a crucial role (such as the voice of the mirror in *Snow White*).

Theatre has, from its earliest times, been a psychospiritual forum where sanity and madness are explored: in Aeschylus' *Eurines* Orestes is pursued by Furies recalling his guilt of matricide, their voices tormenting him. The chorus of Furies sing:

> Over our victim
> we sing this song, maddening the brain,
> carrying away the sense, destroying the mind
> (Lloyd-Jones, 1979: 32)

Macbeth also has guilt induced hallucinations, both visual (of a dagger and ghost) and auditory:

Macbeth: Methought I heard a voice cry, Sleep no more!
  Macbeth doth murder sleep

(Macbeth, Act II, Sc. 2)

Hamlet sees the ghost of his dead father and hears his voice. Hearing the voice of the deceased is a normal experience in bereavement (Slade and Bentall, 1988:

88). The ghost's words motivate Hamlet throughout the play towards decisive action. Indeed the hearing of voices in Shakespeare is not without benefits: Prospero's familiar spirit Ariel is positively helpful to his master, and Caliban, who is tormented by the voices, also delights in them:

> Be not afeard; the isle is full of noises,
> Sounds and sweet airs, that give delight and hurt not.
> Sometimes a thousand twangling instruments
> Will hum about my ears; and sometimes voices,
> That, if I had wak'd after long sleep,
> Will make me sleep again
> (*The Tempest*, Act III, Sc. 2)

Pericles sees a vision and hears the voice of the goddess Diana when overwhelmed by the joy of finding his lost daughter, Marina. Interestingly he asks to be wounded as the intensity of feeling is too great for him to bear:

> O Helicanus, strike me, honoured sir;
> Give me a gash, put me to present pain;
> Lest this great sea of joys rushing upon me
> O'erbear the shores of my mortality,
> And drown me with their sweetness.
> (*Pericles*, Act IV, Sc. 1)

Shakespeare places the voice hearing experience in the context of overwhelming experience and uses water metaphors, which, as we shall see in Chapter 7, are perennial in this context. What the goddess says to Pericles is meaningful, beneficial and directs his future actions. Pericles hears heavenly music before the voice: in my research **Gloria** heard music before she heard voices. It is interesting to note that no character in Shakespeare hears voices or goes mad without there being an explanation in the play as to the meaning of the experience.

Voices may impel people towards destructive acts. In 1836 G. Buchner (1813–1837) wrote the play *Woyzeck* (published in 1879). It is the first modern portrait of a man who today might be diagnosed as paranoid schizophrenic, who hears a voice that prompts him to kill his partner. The play puts Woyzeck's voice hearing experience in the context of his oppressed position in society.

A number of twentieth-century plays incorporated the experience of hearing voices: Carney's *The Righteous are Bold*; Beckett's *Waiting for Godot*; Ayckbourn's *Woman in Mind*; Kushner's *Angels in America*; Dowie's *Adult Child/Dead Child*, Carriere's *Mahabharata*.

Carney's play, set in 1945 and first performed in 1946, is about the return of an émigré woman to her Irish home: she is hearing the voice of the Devil and is exorcised by the local priest.

Priest: The reality of possession is vouched for by Christ himself. He gave power to His followers to expel evil spirits in His name and the Church continued to use this power without interruption to the present day. History records many examples of possession and these records are in many cases compiled by non-Catholic writers.

Doctor: I imagine it could all be explained away by epilepsy or plain lunacy or this newfangled thing they talk about – schizophrenia.

(Carney, 1952: 45)

Carney does not align himself with these views but shows us how oppressed the family are by poverty, religion and fear; and we learn that the woman was used as a spirit medium by her employers in England to receive messages from the dead.

Nora: They said I was a simple girl and would be of use to them. When the day's work was over I'd come home and they'd start. La Cardami used to speak through me. She was a gypsy in Spain two hundred years ago. After a while I got frightened and wouldn't do it any more. And then it happened . . .

Priest: Yes?

Nora: One night in bed I dreamt that bombs were falling. The bricks of the house, the roof and the tiles were scattering in pieces about me. I wakened up in terror to find there was no raid but the room was full of noise of banging and rapping on the wall. I put on the light but there was no one there.

(Carney, 1952: 42)

Chadwick (1997: 25–61) similarly provided an account of his psychotic illness including a belief in possession by the Devil and mysterious noises in the walls. In Chapter 5 I report that Peter Slade worked with a woman who heard voices following her involvement in spirit mediumship in the 1930s.

Carney shows us that no one explanation describes the full complexity of Nora's experience and hints at many forces behind the onset of the voices, including the isolation and stresses of being a poor Irish woman in England during the blitz, discovering that her dream of greater success was not possible. (See Romme, 1993: 178 about the onset of voices in relation to disappointed aspirations.)

Ayckbourn's play *Woman in Mind* shows us the onset of voices after a head injury in the context of marital/family dysfunction. (I know two men whose voices started after head injuries.) Susan is the woman who hallucinates an alternative family; Bill is the GP.

Susan: I know that somehow, like those genies that live in bottles, you know, if I could only keep them from getting out I'll be alright. They mustn't get out whatever happens.

Bill: Do you think that's wise?

Susan: Why not?

Bill: Well, surely, don't you feel that these – whatever they are – are merely a symptom of something else?

Susan: They are?

Bill: Almost certainly. And with any symptom – I'm not a psychiatrist – but with any medical symptom, it can be a dangerous thing to suppress it. Or try and ignore it. A symptom is simply something trying to signal . . . Try to suppress it and you're putting your thumb over the valve of a pressure cooker.

(Ayckbourn, 1989: 67)

In *Adult Child/Dead Child* Dowie provides a theory of the origin and development of voice hearing experiences:

My invisible friend
A voice in my head
I could talk to her
I played with her
we understood each other
she was reliable.
She came I think when I was four or five
or maybe earlier, who knows
but by the age of seven
she was with me always
chattering away, making jokes
telling stories
poking fun at family and visitors
making me laugh at all times
at lonely times, good times,
boring times, embarrassing times
and awkward times
(Dowie, 1987: 54–55)

In my research this was exactly the experience of **Sheila**, who had an imaginary friend from the age of 3 that became a voice (see Chapter 2).

In all these plays the voice hearing experience has meaning and is explicable in terms of interpersonal and intrapsychic pressures.

Theatre and healing

In earlier writing I have traced a continuing tradition of healing theatre from shamanic ritual through Greek tragedy, Shakespeare, Goethe and others to the development of dramatherapy and psychodrama (Casson, 1979, 1984, 1997–1998, 1997b, 1999a, 2000a, 2001a).

Theatre, since its shamanic origins in healing ritual, has been a place of the psyche; the theatrical space has always been psychological, spiritual and symbolic. Moreno did reflect on the classical theatre of Greece and acknowledged the value of catharsis: a purging of emotions. In Sophocles' play *Antigone*, the Chorus sing a hymn to Dionysus invoking his 'swift healing': 'katharsios' (Sophocles 1994: 39 and note 163). Aristotle in his Poetics recognised catharsis as an effect of tragedy (Fyfe 1967: 16).

Shakespeare also knew of the healing potential of drama. In *King Lear* there is a scene in which the King addresses an empty stool as his daughter Goneril in a 'psychodramatic' trial. Later in the play Edgar uses a guided fantasy and enactment to help his suicidal father (Gloucester). He states:

> Why I do trifle thus with his despair is done to cure it.
>
> *(King Lear*, Act IV, Sc. 6)

In both these psychodramatic scenes other characters play auxiliary roles (Casson, 1998: 71).

Shakespeare's ideas may well have been based on the clinical practice of his time. In 1668 Grimmelshausen wrote in his *Simplicissimus* (Book 2, Ch. 13) that doctors used symbolic enactments in the treatment of delusions: one man

> thought he had already died and wandered around as a ghost, refusing both medicine and food and drink until a clever doctor paid two men to pretend they were ghosts, but ones who loved to drink. They joined the other and persuaded him that modern ghosts were in the habit of eating and drinking, through which he was cured.
>
> (Grimmelshausen, 1999)

Just over one hundred years later (*c*.1775–1777), Goethe wrote *Lila*, about the healing, through dramatic action, of a woman suffering a psychotic grief reaction. In the play a Dr Verazio directs improvised drama in which friends and relatives play the roles of Lila's delusions and hallucinations. Through this enacted fantasy Lila is brought back into contact with reality and accepts her husband is not dead (or in thrall to a demon), as she had feared when hearing a rumour of his death in the war.

Count Altenstein: It is your belief, doctor, that we may gain some influence over her if we play up to our niece's fantasies.

Dr Verazio: In the end fantasy and reality will meet. When she holds in her arms the husband she herself has regained, she will have to believe that he is back again.

Count Altenstein: She talks about ogres who want to rob her of her freedom. I want to act the Ogre. Something wild always suited me.

(Goethe, 1973: 21)

Goethe's Dr Verazio is echoed by **Cheryll**, a voice hearer, who said about her individual dramatherapy:

Cheryll: I come up here in a fantasy world – so we could express that fantasy and connect with reality.

Count Altenstein's response can also be set alongside the following:

Gloria: When I was raped the voices represented the **ogres** – the opinions of people who thought there's nothing wrong with rape, mocking me – and came with a loss of power, that it served me right: I was in the wrong place – my own fault. Someone had a troubled life and took it out on me.

Moreno, commenting on a study of the play by Diener and Moreno (1972: 11), quotes a letter from Goethe written in 1818: 'The play "Lila" is actually a psychological cure in which one allows the madness to come to the fore (that is, goes along with it, even intensifying it) in order to cure it.'

At about the same time as he wrote *Lila*, Goethe was writing the first version of his *Wilhelm Meister's Apprenticeship* in which he recommends spontaneous theatre for the benefit of the public (Book 2, Chapter 9). He clearly had drama-therapeutic ideas:

> 'So – what do we do now?' said Philine when they had all found somewhere to sit.
>
> 'The simplest thing would be to extemporise a play,' said Laertes. 'Let everyone pick a role that suits his character, and we'll see how it turns out.'
>
> 'Excellent idea!' said Wilhelm. 'If people don't dissemble at all but simply act according to their own impulses, harmony and contentment will not be theirs for long; and never, if they dissemble all the time. It will be not a bad idea if we assume a personality at the beginning and then show as much as we wish of the real self hidden beneath the mask.'

On the next page Goethe writes:

> 'I think this kind of exercise amongst actors, especially when in the company of friends and acquaintances, is extremely useful,' said the stranger. 'It is the very best way to take people out of themselves and, by way of a detour, return them to themselves. It should be introduced in all theatrical companies. They should practice in this way, and the public would surely profit greatly if every month or so an unwritten play were performed, though the actors would have to prepare for this by several rehearsals.'
>
> (Goethe, 1989: 66–67)

Thus in the play and the novel, Goethe is suggesting that not only might a psychotic woman be healed, but also actors and audiences might also benefit from spontaneous theatre. Count Altenstein realises he is attracted to the role of Ogre: dramatherapists and psychodramatists appreciate his insight that symbolic roles may allow us to temporarily inhabit aspects of ourselves which reality does not normally allow us to play.

Moreno was aware of Goethe's play and quoted the stranger's speech from the novel in reference to his own development of spontaneity theatre and psychodrama. Even as Moreno was developing psychodrama, Artaud, prophet of the theatre, wrote in 1938: 'I propose to bring back into the theatre this elementary magical idea, taken up by modern psychoanalysis, which consists in effecting a patient's cure by making him assume the apparent and exterior attitudes of the desired condition' (Artaud, 1958: 80).

Theatre is, to this day, acknowledged by actors, audiences and therapists as having healing power: 'Theatre is exorcising demons' (Miller, 2000). I have written on the therapeutic benefits of theatre for actors and audiences (Casson, 1994, 1995, 1997c) and the therapeutic impact of the visits of the National Theatre and Royal Shakespeare Company to special hospitals is chronicled by Cox (1992). Internationally, dramatherapists are practising therapeutic theatre; Playback Theatre, Boal's Theatre of the Oppressed, Psychodrama are all therapeutic theatres.

Therapeutic theatre

As psychiatry began to develop in the eighteenth century ideas about the meaning of madness and the possibility of healing through theatre emerge at the same time. Spontaneous, creative acts were found to benefit patients. When Philippe Pinel, a Parisian psychiatrist (who is considered by some as the founder of modern psychiatry), visited Bicetre Asylum, sometime in the period 1793–1795, he witnessed Madame Pussin, wife of the administrator, doing her version of psychotherapy.

> I was astonished at Bicetre to see her approach the most furious maniacs, to calm them with words of consolation and to get them to eat meals that they would obstinately have rejected from any other hand. One day an insane patient, reduced to danger of starvation from his stubborn refusal to eat, revolted against her and, in pushing away the food she was serving him, reviled her in the most outrageous terms. This quick witted woman put herself in unison with his delusional notions, she jumped and danced about in front of him, talked back to him in kind and succeeded in making him smile. Taking advantage of this opportune moment to get him to eat, she saved his life.
>
> (Pinel, 1801: 219, cited in Shorter, 1997: 21)

This can be likened to the psychodrama techniques of doubling and mirroring: the act is not ridicule, it comes from the woman's compassion and is received as empathic. The patient is audience to his own behaviour: his observer ego is suddenly engaged and the smile of recognition shows some insight was achieved through comic effect. These spontaneous acts were to be harnessed in the development of therapeutic theatre, recommended as part of the treatment of people with mental illness by Reil.

Johann Christian Reil (1759–1813) was a student of brain anatomy and one of the foremost clinicians of his time. Kirchhoff called him the conscious discoverer and founder of rational psychotherapy. In 1800 he coined the term 'psychiatry' (Mitchell, 1987: 258; Warmsley, 1984: 109). In 1803, in his book *Rhapsodies on the Application of Psychic Cure Method of Mental Disorders*, Reil elaborates an entire programme for the treatment of mental illness. Reil distinguishes three types of cures: chemical cures (which include dietetics and drug treatment), mechanical and physical cures (which include surgery) and psychic cures which, Reil emphasises, is a branch of therapy in its own right as important as surgery or pharmacology. Reil distinguishes three classes of psychic means of cure:

> 1) Bodily stimulations aimed at a modification of the general bodily feeling. These stimulations, depending on the case, will be pleasurable or unpleasurable in order to correct what we call today the 'vital tonus'.
> 2) Sensory stimulations, including a whole gamut of procedures that would be called today 'reeducation of perception'. Every one of the senses is the object of reeducation through specific methods of training. Among these methods is that of the 'therapeutic theatre' in which the employees of the institution will play various roles and where the patients will also be given parts in accordance with their specific conditions.
> 3) The method of 'signs and symbols' is a kind of school based on reading and writing. It also includes a variety of occupational therapies comprising of physical work, exercise, and art therapy.
>
> (Ellenberger, 1994: 211)

Harms quotes directly from Reil:

> Each mental institution ought to have a specially arranged theatre with the necessary machinery to present various settings. The employees of the institutions should be trained to play various roles – that of judge, an executor, physician or an angel who comes from heaven, or the dead who has risen from the grave – all concepts which might play a serious role in the mental status of this or that patient and what might impress his imagination therapeutically. Such a theatre should be able to present scenes from a prison, the lions' den, a place of execution, and an operating room. There

would be Don Quixote knighted, imaginary pregnant women freed from their load, fools skinned, repenting sinners absolved in a ceremonial play. In short, such a therapeutic theatre could aid individual cases in a variety of diseases, awaken the phantasy and the speculation, call for the most contradictory emotions, such as fear, fright, astonishment, anxiety or mental calm, according to what may help the patient to eliminate his fixed ideas or his misdirected emotions . . . Why could there not be written real plays for the purpose of the work with mental patients, to be performed by the patients themselves. Some may be acting and some watching. The roles would be distributed according to the individual therapeutic needs. The fool for instance, could be given a role making him aware of the foolishness of his way of behaving, and so on.

(Harms, 1957: 806–807)

From 1795 Goethe was aware of Reil; they met in 1802 when Goethe visited Halle and attended Bad Lauchstadt where he opened a new theatre. Goethe used the opportunity for scientific discussions and to consult Reil about an eye condition. There can be little doubt then that Reil would be aware of Goethe's ideas, if not before 1802, then from that time: his own book in which he expounds the idea of therapeutic theatre was published in 1803. Reil's ideas emerged in the context of a Europe-wide development of therapeutic theatre: in 1788 'in the large Lunatic Hospital near Paris, the Patients were encouraged to Act Plays, this pleasing remedy has been found to be very conducive to their recovery' (Hunter and Macalpine, 1964: 644). From 1797 to 1811 Coulmier, at Charenton Asylum, France, encouraged patients, including De Sade, to make theatre. From 1813 theatres were built in psychiatric hospitals in Italy at Aversa, Naples and Palermo. In 1843 William Browne encouraged psychiatric patients to perform plays at the Crichton Royal Institution, Dumfries, Scotland. James Kenney's farce *Raising the Wind* and Shakespeare's *Twelfth Night* were performed by the patients. Stone (1998: 109) calls Browne's creative innovation drama therapy. Interestingly, Browne was a former student of Esquirol at the Charenton Hospital where forty years earlier patients had been encouraged to create theatre. Browne encouraged creative activities and outings to the theatre. At first he was doubtful of the benefits of such theatre, writing in 1837:

I cannot speak so decidedly as to the introduction of dramatic representation as a means of cure. The attempt has been made at Charenton unsuccessfully, at Copenhagen without injury; but the inhabitants of this country manifest during health so little taste for such spectacles, and depend so little upon them as sources of amusement, that it would be injurious to resort to them in order to arouse, or attract, or amuse the insane, while we have so many better modes of abstraction at our disposal.

(Browne, 1837, reprinted in Scull, 1991)

Initially theatre and other entertainments were used as rewards, encouragement and distraction. But soon the therapeutic benefits of involvement in theatre became apparent. Richard Chateris, who had spent much of the previous five years rolled in a carpet, believing he was the King of India, was encouraged to become involved in theatre in 1843. Within a year:

> A total revolution has taken place in this individual's mind. Progress has been slow but the triumph is complete. He reposed great confidence in the Medical Officer. His studies in the oriental languages were encouraged. Long and laboriously did he labour to produce a PERFECT PLAYBILL for the private theatre couched in Hindustani, Persee, etc. His success and his curiosity prompted him at last to witness the performances he had so splendidly chronicled. He was pleased by the evening's entertainment, thoroughly stimulated and the next step was his enrolment among the actors. He was a most diligent student and enacted a female part with great correctness.
>
> (Browne, 1843: 258)

After achieving 'many triumphs in histrionic and pictorial art', Chateris was discharged in 1846.

The annual reports of the hospital testify to the therapeutic benefits of theatre:

> Theatrical representation, as a means of cure and pleasure to the insane, is not now confined to the Crichton Institution. Melodramas have been acted before the inmates of asylums in this country; and *Tartuffe* has been produced by the patients in Salpetriere with the same poetical justice which suggested the selection of *Redgauntlet* by the company in this asylum. Three pieces were brought out during last season. Of these the *Mock Doctor* was the favourite. It contains some ludicrous allusions to asylums and their governors; and the shouts of laughter and triumph with which the exposure of the savage practices formerly pursued in these places was received indicated how keenly some portion of the audience understood the point and truth of the satire, and how cordially they rejoiced at the revolution which had established the gentler rule under which they then were.
>
> (Crichton, 1844: 22–23)

Eleven patients participated in some degree or other in theatre, of these five benefited sufficiently to be discharged.

> No human mean as yet employed has at so little risk and with so little trouble and expense, communicated so much rational happiness to so many of the insane at the same time, or so completely placed them in circumstances so closely allied to those of sane beings, or so calculated either to remove the

burden of mental disease, or to render it more bearable. The attempt is no longer an experiment. It is a great fact of moral science, and must be accepted and acted upon.

(Crichton, 1844: 23)

What perhaps is most significant for us is that these therapeutic effects of theatre were obtained at a time before the introduction of modern medication.

The development of therapeutic theatre continued across Europe. In 1863 Alexandre Dumas witnessed a therapeutic performance by patients at Aversa, Italy (Jones, 1996: 48). In 1878 'An excellent theatre with scenery' was constructed for the use of patients at Ticehurst Asylum, England (Scull, 1979: 207).

Drama in psychotherapy

In 1891 Janet, French pioneer of psychological analysis, used hypnosis and drama to re-enact traumatic scenes, to achieve catharsis and modify the patient's fixed ideas.

Janet could deal with a man who believed himself to be possessed by a devil by striking up a conversation with the devil to see what it wanted. In time it came out that the man began to see devils after a lapse into infidelity on a business trip away from his wife. He could not deal with his errant behaviour or guilt. The devil was placed in the context of a personal (clinical) history and soon disappeared or, at least became more manageable.

(Eigen, 1993: 71–72)

In *Studies on Hysteria* written in 1895 Freud's colleague and co-author Josef Breuer writes of a spontaneous 'psychodrama' (before Moreno) during Anna O's treatment. In this she 'set the scene' and thereby accessed vivid psychological material relating to the repressed trauma of her father's death: 'by the help of rearranging the room so as to resemble her father's sick room she reproduced the terrifying hallucinations . . . which constituted the root of her whole illness' (Freud and Breuer, 1973: 95).

During my research just such another deathbed scene was re-enacted, the scene setting being especially helpful to access the 'bottled up' emotion.

Sheila: We re-enacted when my mum were dying and we set the chairs out as the bedroom was designed at the time. Leah . . . were lying as my mother in the bed: it was like a flash back to what I was actually going through so it helped because I wasn't having to imagine it: it was actually being role played. I got quite upset, because of the memories. I bottle things up about it anyway. (See Chapter 12.)

Thus as psychotherapy emerged in the eighteenth and nineteenth centuries the possibility of using drama in therapy was already being considered in Britain, Germany, France and Italy. It was in the twentieth century that these developments came to fruition.

Chapter 5

The twentieth century
Theatrotherapy, psychodrama and dramatherapy

Vladimir Iljine, from 1908 to 1917, developed therapeutic theatre with psychiatric patients in Kiev in pre-revolutionary Russia (Petzold, 1973; Jones, 1996). He was influenced by Stanislavski. His was the first such work in the twentieth century. In 1909 Iljine published *Improvising Theatre Play in the Treatment of Mood Disorders* and in 1910 *Patients Play Theatre: A Way of Healing Body and Mind*. After the Russian Revolution Iljine travelled to Constantinople, Budapest, Berlin and then settled in Paris. In 1922 in Budapest, he met Sandor Ferenczi, who was already using role play in psychoanalysis. In 1925 in Berlin, Iljine translated Moreno's *The Theatre of Spontaneity* into Russian and eventually met Moreno in 1964 at the first International Congress of Psychodrama in Paris.

In 1920 Ferenczi had addressed the Sixth International Congress of Psycho-Analysis about his Active Techniques and described encouraging a woman to play the role of her sister:

> At one interview a sweet song occurred to her that her elder sister (who tyrannized over her in every way) was in the habit of singing. After hesitating for a long time she repeated the very ambiguous text of the song and was silent for a long time; I extracted from her that she had thought of the *melody* of the song. I did not delay in asking her to sing the song. It took nearly two hours, however, before she could bring herself to perform the song as she really intended it. She was so embarrassed that she broke off repeatedly in the middle of a verse, and to begin with she sang in a low voice until, encouraged by my persuasions, she began to sing louder, when her voice developed more and more and proved to be an unusually beautiful soprano. This did not overcome the resistance; after some difficulty she confessed that her sister was in the habit of accompanying the song with expressive and indeed quite unambiguous *gestures*, and she made some clumsy arm movements to illustrate her sister's behaviour. Finally I asked her to get up and repeat the song *exactly* as she had seen her sister do it. After endless spiritless partial attempts she showed herself to be a perfect *chanteuse*, with all the coquetry of facial play and movement that she had seen in her sister . . . It was

astonishing how favourably this little interlude affected the work. Presently memories of her early childhood, of which she had never spoken, occurred to her.

(Ferenczi, 1920: 203–204, original emphases)

Ferenczi was not physically active himself, except in encouraging or prohibiting the patient to act in certain ways he believed would be therapeutic. Mindful of the opposition of orthodox Freudians he was cautious and hedged his innovation around with caveats while arguing it was in harmony with mainstream psychoanalytic technique: he declared that 'the active technique . . . ought to bring about in the patient the psychical conditions under which repressed material comes forward more easily' (Ferenczi, 1920: 216). He saw the therapeutic value not only of the confession of deeply concealed impulses but also the enactment of these in the therapist's presence so that the patient had the task of consciously controlling these impulses. He also reported that the active techniques were found to be efficient in shortening the treatment of traumatic war hysterias and were effective in the treatment of catatonic patients (Ferenczi, 1920: 210). He further speculated that they might be effective in working with children and the mentally ill.

Freud however did not encourage action in therapy, seeing any action as 'acting out' and, by definition, avoiding feelings or resistance to the therapist. Such ideas were not acceptable to the psychoanalytic establishment. What is interesting for us about Ferenczi's active technique is that it predates Moreno's invention of psychodrama. I have no evidence that Moreno was influenced by Ferenczi, nor Ferenczi by Iljine. They were all independently discovering the therapeutic potential of drama.

Moreno arrived in the United States (from Austria) in 1925. By the late 1930s and early 1940s he was working with psychotic patients using psychodrama at Beacon, New York. His earliest paper on using psychodrama with psychotic patients is from 1939 (see p. 72).

Nicholas Evreinoff (1879–1953), a Russian theatre director (who in 1920 had directed a spectacular mass re-enactment of the storming of the Winter Palace with 8,000 performers: Cosgrove, 1982: 5) had arrived in New York in 1926, where he was already famous: his play *The Gay Death* had been performed in New York in 1916 (Sayler, 1922: 301). In *The Theatre in Life* Evreinoff (1927: 122–127) recommended the development of 'Theatrotherapy'. Moreno knew of this book and I have written elsewhere of the possible links between them (Casson, 1999a). Evreinoff however did not work with people who had mental illnesses. It is likely that Iljine and Evreinoff knew each other, if not in Russia then as émigrés in Paris where they both lived (Evreinoff 1925–1953; Iljine 1942–1974) and created theatre. (See Chapter 9 concerning Evreinoff's 'theatre for oneself'.)

Peter Slade, the founder of dramatherapy in Britain, did some work with a woman who heard voices as early as 1933.

She had started by trying to get in touch with someone who had died. A voice came to her in answer, then others. Finally she was invaded by what she described as 'Legion', many voices, as in the Bible. She finally did much to cure herself . . . The voices stopped eventually, she said, after prayer.

(P. Slade, personal communication, 30 November 2000)

In this early case Slade did not attempt to use drama and the healing is attributed to the woman's own actions and to prayer (many voice hearers report benefits from prayer, including in my own research). From 1937 to 1939 Slade was using drama to facilitate therapy with adults, working in collaboration with Dr Kraemer (a Jungian psychotherapist) in London (Casson 1997b). He was in touch with Moreno by letter from 1938 and they met on at least two occasions when Moreno visited Britain in 1951 and 1954.

In 1941 Slade had a dramatic encounter in the Military Wing of the Crichton Royal Institution, Dumfries (the very hospital where Browne had used theatre with patients in 1843, see Chapter 4) where he was a patient recovering from post-traumatic shock resultant from an accident while making a training film about dealing with incendiary devices.

Very early in my days there I now remember, another young officer approached me. He was wearing a sheet and flourished a cardboard, or wooden sword. 'I am the Holy Ghost,' he said, 'and I have a message from God to kill all newcomers.' I think I said something like 'You can't kill me, though, because I am the Angel Gabriel.' . . . This man had been badly injured in Africa and certainly heard voices. I was just about able, as Gabriel, to give him a message from on High to calm down. We talked in these characters for a long time and I think he finally went to sleep. I got into bed and felt I would die of fatigue. Whether you would call this treatment, I don't know. It was certainly therapy for him, but certainly not for me. We had further conversations in the following weeks, and as Gabriel I began to suggest and order him not to do things that would upset the ward. He often obeyed Gabriel. It is an example of how, as so often happens, patients can do much to help/cure each other. Although being in a state of wreck myself, I remember intending to help and calm him down. As I gained power, his voices and ideas became more weak . . . When I met him months later . . . he was talking quite sensibly. He no longer heard voices.

(P. Slade, personal communication, 30 November 2000)

In psychodrama terms Slade had been an auxiliary ego to this man (see Chapter 12). He was able to be appropriately spontaneous in response to the situation at a time when he himself was a patient. After this informal 'psychodramatic' encounter, 'doctors asked me to talk to other patients and I began to be in a more constructive and empowered position. Finally I was asked to help in the civilian mental hospital' (P. Slade, personal communication, 30 November 2000).

He then began to direct patients in rehearsals for a theatre performance and on 22 December 1941 there were two performances of *Dear Brutus* by J. M. Barrie (1998, first published 1923).

> One thing that stays in my mind during rehearsals was my desperate sadness for the Count. He was a charming man in lucid moments and great fun. But once a month he would go into deep decline, sometimes hear voices, he told me, and then *become* peculiar objects and be unable to move. He was at these times stuck, as it were [in later Slade terminology] in the embodiment of Projected Play rather than in successful Personal Activity.
>
> (P. Slade, personal communication, 30 November 2000)

From the above examples of practice with people who heard voices, Slade was able to work both psychodramatically (with the officer who believed he was the Holy Ghost) and dramatherapeutically using theatre. The hospital supported and valued his work. His is the earliest such work with auditory hallucinations in Britain.

From 1944 to 1977 theatrotherapy and group psychotherapy were used with psychotic children in Saint Alban state hospital (France) by Dr Francois Tosquelles, a Spanish psychiatrist and psychoanalyst (Fontaine, 1999: 27). In 1956 Anne Schutzenberger began to run psychodrama groups at the University of Paris Mental Health Hospital for people struggling with psychosis (Fontaine, 1999: 26).

In 1952 Dr Rollin, a psychiatrist, invited Elsie Green, a theatre director, to work at Horton Hospital, Epsom, Surrey. For thirty-two years, until 1984, Green conducted play reading, theatre therapy and dramatherapy sessions with patients, many of whom suffered psychotic illnesses and some of whom heard voices. Elsie herself spoke of the normalising effect of her work:

> I deal with patients suffering from all kinds of mental illness; psychotics, for instance, whose hold on reality is very fragile, many of whom are lost in a private world of delusions and hallucinations. My job as a therapist is to help them to strengthen their hold on reality, and to build a bridge between their private world and the allegedly sane world in which most of us live. By taking a dramatic role in a group the patient can adopt a personality to which the other members of the group can respond on a reality level. This helps to strengthen a sense of identity in a patient, and supports his ego. It's positively Pirandellian!
>
> (Thompson, 1998: 30)

Sue Jennings began her work using drama with patients in Hatton Psychiatric Hospital, Warwick in 1955. She was 17 years old at this time and was specifically invited by a psychiatrist, Dr Stern, to do drama with patients: he gave her work as a nursing auxiliary for this purpose as he knew she had been to drama college. He said, 'You're not going to do psychodrama are you?' He thought psychodrama would be too intense for the mentally ill patients, whereas creative drama he thought would be helpful. She replied, 'No' (though at that time she had not heard of psychodrama: S. Jennings, personal communication, 15 December 2000).

During the 1950s Veronica Sherborne was employed at the Withymead Centre, Devon, to offer Laban-based movement therapy to psychiatric patients, working with Irene Champernowne (a Jungian psychotherapist). In 1964 Marian Lindkvist founded the Sesame Institute to train drama movement therapists: her first training course was for occupational therapists at York Clinic, Guy's Hospital, London. She worked with Peter Slade and Audrey Wethered and was influenced by Laban and Jung. She researched dance movement with 'schizophrenics' (see p. 81).

From 1966 to 1986 Dorothy Heathcote (who was influenced by Slade) ran drama groups in hospitals for people with disabilities and mental illnesses in England, the United States, Australia, New Zealand and Norway and made videos of her work.

Dramatherapists have worked with people diagnosed as schizophrenic since the 1940s and so with people who hear voices, but no specific research had been done on the effectiveness of dramatherapy with people who hear voices. Psychodramatists have also worked with people with psychotic illnesses. While Moreno and others have claimed that psychodrama helps people who hallucinate, there has been little published follow-up research of this work, a fact lamented by Zerka Moreno (1978: 163).

Before proceeding further to examine the work done by many pioneers, I offer the following definitions of the terms dramatherapy and psychodrama.

Definitions of dramatherapy and psychodrama

Dramatherapy is the heir to the shamanic and theatre traditions of healing through dramatic action. Dramatherapy can be defined as:

> the specific application of theatre structures and drama processes with a declared intention that it is therapy.
>
> (Jennings, 1992: 229)

It could be argued that this definition of dramatherapy includes psychodrama, an action method created by Moreno in the 1920s to 1940s and now recognised internationally as a form of psychotherapy. Moreno defined psychodrama as:

> the science which explores the 'truth' by dramatic methods. It deals with interpersonal relations and private worlds.
>
> (Moreno, 1993: 53)

Dramatherapy and psychodrama, as creative action methods in psychotherapy, can then be seen to overlap. They facilitate the development of the person through encouraging spontaneity and creativity. They are within the humanistic, existential and phenomenological traditions of therapy. Dramatherapy is influenced as much by developments in twentieth-century theatre and drama as by its inter-face with schools of therapy. This makes generalisations about the methods difficult. One potentially useful distinction between the two methods is the degree of 'distancing' used and I now introduce this issue, which will be further explored in Chapter 7.

Direct and indirect work

Dramatherapists often do not work directly with the difficulty with which the client presents. Dramatherapists work with stories, metaphors and objects, to provide people with a safe distance from material that could be too threatening to be addressed directly. In psychodrama there is a greater likelihood that the therapist will work more directly with the person's difficulties. However, this distinction is not absolute: dramatherapists directly rehearse behaviours and explore the dynamics of people's relationships through sculpting objects or people. Psycho-dramatists encourage groups to explore symbolic material, dreams, metaphors: the methods overlap. In dramatherapy and psychodrama people are not passive patients but active agents and creative artists working to change their lives: the methods are empowering.

How might these methods be applied with people who hear voices?

A dramatherapy group might work with an ancient Greek myth: for example Odysseus, travelling home on his ship from Troy, hears the voices of the Sirens, singing, enticing him onto the rocks and certain death. He resists their calls by having his men tie him to the mast of his ship as they sail onward (the crews' ears are plugged by wax: some voice hearers have found ear plugs helpful, see Slade and Bentall, 1988: 196; Sims, 1991: 70; Watkins, 1998: 211). This image from the ancient Greek myth could provide an epic metaphor for dramatising the dilemma of voice hearers who are uncertain whether to listen to their voices and fear being controlled by them. Odysseus was firmly secured to the mast (at the centre of the boat) so that he could listen to the siren songs without being over-whelmed by them. (See Jennings (1998: 111) for photographs of this scene in a dramatherapy group.) Such a myth provides rich imagery for work: often dramatherapists use the image of a journey to represent the therapeutic process. Dramatising such a journey, with its hazards and struggles, provides a group with a shared exploration of the dilemmas of whether to listen to the voices and be commanded by them or to sail on in their lives, acknowledging the voices but staying clear of the rocks and the danger of floundering. Creating such a drama would provide opportunities for play, creativity, movement, voice, group co-operation and sharing.

Alternatively psychodrama offers an opportunity to externalise inner conflicts and struggles in dramatic action: the voice hearer can explore ways of coping and receive support from other group members. When the drama is all internal and invisible it may control the person. When it is externalised the person can be more in charge of their experience: a creator rather than a victim. People may work more directly on a problem of their choosing: such as asserting themselves, challenging the voices they hear, working through experiences that underlie the voices.

Psychodrama, dramatherapy and the person-centred approach

There is a tension in the methods of psychodrama and dramatherapy between the use of technique and the provision of a person-centred facilitative environment, with a spectrum of practitioners using different approaches with different client groups: there is no one manual of technique that is universally practised. The application of Moreno's (1939) philosophy encourages the psychodramatist to enter the world of the person, see things from their perspective and creatively play: to build bridges between delusional fantasy and reality. It can therefore be in harmony with the person-centred approach.

> Rogers discovered that defensiveness and resistance are obviated when one responds to an individual '*within his own **frame of reference**.*' This phrase means that the psychotherapist's response always refers to something which is directly present in the individual's own momentary awareness.
> (Worchel and Byrne, 1964: 107, italics in original, bold added)

Moreno was willing, with psychotic patients, to enter their *frame of reference* and realise their delusions on the therapeutic stage. Psychodrama is a method which respects and accepts the perception of the client. Roine, a psychodramatist, found herself confronted by a psychiatrist on her first day in a new job:

> he called me into his office and told me about the general policy of Reality Confrontation. 'It's very important with psychotic patients.' He implied that when the patients spoke of hearing voices and seeing strange things I had to reply that this was not my reality. 'Then this job is not for me,' I said, 'because in psychodrama our interest is such that we often ask, "What do you hear? What do you see?" Only then is it possible to enter the patient's world.' After this he smiled and said, 'Do as you like then.'
> (Cox, 1992: 202)

In being willing to enter into people's world view psychodrama is not alone: Jung supported dialogue with hallucinations and delusions (Allen, 1994). Laing takes this further:

> The therapist must have the plasticity to transpose himself into another strange and even alien view of the world. In this act, he draws on his own psychotic possibilities, without forgoing his sanity. Only thus can he arrive at an understanding of the patient's position.
>
> (Laing, 1960: 34)

The therapist's own 'madness' thus becomes a source of empathy, understanding and contact. This perspective then offers an alternative view to that of the medical model. The therapist engages with the person and his/her 'madness' rather than denying or suppressing symptoms or experiences. The therapist takes his/her own 'madness' to supervision and when necessary to personal therapy to ensure this is not projected onto the client (see guidelines for good practice in Chapter 14).

Garry Prouty (1990), a person-centred counsellor, developed 'pre-therapy' to establish contact and thereby a therapeutic relationship, with people who are diagnosed schizophrenic, withdrawn or out of contact with reality. Building on this method he developed 'pre-symbolic experiencing' to facilitate the integration and processing of visual hallucinations. Jill Prouty, a psychodramatist, then broke new ground by applying this method to auditory hallucinations. Thereby she enabled the protagonist in a psychodrama to process voices and to express rage and guilt about sexual abuse, which was the origin of the voices.

The arts, creativity and therapeutic benefit

Dramatherapy is one of the arts therapies (see Killick and Schaverien (1997) for an exploration of the value of art therapy in working with psychotic clients). The arts therapies utilise the healing elements of creative processes. Two surveys in the late 1990s have reported the opinions of people who have psychotic experiences about the benefits of working creatively. In a survey of how people in emotional distress take control of their lives:

> 85% of people who had experience of Art and creative therapies found it helpful or helpful at times. In addition 7% or 24 people named art or creative therapy as their most helpful alternative or complementary therapy overall.
>
> (Mental Health Foundation, 1997: 47)

About 5 per cent found these therapies unhelpful and about 1 per cent damaging. The major ways creative therapies were found to be helpful were as follows:

• facilitating expression of feelings (especially through non-verbal means)
• focusing the mind/distracting

- relaxation
- support/empathy
- improving self-esteem and motivation (a reason to get up in the morning).

Most helpful of all were the talking therapies. However, this survey was a broad one in that the majority of clients identified themselves as depressed 51 per cent, only 13.9 per cent as schizophrenic and 6.6 per cent as suffering a psychosis. Therefore all we can tell is that the vast majority of clients found talking helpful and many found art/creative therapies helpful.

This survey was reinforced by another conducted by the National Schizophrenia Fellowship (NSF), MIND and the Manic Depressive Fellowship, *A Question of Choice*, (Hogman and Sandamas, 2000) which surveyed the opinions of 2,663 people of whom 37 per cent had a diagnosis of schizophrenia, 34 per cent of manic depression and 21 per cent of depression. Asked what they found helpful the responses were as follows:

- 85 per cent found exercise and training/education helpful
- 81 per cent art/music
- 79 per cent talking treatments
- 72 per cent cognitive behaviour therapy
- 70 per cent nutrition/diet.

However, neither of these surveys revealed anything about the impact of these on voice hearing.

Dramatherapy and psychodrama use action in therapy. In an American survey of self-help strategies employed by voice hearers, the largest percentage used some form of action as a coping strategy; the largest single strategy was to talk to the voices (Frederick and Cotanch, 1995).

I now examine the specific literature on psychodrama and dramatherapy to learn what other researchers and practitioners have done in the past. I begin with consideration of Moreno, the founding father of psychodrama.

Psychodrama

Moreno heard voices from childhood. 'He had always kept this secret, thinking that people might laugh at him or find it abnormal' (Marineau, 1989: 62). In 1920 a voice dictated Moreno's seminal work *Words of the Father* which he later regarded as the philosophical source of his ideas. This was written in a creative mania on the walls, in red pencil.

> I suddenly felt reborn. I began then to hear voices, not in the sense of a mental patient, but in the sense of a person beginning to feel that he hears a voice which reaches all beings and which speaks to all beings in the same language, which is understood by all men, and one which gives hope, which gives

our life direction, which gives our cosmos a direction and a meaning, that the universe is not just a jungle and a bundle of wild forces, that it is basically infinite creativity.

(Fox, 1987: 212)

Moreno here links the experience of voices with hope, meaning and creativity. The experience empowered him to innovate methods of psychotherapy and was a lasting psychospiritual inspiration in his life. The way of working with people who were struggling with psychotic experiences that he developed grew out of his own experiences, philosophy, experiments and observations of spontaneity and interpersonal relations.

The psychodrama of hallucinations

In psychodrama Moreno encouraged people to embody their hallucinations:

> The patient enacts the hallucinations and delusions he is at present experiencing . . . [the] Patient portrays the voices he hears, the sounds emanating from the chair he sits on, the visions he has when the trees outside his window turn into monsters which pursue him.
>
> (Z. Moreno, 1966: 8)

In these psychodramas trained professionals or other patients acted as 'auxiliary egos' and played delusional roles from the world of the patient, so that the patient was simultaneously confronted with real people (in role) as well as with the hallucinations. Moreno first presented his theory, which he illustrated with three cases, a schizophrenia, manic-depressive psychosis and a psychoneurosis, in 1939.

> During lucid intervals of the psychotic attack or immediately after it the patient is stimulated by use of a warming up-process to throw himself back into the psychotic world. This upsetting experience is called 'psychodramatic shock' . . . it has a cathartic effect on the patients. It enhances their spontaneity and creates barriers against recurrence.
>
> (Moreno, 1939: 1)

None of these cases apparently involved auditory hallucinations, though tactile and visual hallucinations and delusions are mentioned. Moreno's analysis of these three shows he understood the functional meaning of these psychoses. They all involved extreme interpersonal conflict, loss and trauma. The third case was of a Jewish refugee from Nazi Germany, whose business had been seized and whose colleagues had committed suicide. In 1940 Moreno published *Psychodramatic Treatment of Psychoses* in which he mentions one case of a woman who heard voices (Moreno, 1945b: 16; Fox, 1987). This monograph is based on work with eighteen people diagnosed schizophrenic (of whom twelve were paranoid), ten manic-depressive and five with 'involutional' psychosis. Moreno shows that the psychodramas reveal far more about the patient's mental state than interviews:

> by the use of psychodramatic techniques we were able to inaugurate a systematic course of treatment in which there was a high degree of participation and leadership on the part of patients. The psychodrama provided the patients with an environment in which their egos could expand ... we were in a position to arrest further deterioration into psychosis and in twenty-five cases, to guide the patients into relationships which were better suited to a life outside the institution.
>
> (Moreno, 1945b: 17)

Sadly this monograph is less detailed about the treatment than that of 1939. Another 1945 work (in Moreno and Moreno, 1975: 181–197) describes the treatment of a paranoid woman searching for an imaginary lover. With this woman and professional auxiliaries Moreno co-constructed a psychodramatic fantasy that reflected her delusion: Moreno actualised her inner and interpersonal worlds on the therapeutic stage. The auxiliary egos gradually replaced the delusional figures with their real human presence. Moreno also used the mirror technique to enable the protagonist to observe someone in her role hearing the voice and seeing the hallucination of the lover. Gradually Moreno worked from fantasy towards reality. His aim however was not to disillusion the person but to give them an experience of being able to create at will: to feel in control, empowered to own the products of their imagination, express the feeling contained in the hallucination, to play with them and to develop satisfying interpersonal spontaneity, rather than be controlled by the products of psychotic spontaneity (Moreno, 1945a).

Moreno (1945a) stated that one of the functions of an auxiliary ego was to free a subject from that extreme form of isolation – hallucination. He saw the value of an interpersonal treatment of a condition which isolated the person: by engaging them with others, with auxiliaries in their drama, he enabled the person to emerge from isolation into an encounter of self and other and thus return to a social world. Miller (1972) also stressed the importance of the warm support of the group which replaces the previous experience of cold isolation.

By playing out the psychotic material individuals gradually develop their observer ego, achieving some distance between themselves and the overwhelming psychotic experiences. The person is also free to play through the symbolic drama of the psychotic process to a healthier outcome. Moreno suggested that this led to a greater sense of self-control. Blatner and Blatner agreed:

> The patient is helped to portray the hallucination in concrete form – tone of voice, pace, intensity, phraseology. Alternatively an auxiliary might play the role of the hallucination . . . This character can then be interviewed, and a negotiating encounter might even lead to some modification of the

hallucination's power. When the situation is judiciously chosen, this action will not strengthen the psychotic process because the active engagement with these mechanisms introduces a measure of voluntary control that tends to neutralise some of the sense of victimisation . . . The different sources of voices become personalised and elaborated, and alternative outcomes are explored.

(Blatner and Blatner, 1988: 5, 166)

Thus the externalisation of the hallucination in a dramatic enactment of the person's inner world leads to empowerment and a greater sense of control (Kipper, 1986). It can also lead to the discovery of meaning and insight. Goldman and Morrison tell of a girl who was

hallucinating a horrible green devil who was in control of her. We entered into the hallucination, seeing the devil along with her. We used an auxiliary, the lights and sound to produce her 'devil'. At the appropriate time, we helped her to move from the fantasised green devil to the symbol of being controlled. Finally, when she had the act gratification of the director and team seeing what she saw, we . . . asked who the devil really was, we discovered he was father who had sexually molested the girl since childhood. As we arrived at reality, she no longer needed the hallucination.

(Goldman and Morrison, 1984: 26)

Harrow (1952) investigated the effects of psychodrama on the role behaviour of schizophrenic patients. This study combined quantitative and qualitative methods, psychological and role tests, and the use of a control group.

While the quantitative results presented are inconclusive, the consistent tendency . . . in the direction of 'positive' changes in the treatment groups, as compared to insignificant changes in the control group lends [weight to the findings that psychodrama facilitated the development of social and relationship skills, ability to share feelings, more emotional control, more appropriate behaviour, clearer thinking and perception of reality] greater abilities in dealing with their personal and inter-personal problems. Further the statistically significant Rorschach changes of the treatment group, as compared with the control group, suggest that psychodramatic treatment may affect some fundamental personality processes as well as overt role-taking behaviour . . . The findings of the study seem to support the assumption that role-taking behaviour is not a mechanical skill superimposed upon personality, but an essential part of personality formation and adjustment; that the development of role-taking ability, especially for individuals in whom the skill was never adequately developed or has broken down, may be as important an aspect of treatment as the development of strictly emotional processes.

[Psychodrama] leads to better personality integration and a gradual working through of problems.

(Harrow, 1952: 167–170)

Parrish (1959) conducted research into the effectiveness of psychodrama with a group of thirty-two white female in-patients diagnosed as having chronic schizophrenia. Despite considerable prior treatment including ECT, recreational and occupational therapy and individual psychotherapy, their illness seemed to have increased, rather than decreased: she deliberately chose very sick, hostile and withdrawn patients.

> hostility and feelings of anger emerged during the first session . . . by the third session another factor emerged which proved a common denominator – all were lonely and all dreaded the feeling of aloneness. The patients blamed society for their loneliness, wanted revenge and hostile outbursts were the only revenge they could muster.
>
> (Parrish, 1959: 18–19)

The patients began to discover what they shared and that they could help each other through this sharing: from loneliness came social caring. Parish records the following scene enacted at the request of a patient:

Nurse: Good morning girls. Did you sleep good last night?
Patient #1: Who can sleep around here?
Nurse: What's the matter?
Patient #1: I never get any sleep. Someone is talking all night long. Sometimes it's women, sometimes it's men.
Patient #2: I know what she means.
Patient #1: Why don't they leave me alone?
Patient #2: I used to hear voices too, and I used to think it was God's voice, but I don't hear them anymore. It was just my imagination.
Patient #1: I do. I still hear them all the time.
Nurse: Are you sure it isn't your imagination?
Patient #2: I know it's your imagination because when I heard voices I didn't think it was my imagination either . . . She is always talking to herself; she thinks she is a telephone operator.
Patient #1: I answer the telephone but no one is there, and I don't see anyone, but I know they are around somewhere and they just talk and talk and talk.

At the end of the session the patient made the statement, 'I don't see how it could be my imagination; I hear people talking to me at night.' The only response on the part of the therapist was: 'that would certainly be annoying.' At the beginning of the next session the patient remarked, 'I can't understand it, but I have not heard voices all week. Did you tell them to stop?' (Long pause) 'It might *just have been my imagination.*' Other patients remarked that they had not been as bothered as usual by the voices; within a short time the patients no longer discussed the voices and the ward nurse reported a marked improvement in ward conduct (Parrish, 1959: 20–21).

Parrish concludes her study:

> Considering the degree of illness and the duration of illness of these patients, it is remarkable that twenty of the thirty-two should have improved to such an extent that it is possible for them to live in the community . . . Psychodrama is beneficial to such patients in that it helps them socialise . . . overcome their fear of failure . . . reveal their problems . . . The healing effect is achieved through relieving in action and counteraction important life experiences. Such acting out exerts a profound influence on the unrealistic thinking of the psychotic patient.
>
> (Parrish, 1959: 26)

McGee *et al.* (1965) reported on the combined use of psychodrama and talking group therapy with schizophrenic patients. This study involved thirty-four patients over two years. They found the methods complemented each other to the benefit of patients:

> Psychodrama provided certain patients opportunity to demonstrate to the group their identity freer of its 'sick patient' aspects with an associated increase in self-esteem . . . when a patient was able to enact a role in another group member's problem this provided further opportunity to experience normal aspects of personality functioning.
>
> (McGee *et al.*, 1965: 129–130)

This psychodrama team was able to enact delusional material with the result that previously isolated people experienced greater empathy from others and engagement with the group. Action encouraged engagement as patients could function non-verbally and in concrete ways whereas in the verbal psychotherapy group they 'repeatedly withdrew into silence or steadfast denial' (McGee *et al.*, 1965: 130). There followed an increase in social skills and rehearsals for living: patients especially enacting job interviews before their discharge from the unit. The combination therapy

> had a salutary effect on the discharge rate of patients treated. These were schizophrenic individuals in the early stages of chronicity who had experienced multiple prior hospitalisations and for whom the prognosis were poor.
>
> (McGee *et al.*, 1965: 134–135)

Deane and Hanks (1967) described a psychodrama with a man who believed he was accompanied by a ghost which spoke to him. They were able to discover that the ghost appeared after his father's death when he was 5 years old. They psychodramatised this figure but their technique was highly confronting, even aggressive. This paper claims to show benefit from psychodrama; it also shows the method could be used in quite a brutal way. Moreno, who could be directive and controlling, used his power in appropriate, therapeutic ways. There is a danger that such power can be abused. Honig reported working as an ally in a continuous battle with destructive command hallucinations using many different action techniques. He was cautious about their effectiveness but suggested that confronting a command hallucination and defying it 'will empower that person to further defiance and set up a chain of behaviours towards recovery' (Honig, 1992: 33). Honig has been exposed by Masson for his sadistic, controlling, abusive techniques including the use of cattle prods to shock people. Masson (1989) also reported that Honig's staff sexually abused and humiliated patients.

John Rosen, who in the early 1950s developed a technique for the treatment of psychotic patients which he termed 'direct psychoanalysis' (Greenberg: 1975, 387–393), was likewise criticised by Zerka Moreno (1978) and was also exposed by Masson (1989) for his abusive use of action methods. It is important to note that neither Honig nor Rosen were qualified psychodramatists.

Other creative action methods

Creative action methods are not the exclusive preserve of dramatherapy and psychodrama but have been used by therapists of other orientations. Harris (1997), a gestalt therapist, invited a client who heard a voice to *be* the voice (in effect inviting the client to role reverse). After speaking as his angry voice the client reported that he did not hear the voice again. Fritz Perls, who developed gestalt therapy, was influenced by Moreno.

Stone and Winkelman (1987) developed 'Voice Dialogue' therapy in which the

> patient is invited to move physical position and act as if personifying . . . to dramatise various sides of an internal conflict in order to facilitate inner dialogue . . . the approach is unashamedly dramatic, using dissociation deliberately . . . as a prelude to greater communication and integration.
>
> (Mollon, 1996: 107; see also Romme and Escher, 1993: 220)

Therapists of other orientations are using creative action methods: their discoveries and practices complement those of psychodramatists and dramatherapists. I now proceed to consider the work of the latter.

Dramatherapy

In examining the literature I have been able to discover no other dramatherapist who has specifically worked with people who hear voices on their hallucinatory experiences, though many have worked with people diagnosed as schizophrenic, psychotic or struggling with other experiences such as abuse or bereavement when they may hear voices. The words 'voices' or 'auditory hallucinations' do not occur in the indexes of dramatherapy books (except in Schattner and Courtney (1981) in which there are two brief passing references to schizophrenic symptoms). I have found just one instance of a dramatherapist working with a psychotic teenager who heard voices: 'Johan', a 15-year-old Colombian immigrant adopted at 2 years old, who heard voices in his head commenting negatively on his actions or on things he said (van der Wijk, 1996: 247). He was diagnosed as suffering from a schizophrenic developmental disorder. In a brief therapy intervention (twelve 45-minute sessions) the theme of strengthening his assertiveness became a focus. He found it difficult to say 'No'. After dramatherapy sessions Johan's condition had improved so much that the treatment team was able to refer him to a social skills therapy group. Van der Wijk used story and enactment but in this brief intervention did not explore the meaning of the voice. He notes the loss and dislocation of this shy immigrant boy but does not mention whether he suffered from racism or bullying.

A number of dramatherapists have reported their work with people who were diagnosed schizophrenic or who were thought disordered. Langley (1983) advised that the dramatherapy group maximise a sense of safety, trust and relaxation through a slow, gentle pace: repetition was comforting and provided some security. She stated that the therapist should give reassurance, praise and encouragement. Although Langley twice mentioned hearing voices as a symptom of schizophrenia, at no time did she suggest working specifically with the voices. However, she reported that: 'When the members feel free to talk about their psychotic fantasies there is often a sense of relief at having shared a terrible burden' (Langley, 1983: 61). This was confirmed by participants in my study: it was a relief to them to be able to share experiences and find they were not alone, nor judged by their peers.

Grainger's (1990: 141) research showed that a small group of people with thought disorder did benefit from dramatherapy. He used repertory grid tests before and after the therapy and his results 'seemed to provide evidence of the integrating effect of drama upon fragmented human awareness.' He suggested that dramatherapy is appropriate for people diagnosed as schizophrenic because of the provision of a secure, boundaried, structured yet free, playful space where there is relaxation, rehearsal and validation: 'drama is a playground for the release of interpersonal tension and a laboratory for the safe anticipation of events' (Grainger, 1992: 165). Dramatherapy strengthens the person 'by using imaginative involvement in *other* people's lives as a way of validating the *self*' (Grainger, 1992: 177, added emphases). This last statement was anticipated by Moreno who, founding his method on the encounter between people, encouraged them to share life experiences and achieve: 'a realisation of the self through the other' (Moreno and Moreno, 1970: 9).

Embodiment play

Dramatherapists and psychodramatists encourage bodily movement and physical play.

Movement and improvised drama

The earliest study comparing dramatherapy with 'modified group (verbal) psychotherapy' with 'long-stay schizophrenics' was published in 1974 by Nitsun *et al.* From the Sesame Institute (Pearson, 1996), they applied Slade's child drama principles and practice and distanced themselves from psychodrama.

> The situations explored were mainly imaginary in content and involved physical movement . . . such as throwing and catching a ball to quite complicated dramatic improvisations, such as a voyage by sea, leading to a storm, ship-wreck, and a return to safety. Some everyday situations were also enacted, e.g. meeting friends in the street, shopping.
>
> (Nitsun *et al.*, 1974: 103)

In the dramatherapy group people 'showed increasing spontaneity and their improvisations became more complex' (Nitsun *et al.*, 1974: 104). The therapists deliberately offered opportunities to enact aggressive scenes.

> While some showed initial fear of involvement, they generally became increasingly capable of expressing aggression in a dramatic situation. The fear that some patients, especially those with histories of violence, would be provoked into actual aggression, was not borne out in the group. Most patients expressed themselves freely in these situations and were able to keep the aggression at the level of a dramatic improvisation . . . while the expression of aggression in the group produced no change or less overt aggression and increased cooperativeness in some patients, there were also some who showed signs of more independent and assertive behaviour on and off the wards.
>
> (Nitsun *et al.*, 1974: 105)

A decade later McLuskie (1983) followed Nitsun *et al.* (1974) in demonstrating that dramatherapy offered psychiatric patients an opportunity to show active assertiveness and release feelings of aggression which might otherwise explode into anti-social behaviour. These studies are complemented by Logan's (1971) psychodrama research which reported on the role of catharsis in reducing aggressive behaviour.

Nitsun *et al.* (1974: 105) asked the patients for their views: they reported that participants tended to emphasise increased ease of movement and expression. One woman said, 'It put life back into my body.'

Using many assessment methods, psychological rating scales, Rorschach and Draw-a-Person they were able to show that:

> movement and drama has the effect of promoting increased bodily aware-
> ness . . . vitality . . . decrease in restlessness and overactive movements . . .
> improvements on incoherence of speech . . . The change in coherent delusions
> . . . is an interesting finding in view of the fact that no discussion of personal
> beliefs was entered into in this treatment. It is possible that the opportunity
> for enacting varying fantasy situations and roles enabled these patients to test
> against reality their own idiosyncratic beliefs.
>
> (Nitsun *et al.*, 1974: 115–116)

Further, people showed an **'increased capacity for socially appropriate behaviour'** (Nitsun *et al.*, 1974: 117). The benefits from the movement and drama were
shown to be greater than those from purely verbal group psychotherapy.

From 1974 Scoble worked with a team of drama students and nurses in a hospital
with institutionalised patients and found that, with care and sensitive adaptation,
drama activities could aid recovery:

> At the very least they found momentary enjoyment, relaxation and a willing-
> ness to participate and communicate with fellow humans. At its best, drama
> appears to have **increased the capacity for socially appropriate behaviour**
> to such an extent that patients were discharged before the close of the project.
>
> (Scoble, 1978: 16)

It is interesting to note the similarity of language (highlighted in bold) in these two
reports: dramatherapy enabled people to behave in more socially appropriate ways.
This finding, of the development in social skills through drama, is borne out in my
study. This is also confirmed by McLuskie (1983: 23): **'Drama is a useful tool
for rehearsing social skills.'**

Baarrs (1996: 248–249) showed that movement and dramatherapy resulted
in therapeutic benefit for Maud, an elderly woman, institutionalised for forty
years as a schizophrenic, who also suffered from tardive dyskinesia (a condition
of involuntary movements induced by neuroleptic medication). She became
more spontaneous, taking the initiative in more appropriate and creative ways,
showed more humour, trust and confidence. This was a gradual process over
two years. McLuskie (1983: 24) also stated that dramatherapy could counter the
effects of institutionalisation by encouraging autonomous decision making in
improvisations and rehearsals.

Lawrence (in Schattner and Courtney, 1981) reported considerable benefit from
drama in a group of 'severely disturbed' schizophrenic patients who were

> able to take the responsibility that goes with sharing, accepting and receiving,
> and with expressing oneself and supporting others. The Drama Club has come

a long way. It has made people feel better about themselves, with the help of other members. It has made people feel comfortable and human.

(Schattner and Courtney, 1981: 98)

This dramatherapy helped withdrawn, even catatonic and paranoid people to establish and enjoy relationships and it raised their self-esteem. This was also evident in my study.

The value of non-verbal methods

Parrish (1959) stressed the value of the non-verbal active aspects of psychodrama to enable less verbally skilled people to express themselves.

> chronic schizophrenics may in fact feel more at ease with movement and action than with verbal discussion . . . the emphasis on non-verbal interaction and bodily movement . . . seem to be satisfying to the needs of chronic patients.
> (Nitsun *et al.*, 1974: 117; see also McLuskie, 1983: 24)

Johnson (1984) emphasised the importance of movement, symbolic gesture and improvisation:

> Because of its encouragement of sensorimotor and symbolic modes of representation dramatherapy has been found to be especially useful with severely disturbed and ego-impaired patients, such as those suffering from schizophrenia.
> (Johnson, 1984: 299, cited in Allen, 1994: 18)

Lindkvist (1998) explored the use of stamping dances with people with chronic schizophrenia in South Africa. She noticed that the rhythmic stamping, with clapping and drumming, led to people becoming more co-ordinated and able to take part in creative activities. She hypothesised that this stamping stimulated the sensorimotor part of the brain and led to the release of endorphins. These would naturally improve the dancer's mood!

Mitchell (1987: 263) reported that work 'with acutely disturbed patients is most concerned with finding ways of self-expression . . . Mime and sculpting are equally valid ways to self discovery and self awareness when words are not possible.'

Sachs pointed out that:

> body-image is not fixed, as a mechanical static neurology would suppose; body-image is dynamic and plastic – it must be remodelled, updated all the time, and can reorganise itself radically with the contingencies of experience. Body-image is not something fixed a priori in the brain, but is a process adapting itself all the time to experience.
> (Sachs, 1991: 180)

Dramatherapy can, therefore, enable people to explore through movement and action and so clarify their body image: their sense of self: '"The ego is first and foremost a body-ego," as Freud writes' (Sachs, 1991: 189). For people who have difficulty with boundaries and other physical manifestations of psychological distress this can be of considerable therapeutic value.

Voice work

Voice work, specifically working with sound, vocal creativity, speech and song, has been an important activity for dramatherapists. Langley (1983) recognised the communication about self in the style and tone of a person's voice:

> Lowered voice is almost synonymous with self-effacement. Anxiety is expressed by a wavering voice and breathlessness. How we speak is usually an indication of how we feel about ourselves unless we make a conscious effort to conceal our feelings. Appropriate use of voice is something we learn.
>
> (Langley, 1983: 115)

Newham (1993) stated:

> the sounds of the human voice act as a metaphor for the dynamics of the human psyche . . . in the voice you can hear the psyche . . . The quality that gives a voice its unique character serves an important function in maintaining a sense of identity, for the sound of our voice reminds us of who we are; it affirms and re-inforces our self-image.
>
> (Newham, 1993: 200, 213, 218)

Martin (1996) confirmed this, observing that our voice is bound up with our self-esteem. Loss of voice can mean not merely to be disempowered but even to lose a sense of self. Martin (1996: 265) further reported that an acting teacher was thrown into deep depression when his voice was permanently altered by radiation treatment. He felt that he '*no longer existed*' because he had lost his voice. (I further explore the issues of loss of voice and self in Chapter 6.)

Voice work then can aid the recovery of the self. Langley (1983: 116–122, 127–132) suggested that dramatherapeutic voice work can retrain the voice, promote relaxation, breathing, enable emotional expression, raise self-esteem, develop social skills and assertiveness. Mitchell (1994: 155–156) used voice exercises developed by Jerzy Grotowski, beginning the work by teaching specific breathing exercises. Andersen-Warren (1996: 112, 131–132) did voice work in therapeutic theatre rehearsals to promote breathing, relaxation, creativity and the ability to express anger. Through dramatherapeutic use of space, body and movement Johnson enabled a mute, catatonic schizophrenic young man to speak (Emunah, 1994: 158). Using an exercise of pushing against a partner combined with 'Yes' and 'No', Daniel, with great delight and energy shouted 'No' after each time I shouted 'Yes'. When we attempted this without pushing Daniel was mute and seemed anxious.

(Johnson, 1984: 304, cited in Allen, 1994: 18; see also McLuskie, 1983)

Tselikas and Burmeister (1997) reported dramatherapeutic success with a mute, catatonic, paranoid schizophrenic young man. Tselikas used the relationship (including psychodramatic doubling), a drum (a containing ritual), a toy mouse (a transitional object), a story: metaphor and distance.

> Peter not only reacted to the stimuli he was exposed to, he also talked to the therapist . . . He became more lively and moving, communicating also more intensively with the caring staff, and even taking care of himself.
>
> (Tselikas and Burmeister, 1997: 171)

This remarkable transformation was achieved over brief (up to twenty minutes) sessions three times a week for a total of ten hours.

There are numerous drama activities which encourage voice work (see Langley, 1983; Emunah, 1994; Jones, 1996; Andersen-Warren and Grainger, 2000; Armstrong, 1996. See also Chapter 6 in this volume).

The only voice work I have been able to identify related to hallucinations is that of Alfred Wolfsohn. During the First World War, he had listened in horror to the screams of the dying. In 1917, lost in a muddy, shell-cratered wilderness, he chose not to go to the aid of a dying man who was moaning, 'Help, help, help.' After the war he was:

> plagued by aural hallucinations of the extreme vocal sounds which he had heard in the trenches . . . Wolfsohn became convinced that his illness arose from the intense feeling of guilt at having denied help to his dying comrade.
>
> (Newham, 1993: 84)

Wolfsohn wondered if his hallucinations were the expression of the accumulated emotional energy, of terror and guilt, which, in order to cope and survive, he had not been able to express. He became convinced that if he could actually sing the sounds that haunted his mind he would be able to stop them. As a result of this process, Wolfsohn did recover from his illness. He went on to teach his method of voice work to others. His work was developed in the theatre by Roy Hart and others and by Newham in voice movement therapy. Newham (1993: 62) refers back to Jung who 'noticed how schizophrenics often talked to themselves in voices with very different qualities.'

> The schizophrenic does not hear the jumbled word fragments in monotone but in pitches and qualities expressive of the affect of the complex. One is

aggressive, spiteful and provocative, the other luring, shy and seductive; another is Italian, confident and full of bravado, the other English, polite and reserved. The voices of the schizophrenic each have characteristics expressed vocally through an acoustic tone . . . the affective nucleus of a complex as expressed through the acoustic quality of the voice.

(Newham, 1993: 63)

Asking then what the tone of an hallucinated voice is will provide evidence of the feelings needing expression.

Projected play

Dramatherapists use numerous methods of projected play in therapy. These methods have a long history: symbolic objects, masks and puppets have been used in healing ceremonies by shamans for millennia (Casson, 1997–1998). In 1911 H. G. Wells published *Floor Games* about playing with children on the floor with toys. In 1917 Caldwell Cook published *The Play Way*, recommending drama in schools as a rehearsal for living. His methods also included the creation of miniature worlds with toys. Margaret Lowenfeld (1935), child psychotherapist, the creator of Jungian Sandplay, was inspired by Wells and from 1929 developed this as her therapeutic play method. Slade (1980, 1995) named these activities 'projected play'. The following is a survey of their use in the twentieth century dramatherapy.

Use of objects

In 1937 Rosenzweig and Shakow used toy furniture and bricks in a controlled experiment using play techniques with patients diagnosed with schizophrenia and other psychoses. They concluded that:

patients may be able to act out in pantomime what they are not ready to put into words, or they may be able to convey more quickly in a material medium of representation what words would disclose only after a consider- ably longer time . . . there is even the possibility that the technique could be successfully applied to mute individuals with whom verbal communication is not feasible . . . play is a better adapted means than conversation to elicit personal content from patients.

(Rosenzweig and Shakow, 1937: 33, 34, 42)

McLuskie used:

sets of Matrioshka dolls – wooden dolls getting smaller and smaller, one inside the other. They can be set up by the group and given identities, especially as families. By putting a finger on a doll, anyone in the group can speak for that character. Sometimes people find it a lot easier to show their feelings and problems sideways.

(McLuskie, 1983: 25)

Miniature toys and objects seem to empower people by putting them in control. Bannister (2000: 103) stated that puppets provide safe distance and such miniaturisation makes action more manageable.

Langley (1983) advised that working with objects can be helpful in drama-therapy with people struggling with schizophrenia:

> Constant, inanimate objects are less threatening than people. The object fulfils the role projected onto it, unlike people who do not always accept projections . . . I find it useful to start new groups by asking clients to relate to objects rather than a person.
>
> (Langley 1983: 65)

Grainger (1990) saw the potential therapeutic value of such transitional objects which enable people to play, experimenting with various possibilities which are not apparent to them until the ideas involved are externalised. My own use of toys, objects and the invention of the Five Story Self Structure (see Chapter 6) have shown this to be the case. Voices can be represented by buttons, toy chairs or animals.

Story

Playing with objects can lead into storytelling. Brun *et al.* (1993: 32) reported working with a young woman who heard voices using the fairy tale of Thumbelina to enable her to gain some distance, express feelings and talk about her experiences as a child. The woman's voice (a negative old woman, like a witch) had meaning and related to when, aged 4, she had been frightened by a woman. The story functioned as a intermediary object between therapist and client, a projective container for feelings and the nurturing relationship.

Stories often have voices within them: 'The Story Bag' (Gersie, 1990: 131) tells of how a boy collects the spirits of all the stories he has been told in an old bag. As he does not share his stories with others, the spirits, trapped in the bag, become malevolent. Energies that could have been a source of connection with others, being withheld, are turned against the self. In the story the spirits speak of their poisonous, murderous plans: they are angry. The story is itself a metaphoric container. Dramatherapists use stories because they provide structure and multiple levels of meaning: a container for projections and communication at a safe distance, and as a source of healing wisdom (Gersie, 1997).

Role: personal play

Dramatherapists use theatre texts and encourage clients to explore and expand their role repertoire. This work follows on from that of Goethe, Reil, Browne and Slade described in the previous chapter and is part of a continuing tradition of therapeutic theatre.

Theatre therapy

In 1968 in Portugal, at Lisbon's Julio de Matos Hospital, theatre was created by patients, many of whom were diagnosed schizophrenic or psychotic, under the direction of Joao Silva (theatre director) and psychiatrists. They began performing plays by O'Neill and Pirandello for recreational purposes. In 1970 one of the patients, Eduardo Gama, wrote a play critical of his treatment and of the authorities (Jones, 1996: 49). The main effect of this seems to have been to bring down the wrath of the military government censor on the hospital.

The longest running therapeutic theatre in Britain was facilitated by Madeline Andersen-Warren, dramatherapist, from 1986 to 2001. The group devised and performed numerous plays, several of which I have seen. I have been a visiting facilitator, brought in particularly to help with the creation and use of puppets. The group members, aged from early twenties to sixties, had diagnoses of psychotic disorders:

> none were in an acute, florid stage but all had some evidence of psycho-motor retardation and rigidity, concrete thinking, and thought disorder . . . Dramatherapy had already helped to extend the clients' awareness of body boundaries, the relationships between their own body parts and between *self and other*.
>
> (Andersen-Warren, 1992: 4, added emphasis)

One group visited Stratford to see *The Revenger's Tragedy* and worked with images, themes and characters from the play. This drama 'permitted a sharing of different forms of reality, an exploration of the group's own terrors' (Andersen-Warren, 1992: 4, 8; Andersen-Warren and Grainger, 2000: 198–208). They created their own play through a dramatherapeutic rehearsal process. She does not report on any effect of this work on voice hearing. However, carers noticed improved fluency in speech, lessened psychomotor retardation, increased spatial awareness and a marked awareness of social skills including dress sense. She also enabled the group to confront oppression and explore political themes (Andersen-Warren, 1996: 110, 126–127). They reported that their performances were important to them because they were giving something to others which they had created.

> In contrast they described their feelings of impotence about their previous experiences which always involved being passive recipients so that they

had learned to feel out of control of their own needs. The experience of being listened to and provoking emotions in others combined with an ownership of their own creation and a sense of responsibility for their own performance in the play as they learned how to be fellow members of the same cast was stimulating and produced a sense of well being.

(Andersen-Warren, 1996, 110–111)

Ernest Becker confirms this: 'In dramatherapy the patient is enabled to create something. Instead of things happening to him, he makes things happen' (quoted in McLuskie, 1983: 20).

I have written elsewhere on the therapeutic benefits of performance (Casson, 1995a). Dramatherapy gives people empowering experiences of being responsible, in control, creative. Bielanska *et al.* used Shakespeare:

It is seen as especially important with patients with schizophrenia to establish as much structure and order without this becoming too threatening or limiting . . . once a familiarity with the script is established, it is possible to develop the relationship between roles and the patients' own lives and experiences . . . dramatic distance serves as a way for patients to establish a tolerable level of involvement in drama, which they use to express their own thoughts and feelings. The authors report success in terms of the small number of patients re-admitted [to hospital].

(Bielanska *et al.*, 1991, cited in Allen, 1994: 20)

Snow supported a psychotic patient who wrote a play: the dramatherapy

group improvised on Peter's themes. Peter's fantasies and delusions were not challenged. In the sessions, Peter could deconstruct and reconstruct himself at will . . . The play that gradually emerged . . . was itself a kind of transitional object. Eventually, the support staff team was able to help Peter produce this play for the ward and hospital staff. This was an enormously validating experience for him. Through the vehicle of the play, he was able to share parts of himself with others, with the external world. In this way, the construction and performance of the play served as a transitional space, a bridge between the isolation of Peter's inner fantasy life and the external world – his fantasies became part of objective existence.

(Snow, 1996: 229)

Distance and mirror

Scheff (1979) is the original source of ideas about *distance*, developed by Landy (1986), Grainger (1990), Jennings (1990) and others in dramatherapy. I have further adapted this concept to working with people who hear voices (see Chapter 7). Grainger found that:

it was among individuals whose personalities seemed the most 'schizoid' that the treatment (dramatherapy) had most effect. These were people who felt themselves to be alienated from others or engulfed by them. Drama itself is largely concerned with the experience of separation and involvement (or alienation and engulfment) and with the achievement of a healthy balance between them.

(Grainger, 1992: 177)

Grainger had earlier written:

aesthetic distance promotes involvement rather than inhibiting it . . . Involvement to achieve autonomy . . . dramatherapy is largely based on the purposeful manipulation of aesthetic distance, carried out to allow those involved the freedom to experiment with their own image of themselves especially with regard to the crucial boundary between *self and other*.

(Grainger, 1990: 49, added emphasis)

Andersen-Warren (1992, 1996) applied the concept of modulating distance in dramatherapy with people struggling with psychotic illnesses. She used various distancing techniques to ensure clients were not engulfed by emotion but were able to safely experience and express darkness, chaos, oppression, death and transform these into shared experiences of joy, creativity and power. She used mime, sculpts and tableaux, melodrama, 'becoming an object', masks, observer characters (such as country dwellers who observe the actions of tragedy from a distance), theatre practices of Brecht and Boal to enable clients to explore issues at one remove.

Birdfield (1994: 16) stated that it was important to recognise that the schizoid person may sometimes feel overwhelmed, and to intervene in a way which does not threaten to engulf but ultimately to maximise his/her autonomy. He used the psychodrama mirror technique, distancing Doug by placing him in an audience role. The method empowered Doug to work projectively, symbolising his fears instead of being overwhelmed by them, to have some control and to play with others.

Langley (1983) found the mirror technique helpful in that it created sufficient distance:

Sometimes re-enactment of an emotional scene helps to clarify it. Usually this is a family row or angry verbal conflict, but the act of replaying the scene without emotion can give insight. I find it is more successful to have another group member mirror behaviour rather than using the role reversal technique because of the schizophrenic confusion about personal identity. Some clients find it not only threatening but also impossible to do.

(Langley, 1983: 72)

I have found the mirror does provide useful distance for someone to gain insight and it strengthens the observer ego. Difficulty in role reversing does occur however in people who are not diagnosed schizophrenic and is indicative of a developmental impairment: the person may need to experience sufficient doubling and mirroring (empathic validation and witnessing of self/ego) before they are able to role reverse (become/appreciate the other) (see Bannister, 2000: 103).

Moreno suggested three stages of child development:

1   identity: the double method
2   recognition of the self: the mirror
3   recognition of the other: role reversal.

He realised that when people were impaired the recapitulation of these developmental stages may produce therapeutic results:

> when we meet a person who has deteriorated considerably along a psychotic line of experience, unable to communicate, the double technique can be applied with the aid of a specially trained auxiliary ego, the double ego.
>
> (Moreno, 1952, cited in Fox, 1987: 131)

Prouty's 'pre-therapy' is in effect doubling through reflecting and thereby validating the client's experience. He also considers that 'Pre-Therapy facilitates self-integration at a "mirror stage" of development' (Prouty, 2000: 74). He relates this to Lacan's (1997) theory of a 'mirror stage' of 'I' (self) development.

> Moreno's invention of the mirror technique in Psychodrama predates Lacan's first lecture on the Mirror stage of development (1936). He was already using the technique in the early 1930s.
>
> (Casson, 1998b: 11)

Dramatherapists use the mirroring exercise from theatre as a warm-up. McLuskie used it in her work with chronic long-stay psychiatric patients:

> Mirroring a partner's movements in varying degrees of complexity involves decision-making, concentration, trust, eye contact, copying skills, and an acute awareness of another person.
>
> (McLuskie, 1983: 22)

Such mirroring brings people into playful relation with each other, into interpersonal contact at a safe distance. The self meets the other as self. Accurate mirroring becomes a source of empathy (see Casson, 1998b; Slade, 1995: 217; Spolin, 1996: 60).

Safety: contra-indicated dramatherapy techniques

Professional ethics and their code of practice, which above all prize the safety of the client, have led dramatherapists to be cautious in this area. Langley considered dramatherapy most beneficial as a form of rehabilitative therapy with 'chronic' schizophrenia (Allen, 1994: 17). She warned against the use of dramatherapy in acute episodes of schizophrenia and was concerned lest dramatherapy precipitate a psychotic episode (Langley, 1983: 59). She stressed the importance of dramatherapy being voluntary and the client being allowed to withdraw, even leave the room if the session proved too much for them. My use of an audience space has reduced the need for people to actually leave the room (see Chapter 10). This ethical concern for the autonomy and freedom of the client relates to the central issue of power and control. Bolton (1979) worked for three years (c.1975–1978) with adults (selected by a psychiatrist, some of whom were diagnosed schizophrenic) in a large psychiatric hospital. He was concerned that the leader's influence could be dangerous, if patients were to try to please him or her, or the leader imposed his or her values on the group (Bolton, 1979: 13). To counteract the possibility of the abuse of power by therapists who use action methods it is essential to give participants the right to say 'No' or 'Stop' to any technique. Moreno stated:

> There is no moment during the procedure in which the psychiatrist and the patient cannot say 'Stop'. Immediately or a few seconds after the order is given the patient may break up the procedure and act as if nothing had happened. These stop orders produce in the patient a significant co-experience. Acting on a psychotic level at a time when he is extremely sensitive, he learns to check himself. It is training in mastery of psychotic invasions, not through intellectual means, but through a sort of spontaneity training.
>
> (Moreno, 1939: 6)

Estall and Read (1981: 10) ensured that within any dramatherapy structure patients took responsibility for themselves through being able to assert the 'right to say "no" to involvement at any point.' In my research and practice I have rehearsed saying 'No' and 'Stop' with clients to empower them in the process. Because of the importance of this I further explore the issues of power and control in Chapters 6, 7, 8 and 11.

Emunah (1994: 174) advised that a drama game which involves disorienting blindfolded people should not be used with clients who are psychotic. She further advised that a game of true and false statements was 'not recommended for use with schizophrenic clients who have difficulty distinguishing between fantasy and reality (or lies and truth), as they may find the false statements disturbing and threatening' (Emunah, 1994: 239).

Bolton (1979) was also concerned that role play might be 'ineffective if not harmful with those patients who cannot distinguish between fiction and reality.' He recommended a period of reflection after role play.

Tselikas and Burmeister (1997), van der Wijk (1996) and Snow (1996) have conducted very brief therapy with people with psychotic experiences. While these interventions may have been effective at the time, my own research suggests that too brief an intervention may leave people feeling abandoned just as they emerge in the therapeutic relationship.

Summary

This review of the literature has revealed the possibility and the paucity of therapeutic work with people who hear voices. For two hundred years people have been considering the psychological nature of psychosis and possible treatments, including therapeutic theatre. In my view Moreno's creative innovations have not been followed up sufficiently, possibly due to the dominant biological culture of psychiatry and a failure to grasp his courageous insights. Dramatherapists have meanwhile continued to develop safe practice. The new thinking begun by the Hearing Voices Network and cognitive behavioural therapists offers an opening for a creative response to psychosis and voice hearing to which dramatherapy and psychodrama can contribute and the literature has given some indications of what people who hear voices may find helpful or not helpful in these creative action methods. In the next chapter I describe my own dramatherapy practice with individuals.

Chapter 6

Dramatherapy with individuals

Finding a voice and telling stories

Even when assessing and preparing people for group therapy, some individual sessions are essential and I now turn to exploring the theory and practice of individual dramatherapy with people who have psychotic experiences and who hear voices. Individual therapy is particularly indicated for those who are too anxious for a group, are anti-social or have particular, profound difficulties that might be impossible to address in a group. However individual therapy may reinforce isolation and needs to be balanced by a programme of care that offers social activities. A period of individual therapy before a group enables people to make better use of the group when they do eventually join. The relationship with the therapist achieved in pre-group individual work helps to sustain people through the first weeks of the group when they were settling into new relationships.

Establishing the therapeutic relationship

The first session of individual work is an *encounter* to establish the beginnings of a *relationship*. It is an opportunity to *talk*. This is the essential basis for whatever therapy may follow. However for people who are very anxious, talking, establishing and maintaining a trusting relationship can be extremely difficult. Roth and Fonagy (1996: 204) reported that: 'Patients with a diagnosis of paranoid personality disorder tended to drop out of treatment earlier. Nine out of 10 subjects with this condition left treatment prematurely.'

In the first dramatherapy study conducted in Britain with 'schizophrenics', Nitsun *et al.* (1974) reported that a 39-year-old female became very paranoid and refused to come after the fourth session. The only person to drop out of individual therapy (at the thirtieth session) in my study was paranoid. Others who were less paranoid did not drop out. The overall dropout rate for my research was 20 per cent. This is a low dropout rate compared with many studies and I suggest that the long and careful assessment (of six sessions) built up sufficient therapeutic alliance to sustain most participants through the therapy: the development of a warm, holding relationship is essential to effective therapy. This is in accord with client-centred counselling theory and research (Rogers, 1959). For some withdrawn, anxious clients talking itself is difficult.

On being unable to speak

I began my research with an intuition that people who hear voices have, at some time in their lives, been *unable to voice* what they have experienced. Unable to speak of it, their experience has become unspeakable. The voices they hear are testimony to that experience and therefore are meaningful.

As **Gloria** said: I felt overwhelmed, overpowered by my father *so could not voice my feelings, opinions* . . .

It is therefore essential to consider what blocks speech and how the ability to speak may be regained: how people who hear voices may be empowered to speak of their experience. They may not be able to speak of their experience because others: family, abusers, professionals, society, do not give them permission to speak or refuse to listen (see Watkins, 1998: 273; Leudar and Thomas, 2000: 77–81, 127).

In **Ben**'s life and in the lives of **Gloria**'s and **Roger**'s fathers and **Dillon**'s grandfather there had been times when to speak out would literally have cost them their lives. All these had experienced wars or civil conflicts. **Ben** was unable to speak when his father was executed in front of him: survival meant passive, silent acceptance and his traumatic experience became unspeakable, locked within his psychotic illness. An example of the loss of the ability to speak in traumatic experience was reported by Muna Khleifi, a Palestinian inhabitant of Ramallah, during the siege by Israeli soldiers:

> Last night it got worse, five tanks stopped 200m away from our house and started to bomb and shoot . . . helicopters were shelling from above . . . I found my daughter awake in her bed, unable to speak, her eyes full of fear. I carried her in my arms and took her to our bed. She could not speak at all.
>
> (*Guardian* Real Lives, 4 April 2002, p. 6)

Abuse and loss of voice

Many of the people in my research were survivors of abuse. Abusers silence children with threats (Warner, 2000). In Paris, 1882, Dr Bourdon reported on a mute child who eventually disclosed that: 'He kept silent because his father told him he would kill him if he said a single word' (Masson, 1992: 47).

Similarly, a convicted sexual abuser

> repeatedly attacked schoolgirls . . . then warned them not to breathe a word. He would threaten the children and tell them that no-one would believe them if they ever told their parents. He also said the abuse would be their 'little secret'.
>
> (*Oldham Advertiser*, 21 December 2000, p. 13)

Coleman (1998) stated that **Abuse means loss of** (your) **voice.**

This may not only be a matter of inhibition but as a result of the impact of traumatic experience on the brain. Bremner *et al.* (1996) reported PET (positron-emission tomography) scans of the brain suggested that trauma survivors remember their past horrors in a state of 'speechless terror' (see also Rauch *et al.* 1996; Shin *et al.* 1997). During flashbacks, the part of the brain known to play a role in the verbal articulation of experience – Broca's area – was relatively quiescent on the scans. **Leah** however gave very practical reasons for not being able to speak, saying that her father *beat me every day . . . I was too scared to tell . . .* Father strangled her, tied her up and battered her, put tape over her mouth . . . *I couldn't talk to anyone lest father hear about it and punish me.* She also couldn't talk to her father as he hit her worse. Her mother was depressed and they were in the habit of not talking, reinforcing each other's silence. When on section in hospital she was mute. She did not disclose her father's abusive behaviour of which there was no mention in her hospital notes. She said that she stopped speaking because she did not know what to say, was frightened and couldn't get her mouth open.

Diane, in projected play, chose a zipper to represent herself because she had zipped her mouth closed and did not speak about her sexual abuse: she feared people would not believe her.

One woman said: *No one knew about the rape, I was dumb, I had no mind at that age* (15). **Gloria**'s mother discouraged her from speaking to the police about the rape. Another woman said that she carried a secret, which was *unspeakable*.

What makes the patient ill is silence.

(Forrester, 1980: 31)

Intrapsychic forces, emotion, depression, voices also prevent people speaking: **Cheryll** said one of her voices stopped her speaking and that pain also blocked her ability to speak. **Jimmy** said: *the voice blocks a word, they take a word out of a sentence . . .* This could be described as 'thought blocking or extraction' and attributed to a biochemical event in the brain due to schizophrenia. However it may alternatively be described as resulting from trauma:

> People under severe stress secrete neurohormones that affect the way their memories are stored . . . high levels of glucocorticoids secreted during stress impair the functioning of the hippocampus . . . This may partially or totally disable the ability of the brain to verbally categorise incoming information. At the same time, during states of high fear, the amygdala is extremely active and interferes with hippocampal functioning. The result is a partial or complete loss of the ability to assign words to incoming experience, the biological equivalent of 'speechless terror'. Dependent upon words, our capacity to logically think through a problem is diminished or entirely shut down and our minds shift to a mode of consciousness that is characterised by visual, auditory, kinaesthetic images and physical sensations as well as strong feelings.
>
> (Bloom, 1997: 28)

The inability to speak may be due to a specific trauma or to temperament: some children are timid from their infancy (such vulnerability may mean they are more targeted for abuse).

> Silence is another barometer of timidity. Whenever Kagan's team observed shy and bold children . . . the timid children talked less. One timid kindergartener would say nothing when other children spoke to her, and spent most of her day just watching others play. Kagan speculates that a timid silence in the face of novelty or a perceived threat is a sign of the activity of a neural circuit running between the forebrain, the amygdala, and nearby limbic structures that control the ability to vocalise (these same circuits make us 'choke up' under stress).
>
> (Kagan, 1994, quoted by Goleman, 1996: 218)

Timidity and anxiety can be learned and instilled in a child by a parent or other person. **Cheryll**'s dysfunctional relationship with her mother began before her birth and she was traumatised before she learned to speak. Later as an adult she was terrorised by a psychopathic partner:

Cheryll: I lost my voice and felt like a ventriloquist's dummy, you try to speak and you can hear a disturbing sound of nothing, you want to relax your voice place, but the perverseness is there screaming at you to speak but . . . my mouth felt wooded . . . I tend to be withdrawn when they (voices) are speaking and don't reply out loud sometimes because I can't because my own voice goes really in. Once I lost my voice altogether . . . When I feel anger, it's extreme – *I can't speak* . . .

Tina: I couldn't talk or communicate with people . . . not for years, about three years . . . I was like a zombie . . . *never spoke, I couldn't talk* . . .

Another woman was an elective mute: she had not spoken for several years. Her voices had started after she had stopped speaking. She had gradually withdrawn from the world. She stopped speaking after she disclosed childhood sexual abuse. Her voices spoke of significant psychological distress that she had been unable to process, her hopelessness and guilt.

When someone cannot speak out, their only option may be 'inner speech' (which Leudar and Thomas (2000) suggest is the nature of voice hearing). Not able to communicate directly with him, **Diane** identified one of her voices as her father, communicating telepathically. She was in effect talking to father inside her head when she couldn't talk to him in reality: I know that I can hear my dad in my head, I know that he is talking to me . . . I needed a mother figure, I still do. My mother can't meet my needs I don't think she's ever been able to . . . I feel really depressed because my mum doesn't talk to me . . . I feel so lonely and unwanted.

Not being able to speak may be endemic in some families: a lack of family communication may result in a young person not being emotionally articulate. **Dave** said he was disappointed because mother was always busy and he couldn't talk to her: With Dad it's *unsaid* . . . (He also wrote of his grandfather as the) man who smoked his pipe *saying nothing* . . . With such role models Dave was unable to speak out directly: he remembered sending psychic message at the age of 16 to a girl I fancied. Later he heard voices in reply.

Leah said she couldn't really speak to her family: I couldn't talk in those days, didn't know how to talk about voices, how I suffered. Couldn't talk to the doctor . . .

Jenny said it was difficult to speak, she was often not allowed to: in the face of criticisms from her voice and husband: *I keep my mouth shut.*

In her family **Pat** said: *I'm not allowed to talk* about it (voice hearing) because it upsets everybody . . . **Pat** had not been able to talk about her mother's mental illness when she was a child. It was a shock when she went to school and found that other mothers did not behave like her mother (sitting on the roof, locking herself in the bedroom). Embarrassed, **Pat** felt she had to keep quiet then.

Talking sometimes is difficult. As **Ben** said: Some problems were private that it was difficult to talk about. Here **Ben** is referring to sexual aspects of his psychotic experience. Embarrassment and shame may prevent people speaking. The culture of the wider society may also prohibit speech.

Dave: Isolation can be due to the *taboo of talking* about mental illness . . .

Dillon: Many people with these problems *can't speak publicly*, they feel they will be attacked/joked about . . .

The inhibition of refugees to speak their own language is likely to be due to the dominance of the culture they have entered: there is pressure to assimilate and they may be isolated from others who speak their language. The voices may be the only ones who speak the old language, as **Gloria** and **Ben** experienced. **Gloria** felt empowered when I said she could speak in any language she wanted to: she occasionally spoke her ancestral tongue. I also encouraged **Ben** to speak his native language.

The culture of medical model psychiatry may also inhibit speech. One woman said: *I don't open my mouth* to tell psychiatrists about what I see or hear as they don't want to know. **Roger** also had this experience of not being listened to by psychiatrists. He wrote a poem of wanting to scream but no one hearing. (See Thomas (1997) on psychiatrists' unwillingness to listen to those who suffer from schizophrenia.)

> **Cheryll** wrote: I went into psychiatric units wondering where is treatment . . . I think I must have screamed but nothing ever came through my lips, my voice escaped to the back of my head under all the depression and subdued restraints that society had imposed on me . . .

Likewise **Harry** also felt unable to openly express how he felt: *At one time I used to sit on a chair screaming inside my head . . .* This inability to scream may be due to the impossibility of doing so when the abuse had originally occurred. **Sheila** said: *I wanted to yell but couldn't when the man abused me.*

Institutional culture can inhibit even those who, in hierarchical terms, may be considered powerful: a consultant psychiatrist told me that when he was in hospital with encephalitis he could not tell the nurses that he was hearing voices, as they were busy. The 'positive' ward culture, their hope that he was feeling better, did not give him permission to speak.

In summary, not being able to talk, whether this is due to temperament, brain chemistry, interpersonal relations, culture, appears to prevent people from healing, from processing experience and receiving support. It isolates and may mean that inner speech (voices) becomes the preferred or only means of much needed dialogue.

Therapy: an opportunity to talk

Therapy, an antidote to silence and isolation, offers people an opportunity to talk, communicate and relate to others. The Hearing Voices Network and others have found that people can benefit from talking about the voices. It is possible to start a therapeutic relationship with someone who is unable to talk as Tselikas and Burmeister (1997; see also Chapter 5 in this volume) and Prouty (1990, 2000) have demonstrated. Therapy then can enable people to regain their voice: to speak of their experiences.

For **Jenny** talking brought her relief from tension and some peace:

> I've found (a) that something's been said and (b) that somebody's listened and not been judgmental . . . It's a relief that somebody knows other than me: I'm not alone anymore: you do get isolated with things like that: you think you're the only one . . . even though I got upset later on it was a bit more peaceful, after I'd calmed down. I felt that very strongly the last few times we met: a more peaceful feeling than I've felt for years.

As **Jenny** said, having a voice is useless unless one is not only listened to but also *heard*. If someone feels not heard by the other they would in effect not have a voice: having a voice is an interpersonal process whereby self relates to other in an intersubjective reflexivity. Having a voice is also a source of power: 'voicing is a process of empowerment' (Martin, 1996: 264).

Voice work

To counter the disempowerment and silencing of the person's own voice I encouraged all kinds of voice work in dramatherapy sessions: speaking, shouting, swearing, laughing, growling, humming, singing: aiming to enable people to own their voice, to empower them. When someone is hearing voices there are subvocal movements of the vocal cords and brain scans have revealed that the speech area of the brain is active. Some people have stated that they are less able to speak when the voices are active. This suggests that vocalising (and thereby otherwise using the area of the brain producing the voices) could reduce the voices. I have therefore encouraged people to rediscover their voice, whatever their ability is: to make a sound, to gain strength from being loud! One feels less self-conscious/inhibited using the voice if there's other sound: yelling together (when **Harry** wanted to shout I shouted with him) or at the same time as drumming, gives people permission to be vocally powerful. These activities release tension, promote breathing and relaxation.

Gloria said that for three months in hospital she did not speak because she was so angry. She had been training as a singer and had a beautiful voice. She had stopped singing: she felt she had lost her voice and could not sing any more. I found the medication I was taking flattened my mood and as a result I didn't like the way I sounded. She felt deeply disappointed, guilty and ashamed. She said she had come from a male-dominated society where women and children did not get heard. Her father had once told her she was stupid: she felt she could not speak for fear of appearing foolish and so had lost the ability to express herself. I felt overwhelmed, overpowered by my father so could not voice my feelings, opinions . . . She said she couldn't let the words out of (her) mouth. Her boss had bullied, exploited and trapped her: she felt she could not speak out against him. The man who had raped her had also trapped her into silence. We did breathing exercises, relaxation and letting a sound out without pushing. Slowly her beautiful singing voice emerged. As she rediscovered her voice she wept tears of joy, and said she had a sense of regaining a part of herself.

Gloria: Singing made me feel happier . . . I found it very helpful in giving me a voice, especially when I was blaming myself . . . Only when I started dramatherapy I was able to state how I felt . . . If I hadn't been given back a voice I wouldn't have tried (to assert herself with doctor, social worker and the benefits agency).

To use the voice one must be able to breathe. The shock of abuse can literally take one's breath away and freezing as a survival strategy may include not breathing. Hyperventilation can also result in hallucinations (Slade and Bentall, 1988: 33). We have therefore practised calm breathing, movement, relaxation to empower the person, achieve voluntary self-control of the body and prepare for further action in role play.

Individual assessment sessions

I now turn to the practice of individual dramatherapy, beginning with the assessment sessions which are concerned essentially with the relationship, an exchange of necessary information and establishing an empowering, therapeutic alliance and creative culture.

Relationship

The first meeting, which might be in the person's home or in a professional setting, is an encounter to establish the beginnings of a relationship. Coleman (1998) asserted that *Recovery is rooted in the relationship not biology*.

Perry (1986: 35) confirmed this: 'The most fragmented "thought disorder" can become quite coherent and orderly within a short time if someone is present to respond to it with compassion. Such a relationship is far better than a tranquilliser in most instances.'

I believe that whatever method of therapy is used, the prime healing forces are within the client and in the relationship between the client and the therapist: without a safe, empathic relationship there is less likely to be therapeutic benefit for the client. There are non-verbal aspects to this relationship: emotional holding, mirroring, warmth, eye contact, smiles, noticing/witnessing and listening. Once the therapeutic relationship is established the methods offered to the client by the therapist might have some value, if they are appropriate to the client's needs and are offered at the right time, in the right way. No one prescription could suit all clients. This is central to the philosophy underpinning Moreno's psychodrama: the encounter between people is the basis for healing and growth. It is also the central tenet of Rogers' person-centred approach. Before a therapist uses any technique there are, at least, two people in the room: two human beings. They are in different, complementary roles but beneath the superstructure of any acquired role repertoire there are two people, perhaps frightened, unsure, negotiating a relationship. The therapeutic relationship brings the person (self/client) and another (the therapist) into relationship with the other (the voice) as **Jenny** said: I have sat and talked to him, to John and Mr's (voice) been talking to me and Mr's been going on while John's been going on. Mr sounds weaker and a bit silly sometimes: what Mr goes on about. I feel torn about who to listen to, about loyalties, Oh God: I hope he doesn't hear Mr.

Information

Throughout the assessment sessions there is an exchange of basic information, for the client and the therapist. At the first session I offer a copy of my confidentiality policy. In the second session I use a shortened version of the Romme (1994) voice interview (see Appendix 1). Sometimes it may take two sessions to complete. It can be useful also to draw the client's family tree which, annotated with the psychological, social, economic and cultural history of the family, becomes a 'genosociogram' (Schutzenberger, 1998). This can provide vital information in understanding the development of the psychosis. The family scripts, messages and secrets passed down the generations, can thus be discovered: these may well relate to the voices. While compiling such a genosociogram one man's voice kept interrupting the process: the timing, process and content of these interruptions provided us with useful insights into the function of the voice. I have written elsewhere of the revelatory value of the genosociogram (Casson, 2000b).

I also answer any questions clients may have about therapy, my practice and professional experience and give them information about what I know about voices in response to their questions: information is power. In the final assessment session, if we decide to contract for a period of therapy, I offer an agreement for therapy and copies of my professional codes of practice.

Creative methods

At the third session I offer a first experience of dramatherapy. I use mostly projective techniques, giving the person a choice of the following:

- Storymaking (Six Piece Story Making: see Lahad, 1992) in which the client draws or writes a short story about a hero/heroine, their mission, helper, the obstacles they encounter and the way they overcome these.

Leah: I liked it when John and I did an exercise together with an imaginative story; anyway this (**story**) did me good and my mind was refreshing after I did it, but first nervous and surprised with myself . . .

- Work with a small container (inside which were Guatemalan 'worry dolls': half-inch figures in different costumes): there may be storymaking about the container and/or the figures which can also be sculpted (arranged in symbolic order). **Diane** found it helpful working with the Guatemalan worry dolls as her voices. One of the 'good voices' said that she was not alone, other people had bad experiences: this she found helpful.
- Work with a small toy house (inside which were Guatemalan worry dolls): again storymaking and sculpting. **Gloria** found working with the worry dolls empowering.
- Work with the Chinese Tangram puzzle (which I called 'a pattern'): this method involves the client arranging the pieces in new patterns, saying what they see and possibly developing a story (see Chapter 8).
- Role work: creating a friend. The client chooses a real or imaginary friend and role reversing with that person says what he/she, as a friend, likes and appreciates about the client.

Tom: You imagine yourself in your friend's shoes or what would a friend do in this position? . . . It eased me, before you start anything you always have butterflies, I thought, 'That's easy, I can do it.' I know friends of mine, I know my good points, I can speak up for myself . . .

This exercise raises self-esteem as people say positive, friendly things about themselves.

The choice of which of these methods to use is made either by myself, whichever seems to grow naturally out of the process of the interview (such as a discussion about friends/loneliness leading to the creation of an imaginary friend) or by me making an offer, asking the person, 'Which would you like to work with?' Offering of a choice (of two or three methods) is a therapeutic strategy: to empower people to have some agency, control and ownership of the process.

Safe space

Essential to safe and effective therapy is the establishment of a boundaried space that can become a container for therapeutic work. To symbolise this and give the client a greater sense of ownership of the space I invite them to create a 'safe space' with cushions, cloth and other equipment.

Jenny: Making your own space, making it seem a bit more familiar to you, to me, a bit of control, a bit of comfort.

This was in sharp contrast to **Jenny**'s experiences of the formality of other therapy settings where the control stayed with the therapist. For **Diane** being able to create her own safe space in the room was essential to establishing trust with a male therapist. She said: You never invaded my space. This projective action also helped her show me her isolation: when I was in them cushions and that was me that was the way I felt and nobody knew how to reach me and I didn't know how to reach anybody else and I felt great comfort in being isolated but . . . it was painful because people couldn't read my thoughts. People couldn't help me to get out of this cocoon which was a love hate relationship.

During her therapy **Diane** was able to separate from her mother, a love–hate relationship, and leave home: to have her own space.

Saying 'No' or 'Stop'

Experiences of powerlessness, intrapsychic or interpersonal, can lead to depression, loss of motivation, lack of freedom, choice, loss of strength, confidence and self-esteem. Therapy must counter this and not reproduce it: the locus of control might initially be in the hands of the therapist but must be returned gradually to the client. I have done this through enabling the person to choose activities and the focus of sessions, to say 'No' or 'Stop' to any technique or intervention and by not rushing or pushing people. I asked during sessions, 'Do you want to stop now?' My thinking was that not only was this ethical practice but also it was essential to real empowerment. Only when people feel they can say 'No' can they truly say 'Yes'. I was also aware that many were survivors of abuse and this is a normal part of my way of working with survivors: who are people who were not able to say 'No' or 'Stop' to an abuser who had taken their power, their voice, away. Gradually as people have owned their therapy space, time, process and content they have been empowered to say 'No' to the voices, assert themselves with others and gain greater confidence.

Jenny: You gave the option to say, 'Yea or nay,' . . . Even knowing you had that option to say, 'No' . . . if I don't like it I could say, 'No or stop' . . . and sometimes that made me carry on a bit. Well I'll just give it a bit longer and see what happens . . . (Being able to say 'No' is) very helpful: it gives you some control. It allows you to know how far you can go with your feelings. If you start getting over anxious you can say, 'Right that's it, enough's enough.'

Despite my repeated assurances that people had the right to say 'No' some found it difficult to accept this:

Sheila: If you're upset he asks whether you want to carry on or stop: he gives you the choice . . . (Being able to say 'No'): I found that really hard.

Sheila and **Jenny** were sexually abused as children. **Jenny** said that when a man pressed his sexual needs on her she regressed to being a child and agreed to what he wanted: it would be naughty to say 'No'.

Speaking about my invitation to take part **Pat** said: He says, 'Do you want to do it?' in such a way as you feel you can't say, 'No'. That's not a bad thing.

This last statement suggests that either the authority of the therapist can still be felt to be overpowering or that there is a way of offering activities that does not prompt resistance. Pat said: 'That's not a bad thing,' suggesting she did not regard this as problematic. She was capable of saying 'No' at other times. However, this alerts the therapist to be cautious, checking that the person can really say 'No' and does freely consent. I have done exercises which were intended to enable the person to say 'No' and given open choices as to what activities to do and the opportunity to refuse all activities. Such experiences of being in control enabled participants to feel more in control in relation to the voices:

Jenny: I feel a bit stronger, a bit more positive. I were letting people walk all over me again and I were letting Mr Bossy (voice) rabbit on tenfold . . . I've started in the last few weeks to take myself in hand and stand up for myself, be me again . . .

Thus by the end of the assessment people are thoroughly informed, have had numerous opportunities to express their informed consent, know (and have practised) that they can say 'No' to any technique or withdraw from therapy when they chose. The right to say 'No' or 'Stop' continues to be exercised throughout therapy.

Once an agreement for therapy has been made, I work with the client according to their needs, using appropriate dramatherapy methods.

Projected play

In individual therapy I stimulate projected play through visualisation and images on cards; the client may make drawings, including mandalas; tell stories with symbolic objects, containers, toys, buttons, stones, doll's house furniture, toy animals, Babushka dolls, toy theatre; write poems, scenarios and speeches for plays and enact these.

Projection is a normal mental mechanism whereby we put out into the world the unacceptable or ideal contents of our inner reality: we project our feelings or fantasies onto other people or objects. Slade wrote (1980, first published in 1954) about 'projected play' as a normal stage of developmental play which preceded 'personal play': projected play being with objects outside of the self and personal play being with the whole body, in action and role. In psychosis this mechanism is taken to extreme: parts of the self are ejected into the world to become utterly other. Using projective techniques with people struggling with psychosis is a homeopathic treatment: treating like with like. Voices can be seen as the result of the client projecting out into the environment unwanted parts of the self. Therefore to work projectively enables the client to put out of themselves, onto objects, stories, toy theatre and puppets aspects of themselves which they can then relate to, own or reject and over which they can have control. Developmentally projected play comes before personal (role) play and with people who have difficulty with role play or drama, projected play enables them to find safe ways into play. It enables people to externalise and concretise. The process invites the person first to look out into the world, at an object, and associate with it, in effect grounding them in here and now reality and shifting the focus from the anxious self onto some reliable object in the environment. This can have a soothing effect: I often begin with projected play as this is less likely to overwhelm the person. Projected play with miniature objects was found to be especially empowering:

Jenny (working with small objects: animals, buttons): *once you got going and got over the initial nervousness about doing anything like that . . . it just built up and built up your imagination, but it wasn't just imagination it was real life as well, what had happened . . . When I came away I did think about what we'd done. I found it very helpful . . . First thing because they wasn't specific: like using the buttons; it wasn't a specific thing, a person or whatever: you made that person yourself . . . Sometimes you're doing things and not realising quite right away what you are doing and then all of a sudden you find you're doing something you thought would be too intense and you actually enjoy doing it: that going back to being in control like playing with the buttons and visualising. No pressure. No judgement . . .*

The use of buttons and animals (including the giraffe who could look over the scene from above) enabled her to have an overview, strengthening her observer ego.

Babushkas

Another method of projected play is the use of Babushka dolls, which are also containers. The Babushka is a useful symbol as the outer doll contains several inner selves (Illustration 1).

I have a collection, including male and female figures, animals, globes, an egg. **Dave** wrote: *My mind is a broken egg inside a Russian doll reality skull.* Such vulnerability needs a container. The dolls enable one to explore vulnerability and strength. **Leah** (who had been beaten by her father) used the Babushka dolls to create the story of a powerful queen who had control over men and executed them when they didn't do what she wanted. She told the queen to *cool it!*

Tina said, after working with the Babushka dolls: *I used to be small and voices contained little me. Now they are small and I contain them.*

Johnson a dramatherapist, validates **Tina**'s discovery:

> Freed temporarily from the dilemma of deciding who he is in totality, the patient can take one piece of himself at a time, elaborate on it, play with it, and finally learn to control it instead of being controlled by it.
>
> (Johnson, 1981: 60)

Toy animals

Working with toy animals enabled **Pat** to put what she learned in the session into practice at home: to create boundaries and space between herself and her husband when he was angry.

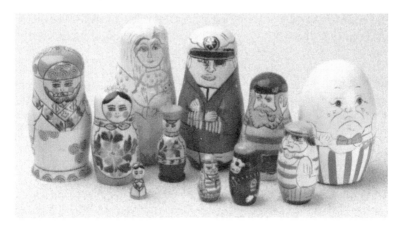

Illustration 1 Babushka collection

Pat: *I did learn that the best thing to do if M. (husband) is in a paddy is to go upstairs and shut the door.* (How did you learn that?) *Through doing the work with animals: animals who are safely in different countries.* (She used walls and fences to represent the boundaries of the countries. When you were doing that exercise were you thinking of M.?) *He came into my mind yeah. Then in the situation I just went upstairs and shut the door . . . After a while I realised I was actually coping. When M. started paddying I turned round and said, 'Ah shut up!' . . . he's not a bad man, he's just very short tempered.*

Jenny found playing with small animals was easier than doing role play: she was able to use projected play rather than personal play:

> *I found role play hard: it was the reasons why I was doing role play: I found it difficult to step outside. We played with little animals once: quite fun really after. I found it funny at first but while we were doing it I didn't think about it, quite enjoyed it. I think role play can be very hard . . .* (Sculpting): *We did that with animals: it were using something you knew what, instead of using empty chairs, something you could see . . .*

The concrete presence of an object was more helpful than the abstract emptiness of a chair.

Anton used an elephant to represent himself and an eagle as a 'buzzing' voice. The elephant he said had a thick hide and told the voice to bugger off: he had allies and a safe place, size and the ability to defend himself.

Gloria shrank her abuser, using a toy gorilla, and confronted him. **Diane** used animal puppets to tell the story of her sexual abuse. Miniature work holds material at a safe distance. **Dirk** was able to explore very distressing material when working with toy animals: they were outside him, at a distance, he was in control of them and he was not flooded with overwhelming feelings. Projected play is playing with distance: the person is able to explore through metaphor.

Buttons

I noticed that button sculpting (a projective method during which people arrange patterns of buttons in symbolic arrangements) was useful and empowering. **Anton** used buttons in his individual therapy: he chose different buttons to be aspects of himself, roles he played and his voices. Looking at the complex arrangement he said: *I'm a whole person, sometimes people judge just one aspect of me.*

Gloria was also surprised, as she looked at her button sculpt, to see how large and complex she was.

The Five Story Self Structure

I went on to develop this method in the Five Story Self Structure which was invented as a direct result of listening to people who hear voices. I noticed that they referred to voices being on different levels: above/below, behind or to one side (see Watkins, 1998: 152, 174; Romme and Escher, 1993: 89). For example **Gloria** said the voices enslaved her, taking up *many levels* that she used to think on, so that she could not think clearly. **Diane** said her voices were on different levels: she pictured them on *a ladder* with the bad voices at the bottom: when she was down there they had control over her. I wondered how to represent the voices being on different levels. I imagined a transparent structure, like the multilevel stages used by the Living Theatre (Brecht, 1969: 61–73) in *Frankenstein* and later in *The Money Tower*. I also recalled that when Moreno built his first psychodrama theatre in 1936, his structure of three concentric stages and a balcony represented different levels of the psyche (thus with the floor of the room where the audience sat, there were five levels: see Figure 2 on p. 107). I built a proto-type and eventually had this transparent five level structure manufactured (see Illustration 2).

I then used this to promote projected play including storymaking and working with voices.

The method is as follows:

1   I show the person the structure and ask them what they see, notice, imagine it is. Often the structure reminded people of the three-dimensional chess set in *Star Trek*, alternatively a multi-storey car park, office block, house. We might explore this image and develop a story. The structure clearly intrigues people and if they are willing to continue to use it, we move on to stage 2.
2   I produce the buttons and offer the opportunity to choose buttons and place them wherever the person wishes. This might also lead to storymaking or to developing a pattern. This step may be useful in enabling the person to use to the structure: it is more distanced than the next step and in not stipulating what the pattern might be, this step gives the person maximum freedom to project whatever they will onto the structure. Alternatively we might pass straight to stage 3.
3   I invite the person to choose one button to represent themselves: 'to be you: place it wherever you feel you are or wish to be.'
4   'Choose other buttons to represent the voices and place those in relation to your button.'
5   'Choose more buttons to represent other aspects of yourself or people or things in your life and place them.'
6   'Step back and look at the pattern you have created, look from above so you can see the whole pattern through the different layers (of the transparent shelves). Are there any changes you want to make?'
7   'Reflect, express how you feel and discuss what you notice.'

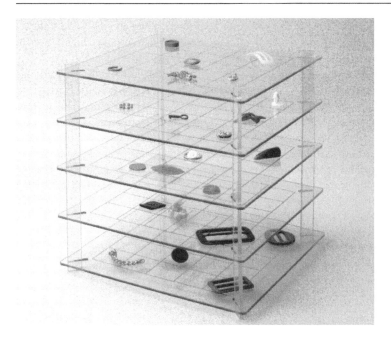

Illustration 2 The Five Story Self Structure

After the session I make a record of where each button is placed so that before the start of the next session I can reproduce the pattern: it is there waiting for the client's return. The structure holds the material at a safe distance and the client can choose whether to return to it, make changes, do further work or leave it to another session.

This has proved an extraordinarily flexible and useful technique. The structure enables play and concentration: it fascinates and focuses (due to its interesting, concentric design). It enables people to explore creatively through stories and patterns (right brain activities) their mental/spiritual 'geography': they can in effect create a three-dimensional model of their voices/psyche and so see structure emerge from chaos. With such structure emerges meaning: it has sometimes been breathtaking to watch this process as people have realised things through placing the buttons in relation to one another. I also thought that miniaturising the voices would place the person in control: buttons can be picked up and moved to other levels. Working on this small scale enables the person to feel powerful. As the person chooses buttons as voices they can talk about each voice and its place in the structure; talk to the voice and explore the conversations between voices and different roles or relationships within the structure; and rearrange these parts in relation to the whole. The structure can be seen as a metaphor for the self.

Diane: That was like my brain, actually I felt it was my brain, and where the voices and people were coming from. It was useful . . .

One woman said it was like my mind. Her arrangement had an empty level above the voices which she said was a blankness, keeping the voices at bay. **Cheryll** also said the central level that was empty was anaesthetic: to not feel/think relieved her of the pain on the lower level but left her vacant and unable to concentrate. She placed a green button (symbolic of her ability to forget distressing experiences) on top: the voices also helped her by distracting her from pain. The lowest level was of sensory pleasures, childhood memories of Christmas, nature and creativity but this level was blocked by the next level of cruelty and depression and this was where she placed her first voice: that of a young man who said, 'What if you shut your eyes and the world did not exist?' Over time he had become persecutory and controlling. **Cheryll** called the structure a wedding cake and linked it with *A Midsummer Night's Dream*, in which there are also levels: the supernatural level of the fairies, the social levels of the Duke's court, above the lovers, above the 'rude mechanicals' (Bottom and Co.). The play ends in marriage. **Cheryll** dreamed of the structure and of marrying herself. As her therapy progressed more evidence of the integration of fragments of her self (marriage) occurred (see Chapter 8 for an account of her therapy).

Speaking of the Five Story Self Structure, **Tina** said:

> That was really good that. It summed up my life; it put my life into proportion . . . You had to put an object on different shelves . . . pick some other objects for the voices then you had to put them where you thought they went. It was very good . . . summed up how I felt, how I felt about my life and the voices.

She chose a diamante brooch to represent the vivacious part of her personality and said: I am a person. I have opinions, my own thoughts, parts of me have been taken from me . . . I feel I've lost part of my personality (after her marriage to a domineering husband). With a hat and gloves she later created a vivacious character, 'Jasmine', who went to weddings and funerals, who wept and laughed. I don't where that come from: it just used to come off the top of my head . . . **Tina** had re-created the lost part of her personality.

Jenny used the structure to tell an epic story of inter-planetary struggles for freedom and justice:

> I had these ambassadors who were going to consolidate this other planet to stop the wars and one of them weren't and I were role playing different ones and by the time I'd finished I'd shifted power to the little ones. But when I started playing this game Mr (voice) was going on, 'Oh stupid, do you realise how silly you look.' I nearly stopped but I carried on and I won. That's the only way I can say it: I didn't let Mr stop me. I didn't let Mr beat me. Because Mr was telling me, 'That one should be Power,' and why, and I did it myself and I was quite pleased about that . . . afterwards . . . thinking about the game we played and what we did with them, it sort of put what had

happened in the past in some sort of context: it didn't seem as scarey after . . . because I was in control of what was happening . . . although it had happened to some of the people I visualised with the buttons had been like I was playing, it didn't seem as scarey because I had control . . .

The structure creates distance, empowers, helps reinforce the observer ego and put things into perspective. One man said: *it clarified things, bringing things that were at the back of my mind to the fore and setting them in relation to each other.*

The structure is archetypal: we often speak of levels of our experience and layers in organising our world view. Many religious images of different spiritual realms, such as the ziggurats of ancient Assyria, the step pyramids of Mexico, the Jewish Kaballah, Dante's Divine Comedy, the Hindu temples of India, the Buddhist temple at Borobudur in Java, are concentric designs which integrate different levels in a mandala.

The different levels, from the top down, might represent:

1	Head	Spirit	Thought/Intellect	Air	Joy	Maturity
2	Chest/Lungs	Heart	Feeling	Fire	Love	Adulthood
3	Belly/Sex	Soul	Imagination/Intuition	Water	Grief	Adolescence
4	Legs	Body	Senses	Earth	Hope	Childhood
5	Feet	Unconscious	Memory	Metal	Despair	Birth/Death

In terms of brain organisation the five levels might be:

1   (top level): consciousness of a personal self/ego
2   larger brain systems (such as the hippocampus, thalamus, amygdala etc.)
3   neurones/cells and their connections
4   chemical/genetic components (hormones, neuro-transmitters, DNA)
5   (lowest level): atomic structure and electrical charge.

Only when all these levels are integrated effectively can the whole be greater than its parts. In offering these ideas I am not suggesting that the different levels of the Five Story Self Structure have particular meanings: they will mean whatever the client using the structure chooses them to mean. It is in effect a toy theatre: a world in miniature.

Working through projected play in miniature promotes symbolisation: the concrete becomes metaphor, a means of communication and relating. Killick (1995: 117) stated that 'the making of visual imagery can assist in this process of reconstituting thinking. It can give form to emotional experience, enabling the patient to develop an increasingly metaphorical language to assist him or her in the effort to convey experience.'

I have further developed the Five Story Self Structure for group work: a co-operative game of free association between the players called Quintessence ©. It has also been used in team building for staff groups and has wider potential uses. (See Appendix 3 for how to purchase.)

Toy theatre

Dirk wanted to be in the audience and found toy theatre helped because it was miniature and at a safe distance: it also recalled happy childhood memories (see Illustration 3).

In using this toy theatre **Anton** said that the focus helped. He gave himself a message of hope and remembered himself at age 7 or 8, in the audience of a religious play, identifying with Christ and wanting to have his miraculous powers, to have significance and importance in life.

Dillon said that the toy theatre was useful . . . He used the toy theatre I had made from a cardboard box to create an epic political play, designing sets, scenarios,

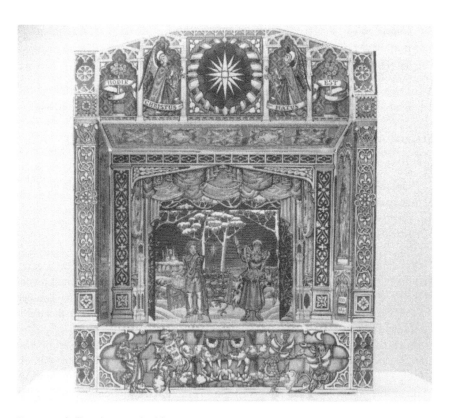

Illustration 3 Toy theatre: the Nativity

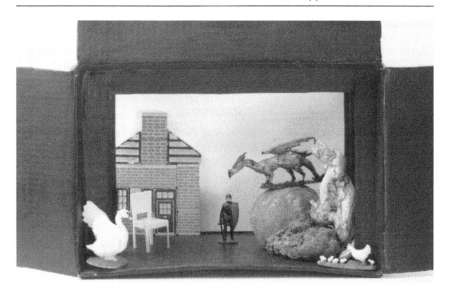

Illustration 4 Multipurpose toy theatre

writing speeches, improvising music over several sessions (Illustration 4). He said the play was to enable people to transcend death, find healing and achieve a transcendental view. He continued to think about this play between sessions and felt better: the creativity gave him a sense of purpose. He wanted the audience to feel the power of the actors and so feel empowered themselves. The play was about power, violence and spirituality. He was able to project his delusional ideas into the drama and get satisfaction from this creativity. His desire for power led him to identify with power figures. For his epic play **Dillon** created a speech by Trotsky: this spontaneity enabled him to flow and to be *heard* (I wrote down the speech to his dictation). He also played the role of Gandhi, asking me just to *listen*. He role played Saddam Hussein: through the role he expressed his contempt and will to power and control, issuing orders to kill. He ordered me to get the guns and swear an oath of allegiance against Hitler. He said I was a Jew in a previous life. Many of **Dillon**'s dramas were about political/spiritual power and control: whether someone could survive through violence. His relatives had died in the Nazi concentration camps. He believed he was controlled by a deity, an extremely hard, violent task master. Theatre offered him the opportunity to explore being powerful without being actually destructive: through creative action he could experience having some control when in life he was powerless, isolated and felt controlled by extra terrestrial deities.

Projected play and storymaking then lead naturally into role play and enactment.

Empowerment through enactment and role play

Gloria brought the text of *Anthony and Cleopatra* to her therapy and we spent the session reading and then improvising on the role of the Queen (I played her servant). This enabled her to feel a sense of dignified power and to express her wishes and feelings: the role enabled her to rehearse asserting herself and feel a dignity which, as a patient and a victim of abuse, she felt she had lost.

Creating a character can also bring wisdom: **Anton** created a character who had survived years of voice hearing, heard more celestial voices and had learned wisdom. His message to **Anton** was to accept his whole self, including the voices and 'bad' parts: he did not have to cut off any part of him. (**Anton** had heard a voice telling him to cut off his genitals. Due to his commitment to religion he felt guilty about his sexual needs.)

Reflecting on how she was treated like a football as a child, **Jenny** created the role of a referee who demanded fair play and said it was not the ball's (child's) fault that others kicked it: the others were responsible for their actions. This referee could be regarded as an emergent observer ego.

Creating and playing roles then can enable people to express and recreate themselves. The therapeutic relationship enabled **Pat** to be more authentic and give up denial as a survival strategy. At her twenty-seventh individual session she said: I've stopped confabulating since I came to see you.

Gloria (at her thirty-second individual session) said: I'm starting to come into my own self. The sessions had helped her focus, gain self-respect and a greater sense of control in her life, regain herself in both a cultural and psychological sense. She was able to assert her rights, let go of past attitudes, losses and feelings, communicate more with others and renew her creative activities. Both **Cheryll** (Chapter 8) and **Harry** (Chapter 10) said they were more able to be authentic, to be themselves, due to their individual therapy.

Individual versus group therapy

Research participants were asked: 'Did you find the individual work more or less helpful/unhelpful, the same or different from group work?'

Ben: Individual work was more direct. Group work helped me to learn to listen to others.

Anton said it was easier to concentrate in individual therapy (one hour): the longer group time (two hours) and the number of people made it difficult for him to concentrate.

People must be offered a choice. It may be that a period of individual therapy before and after group therapy can promote and consolidate growth. **Pat**, **Ben**, **Anton** and **Dillon** found it helpful to move into group therapy after individual therapy: it enabled them to progress, apply their learning about relationships and practice developing social skills in the group.

In Chapter 8 I present a case study of individual dramatherapy, and in Chapter 11 a case study of individual psychodrama.

Chapter 7

The wave and the whelm

Distance and empowerment

From the environmental model (Chapter 3) the development of a psychosis can be seen as a wave slowly gathering momentum. The forces accumulate until they eventually *overwhelm* the person.

Gloria: sometimes things ***overwhelm*** us, even when we've done all we can – it was accepting that . . . I felt ***overwhelmed***, overpowered . . .

I noticed how the word *overwhelmed* recurred in my notes about clients' experiences, in the literature on psychosis and in research participants' statements. I looked the word up in a dictionary:

> **Overwhelm**: To overturn, upset; to turn upside down . . . To cover (anything) as with something turned over and cast upon it; to bury or *drown* beneath this; to *submerge* completely (and ruin or destroy) 1450. To overhang so as to cover more or less SHAKS. To overcome or overpower; to bring to ruin or destruction; to crush 1529. To overpower utterly with some emotion 1535. To *deluge* 1860. 'The *earthquake* . . . overwhelmed a chain of mountains . . . ' 1796. 'I was overwhelmed with the sense of my condition' DE FOE
>
> (Onions, 1988, II: 1486, emphases added)

I wondered what a whelm was.

> **Whelm**: (hwelm) 1576 A wooden drain pipe; orig. a tree-trunk halved vertically, hollowed, and turned with the concavity downwards to form an arched *water*-course.
>
> (Onions, 1988, II: 2533, emphasis added)

Such a *containing channel* might be used to irrigate crops, funnelling the water for the purpose of nurturing creative growth. If the water were to *overwhelm* the channel it would rush over the sides of the drain, flooding the ground. Water is used as a metaphor for emotions. So frequently does the word 'overwhelm' occur in the literature on psychosis that I will not list the references. I have found water metaphors in many authors in this subject area (of psychosis, voice hearing, therapy): 'turbulent and . . . dangerous waters' (Roberts and Holmes, 1999: 160); 'dissolves' (Perry, 1987: 108); 'fluidity' (Rosenzweig and Shakow, 1937: 44); 'flow' (Csikszentmihalyi, 1990); 'ebb and flow' (Minkowski, 1970); 'flood', 'submerging', 'washed away' (Moreno, 1939: 5, 15); 'flooded' (Birdfield, 1998–1999: 25); 'swamped' (Gersie, 1987: 47); 'engulfing' (Laing, 1960: 83); 'engulfed' (Johnson, 1981: 49); 'drowning' (Miller, 1972: 60); 'bridge', 'floating anchor' (Snow, 1996: 233); 'anchorage/anchors', 'channelizing' (Moreno, 1945b: 3); 'bridge' (Z. Moreno, 1978: 165); 'funnel' (Chadwick, 1992: 69).

Here, for example, preserved by Moreno from 1939, is the voice of a psychotic woman:

> 'It is an earthquake. It sounds terrific. I am a great magician. Houses are breaking down. People are dying in the street. This is the end of the world . . . It is a flood. Water must be everywhere . . . ' She dips her fingers into the hallucinatory water. 'I am here on a ship. I am the captain. I hold it tightly. The boat begins to sink. Cold water is all around me. We sink to the bottom of the sea.'
>
> (Moreno, 1939: 11–12)

This imagery is perennial: a century before at the Crichton Royal Institution, Dumfries:

> A terrified melancholic saw the walls tottering which were to crush her – heard the waves rising and rushing which were to engulph her – was alternatively in a room filled with feathers and with water, from which she could not escape.
>
> (Crichton, 1850: 15)

Cheryll felt she was under the sea. **Jimmy** said he felt he was *drowning in a sea of voices* . . . Playing with the globe, **Harry**, who had been unable to grieve, expressed a fear of the polar ice breaking and the ocean overwhelming the land.

Eventually I noticed another word used occasionally by clients about the effect of therapy: after a good session they felt *buoyant* or spoke of a feeling of *buoyancy*. This of course would be the antidote to being *overwhelmed*: to be able to float rather than drown.

> **Buoy**: 1466, Greek βοειαι, straps of ox-leather f. βους ox. A floating object fastened in a particular place to point out the position of things under the water (as anchors, shoals, rocks), or the course for ships . . . that which buoys up a person in the water (= life-b.) . . . that marks out a course, indicates danger, or keeps one afloat.
>
> **Buoyancy**: power of floating . . . the vertical upward pressure of a liquid on a floating body.
>
> (Onions, 1988, I: 252)

Here the water is holding one up: sustaining rather than drowning: the ox hide (an inflated hide is still used in some cultures as a buoy to help people float across a river) holds one up above the surface. Being able to relax helps one breathe, makes one more buoyant through having air in one's lungs; feeling held enables one to relax and float rather than panic and drown. The air in the ox, the light material in the life-belt, holds one up: air and lightness countering heaviness and sinking.

Jimmy, commenting on dramatherapy, said that it was: something new and pleasant each time: creative. A **buoyancy to keep me afloat**, it enabled me to get through the week more easily.

The use of these metaphors in relation to the experience of voice hearing is ancient. Plutarch, writing about Socrates' voice-hearing experiences and the soul, used these water metaphors: 'overwhelmed . . . sink . . . buoy . . . floating . . . submerged in the depths' (Leudar and Thomas, 2000: 19–20).

Following this water metaphor I realised that sufficient containing boundaries, the sides of the whelm (channel), are essential in such work. What the whelm does is to separate the flowing waters from the general environment, contain and channel the flow in a creative way to encourage growth. The whelm channels energy. A boat or life buoy contains and sustains on the flood, making it possible to journey, rather than drown. This metaphor occurred spontaneously in creative work, in a song composed by a men's dramatherapy group:

> We're all in the same boat:
> Probably a Hovercraft,
> Floating on Air,
> Floating on Flux.

Cheryll wrote that her therapist

> was the lifeboat, he kept me from going under the current . . . the rain falls and the river swells . . . I see him there at the riverside with his lifeboat, I become Neptune and make tall violent waves they fall into John's lifeboat and it falls into parts and breaks into scattered pieces, a cold North Easterly wind bites into his face and and the waves wet his socks, he sees not Neptune but me but cannot climb in to reach, I reach for the fish and fling them at him my pride hides a smile but my tears swell the river . . . I go below with the strong current and swim like a fish back to . . . where it's calm and peaceful . . .

The riverbanks are containing boundaries. To counterbalance overwhelming feelings and experiences dramatherapy provides a container and some buoyancy, lifting and supporting people.

Tom: (referring to visualising and role-playing a positive character) Some people *can influence you, make you feel good and when you're in a down spot you always think of them and they **bring you back up again** . . .*

Therapy then must contain, be made of light, buoyant material, rather than be too heavy, and channel energy in creative ways to ensure the person is not overwhelmed. The whelm, boat, buoy, container, separates the person from the engulfing waters/emotions, putting just sufficient distance/boundary between self and other to ensure survival. This accords with the dramatherapy theory concerning the value of dramatic distance (Scheff, 1979). It is the modulation of distance in dramatherapy that is the therapeutic method to prevent people from being overwhelmed.

Another word for overwhelm is overpower. In Chapter 6, the loss of the ability to speak, to voice the self, was related to experiences of being overpowered. The related issues of power and control are central to effective therapy for people who hear voices (see Chapters 2, 3, 5, 6, 8 and 11). The whelm controls the flow of water by containing and channelling it.

The psychotic experience and therapy: the value of distance

How then does a dramatherapist prevent therapy becoming overwhelming for a vulnerable client? Already the metaphors of 'whelm' and 'buoy' have signalled that it is the modulation of distance, the provision of a safe container and sufficient support in dramatherapy that are the therapeutic methods to prevent people from being overwhelmed. Metaphors can provide sufficiently distanced containers/channels for potentially overwhelming material.

Metaphor

In considering the word 'metaphor' I notice another possible, implicit water image: the word itself contains the idea of a bridge or boat. The word 'metaphor' means literally 'to carry across' (meta = across, between; phor = carry – as in aquifer, or ferry). Metaphor 'carries across' an image, which may contain emotion, from the right brain hemisphere to the left brain, where the image is translated into language and thus conveys meaning. Metaphor is a *bridge* between worlds, brain hemispheres, between inner and outer, self and other and occupies the *transitional* space spoken of by Winnicott (1991) as the place where creativity occurs. Note the recurrence of the idea of space: a bridge spans a space. Space is that which creates distance. Spatial awareness is a faculty of the right brain. Jennings (1992: 238–239) has written about trance, metaphor, sculpts and drama-therapy and (in Jennings and Minde, 1995: 133–148) about transitions and bridges. The word 'metamorphose' means to change, and the transformational potential of work with metaphor was noted by Cox and Theilgaard (1987). The occurrence of metaphor signals that the right brain is engaged and a dramatherapist must learn to listen for metaphors and engage with them to facilitate communication and change (see Casson, 1998c). Cox and Theilgaard (1994: 223, 255) state: 'Metaphoric language has far greater possibilities for influencing the unconscious than logical, informative language . . . Images are closer to the inner centre, whereas words are closer to the voice of the ego.'

Furthermore, Jung believed that images were the way the self communicated with the ego. Indeed there is some evidence that the right brain hemisphere is more active during dream sleep (see Cox and Theilgaard, 1994: 215). Freud (1924) suggested that dreams and hallucinations were similar processes. There is also evidence that voices may originate in the right brain (Slade and Bentall, 1988: 37–38, 145–148) though Broca's speech area in the left brain is also shown to be active in scans of hallucinating patients. Gruber *et al.* (1984) found an association between mood and the location of the voices: evidence of a connection between voices and the emotional right brain. The left brain appears to be dominant and may in effect control the emotional right brain through analytic language; the use of metaphoric language and images may 'carry across' more emotion/meaning from the right brain than the left brain would normally 'allow'.

I also note that the word 'transference' has the same meaning as 'metaphor' (Cox and Theilgaard, 1987: xxvii), the former being of Latin root: trans = across; ference = carry or convey, the latter Greek. The Greek root of μετα means:

> 'sharing, *action in common*; pursuit or *quest*; and *esp. change* (of place, order, condition, or nature)
>
> (Onions, 1998: 1313, emphases added).

> in the midst of, among, between . . . in common, along with, by aid of, in co-operation with . . . indicating *community of action* and serving to join two subjects.
>
> (Liddell and Scott, 1996: 108–109, emphasis added)

The therapeutic relationship (which is a '*quest for change*'), within which trans-ference can occur, involves communication during which messages are 'carried across', conveyed from one person to another. Metaphors convey meaning across the space between therapist and client. Such meaning, with the accompanying feelings (even when not interpreted or fully understood) joins therapist and client together, promoting attachment. Transference is also a fantasy relationship that can be metaphoric: 'as if' the therapist were a good parent, a judge, a prophet of life. These different roles may be projected by the client onto the therapist who temporally holds them until the client can reintegrate them. Roles can therefore be seen as metaphors that carry us across from inner (dramatic) to outer (everyday, social) reality. In the above list the roles could be seen to carry needed/feared emotional loads:

good parent   = supportive compassion
judge   = criticism/condemnation or justice
prophet of life = hope and a source of personal vision.

Roles and metaphors can be see then as containers for significant meaning and also 'carry across' not only internally, between brain hemispheres, between self and ego, but also between persons, mediating our relations with self, other and world. In my view when these relations are disturbed there is a need for a way of working that uses the 'whelms' of role and metaphor to re-establish appropriate distance so that the person is neither underdistanced nor overdistanced. (For the etymological connection between the words 'whelm' and 'role' see Appendix 2.)

Furthermore, I suggest that voices and delusions are metaphoric and contain meaning (see Chapter 3). Some voices however seem to generate mindlessness: what is particularly disempowering about them is their apparent lack of meaning. This may be one of their functions: in hindering/destroying the person's ability to think, concentrate, understand, they may effectively protect the person from over-whelming meanings or feelings. The nonsense of madness distances the person from meaning and relatedness, just as a maze may disorient someone so that they give up, lost, alone, unable to find the centre (self) or the way out (other). Disguised in the metaphors of delusions and disembodied voices these meanings are inaccessible at first and may be worked out over time by client and therapist as the whelm of the relationship becomes a channel for such meaning. When clients use language in therapy it is saturated with meaning and complemented by the meaning of body language and non-verbal communication (including costume: dramatherapy and psychodrama both attend not just to words but to their accom-panying actions, the set and design elements; see Cox, 1978a). However, access to this meaning may be blocked, by brain biochemistry (including the effects of medication), by the culture of the medical model of psychiatry, by the inability of those around the person who hears voices to listen and tolerate the emerging meaning. People may need to overdistance themselves from the meaning contained in the psychotic experiences because of the overwhelming feelings and experiences encapsulated in these coded communications. Dramatherapy provides a way of working at sufficient distance for metaphoric material to be safely explored.

Distance theory

We are individuals because we can separate from the other (Landy, 1996: 13). To separate we must have appropriate boundaries and be able to express and assert ourselves in relation to the other, people and the world. To do this we need to achieve a 'middle' distance in our relationships, neither too distant nor too close: we must mediate our closeness, negotiate our intimacy and regulate our distance so as to be neither overwhelmed nor too isolated. We must also mediate our relationship with ourselves: the I–me relationship, so that we are not overwhelmed by our own experience nor too distant from our own needs: self-aware and able to achieve a balanced, self-regulated sense of self. In order to survive we need relationships: we are social creatures. Withdrawal into isolation may be healthy sometimes, giving us time to think, breathe, relax, contemplate, and so moderate the impact of the other, people/world. Letting ourselves be engulfed by others, giving up our separateness may sometimes be healthy: in the ecstasy of love/sex, in football crowds, in political or religious experiences. But between these extremes we need a middle distance, a fulcrum, to hold these polarities, of extreme isolation on the one hand, and merging so we lose identity on the other hand, in balance. Birdfield (1998–1999: 27) proposed a middle path between underdistance and overdistance which he called therapeutic or aesthetic distance. Landy (1993) adapted Scheff's ideas on distance to provide a core concept for dramatherapy:

1   Overdistance . . . is characterised by a minimal degree of affect and a high degree of rational thought that removes one from one's own feelings and those of others.
2   Underdistance . . . is marked by an overabundance of feeling which floods one's objectivity and capabilities.
3   Aesthetic distance . . . is notable for balance of affect and cognition, wherein both feeling and reflection are available.

(Landy, 1993: 25)

Aesthetic distance I prefer to call 'middle' distance. The term 'aesthetic' comes from the origins of the theory in theatre (Scheff, 1979). Landy stated that:

Aesthetic distance is an ideal state in which one is able to think feelingly and feel without the fear of being overwhelmed with passion. Csikszentmihalyi (1990) has conceptualised this state as 'flow', a point of spontaneity that marks effective experiences in problem solving, creativity and human relations. When in 'flow' or at aesthetic distance, an individual is able to be playful.

(Landy, 1993: 149)

Note the water metaphor here: the whelm of distance enables *flow* and *play*. Play gives us the flexibility to more effectively modulate the distance in our relationships: drawing closer to some, creating more distance, separation from others. This is not only an interpersonal skill: we can also apply this to intrapsychic material. We might be overdistanced from our body, neglecting our physical fitness. We might be underdistanced from our nightmares, feeling overwhelmed even during the day by images from the night. We may need to achieve a more balanced middle distance from a compulsion to work: having time off rather than being overwhelmed by work stresses.

Landy (1993) linked this theory with Sarbin's (1954) narrative psychology and role enactment:

Sarbin conceives of a continuum that begins with noninvolvement and proceeds to casual role enactment, ritual acting, engrossed acting, classical hypnotic role taking, histrionic neurosis, ecstasy, and sorcery and witchcraft.

Sarbin's model thus takes into consideration not only the ways in which we play out our ordinary roles, but also those extraordinary states found in worship, sex, mental illness, and trance.

(Landy, 1993: 25)

This suggests that certain roles may provide greater or lesser degrees of distance. Being able to play a role enables the person to discover they can step back, or get closer, depending on their psychological or interpersonal need (see also Landy, 1996: 13–27).

Towards a theory of distance in psychosis

I will now adapt these concepts to psychosis. I define the extreme of overdistance as being characterised by not being able to feel or think: disengaging, dissociating, withdrawal, escaping; for example **Dillon** did not come out of his house except on rare occasions (thus distancing himself from others) and had delusions of inter-galactic deities (at the greatest possible distances) who clearly encapsulated feelings of power and control, rage, aggression and hatred. In Miller's (1972: 63) view the schizophrenic patient, like a master poker-player, has overlearned the apparent security value of keeping his feelings to himself. The task becomes easier as he learns to care less. He is impelled to put more and more *distance* between himself and others. **Gloria** confirmed this with her statement: I thought I would harm my family (in response to voices) so I distanced myself.

I define underdistance as being flooded, overwhelmed by feelings, unconscious contents, fantasy, until the boundaries between self and other, reality and fantasy become swamped. **Dirk** ended his therapy with me when I entered one of his dramatic images in a powerful role. He told his psychiatrist that I had got *too close*. He complained that therapy exacerbated his paranoia: it may be that the therapy was not sufficiently distanced.

Hypomania may be understood as being flooded or taken over by one's feelings. An imbalance which prevents rational thought and reflection. This may be referred to as being underdistanced.

(Birdfield, 1998–1999: 25)

In trauma the victim is underdistanced from their experience and the hostile other: then dissociation, out-of-body experience, altered states of conciousness 'have the effect of creating psychological distance from such experience' (Baars, 1997: 161).

I now offer the following categorisation of the phenomenon of psychotic experience and hearing voices when viewed through the lens of this theory of distance. (The three degrees of distance can be seen to be characterised by the experiences cited below each.)

Overdistance	Middle distance	Underdistance
Isolation	Relationship	Lack of boundaries
Withdrawal/escape	Safe space	Abuse
Split-off feelings	Expressed feelings	Overwhelming feelings
Dissociation	Association	Confluence/symbiosis
Blank	Clarity of thought	Confusion
Forgetting	Remembering	Regression
Speechless	Own voice	Voices as invasive others
Frozen/stuckness	Creative spontaneity	Pathological spontaneity
Delusions	Play/story/myth	Hallucinations
Omnipotence	Sharing/negotiating	Powerlessness
Inflated ego/mania	Functional ego	Imploded ego/depression
Other as persecutory	Self–other	Loss of self
Psychopathic	Empathic	Victim

The *underdistance* and *overdistance* are polarities: psychological health is to be able to vary the distance between ourselves and others appropriate to the circumstances and our needs. The overdistance is in reaction to the underdistance: the lack of safe boundaries results in the person isolating themselves; in an attempt to make sense of hallucinations the person develops delusions (Slade and Bentall, 1988: 54). When the other is persecutory the person loses power and ultimately the sense of self. The more we are distanced from the other the less empathy we may have; the less distance we have from the other the more likely we are to be overwhelmed, be a victim if the other has no empathy. Many psychotic people have not had sufficient experience of an empathic carer. The psychiatric professions may also lack empathy for a psychotic person and this may be one reason for some of the difficulties in providing effective services to people who hear voices. For fear of being flooded by the needs and feelings of the psychotic patient the professionals may overdistance themselves. In so protecting themselves from the psychotic material the professionals may be unable to offer a therapeutic relationship or be in danger of creating an anti-therapeutic relationship: one in which the professional is overdistant, does not express feelings, uses power to control, not listening to the client's voice, regarding the client as stuck, powerless or deluded to the point that they cannot relate. A therapeutic relationship would be one in which the therapist owns his/her own feelings and psychotic material (such as grandiose fantasies of omnipotence or omniscience), has clear boundaries yet is able to offer warmth and empathic responses: in short, a relationship within which it is possible to express feelings in such a way that they are not over-whelming, where there is shared power and play, where the client's voice is heard and the whole person is accepted. During the therapeutic process, significant material or feelings may emerge that are potentially overwhelming and the voice hearer may again need to distance themselves. This they may do by dissociating or leaving therapy. Dramatherapy offers ways to provide safe distance when needed. To discover a balanced, middle distance and healthy relationship of self and other, the person needs a holding relationship where this is modelled and enabled. The person may go from overdistance to underdistance and needs to discover a middle ground, like Winnicott's potential space, where play and creativity are possible, where it is possible to voice feelings and grow as a whole person. The person may then, as **Gloria** said to me, come to see voices as signals that she was stressed and it was time to relax. Coleman confirmed this:

> I still hear them, I just don't see them as a problem any more – in fact, I regard them as [a] positive factor. When I'm overworked and under enormous stress the voices return. They act like alarm bells telling me to slow down.
>
> (Coleman, 2001: 3)

The voices then may be seen as messengers carrying meaning. Note that Coleman here refers to 'overwork and enormous stress': voices come when he is *overwhelmed*.

Applying distance theory to therapy

One aim of therapy then is to enable the person to find a middle distance. **Anton**, for example, sometimes had difficulty when he felt he was merging with others: Sometimes I'm in my father's body when I was conceived . . . I feel my father's heart attack in my own body . . . In this experience he was underdistanced from his father. In one individual therapy session we worked on a continuum: at one end of which was merging, being a doormat, losing his identity (underdistance) and at the other end being sad, abandoned, lonely, dead (overdistance). Moving into the central place he told himself: Stand up for yourself: tell people not to criticise, get lost. Use humour . . . **Anton** was now standing in a middle place between being underdistanced and overdistanced.

Finding the middle distance reduces the need to dissociate, enabling people to stay in the here and now. In interpersonal relationships it promotes tact and the necessary space for reflection and more effective communication. Distance also has a paradoxical effect: it allows distraction from what might be overwhelming and yet enables concentration to therapeutic effect.

Jenny, when speaking of the use of button sculpting, illustrated this effect: It did make it easier. Takes the pressure away from the situation you're talking about . . . it did make me think a bit instead of shutting off . . . It **didn't overwhelm** me . . . Sort of **put some things in perspective**. . . .

Distance creates space for more effective communication: for example **Harry** stated that breathing helped, keeping my **distance** . . . I used to get very close and try and get into her head, I keep my boundaries now . . . so I can talk fluently. (Note the word fluently: he was more able to flow.) Dramatherapy helped him gain distance with adults but also to play and get closer to his children. As an abuse survivor himself, he had become overdistanced from his children for fear of abusing them but was underdistanced from adults, and felt overpowered or abused by them.

Therapy then must provide clear boundaries and enable people to distance themselves sufficiently from material that might otherwise overwhelm and so re-traumatise. Ritual structure and creative methods nurture healthy aspects of the self. Andersen-Warren (1996: 133–134) has written of the multiple ways dramatherapy explores and strengthens a sense of boundaries.

Through playing with toy animals **Pat** was able to gain greater distance from the things that overwhelmed her: her voices, her husband's anger and the family arguments. Her observer ego grew in humour and playfulness. Distance helped **Pat** become more tactful:

> John became me (in a psychodramatic mirror) and I learned how tactless and rather selfish (I was) and my 'brick wall' is aggression . . . in the group (it was helpful/important) to work as a group: for me **to stand back** and think, 'You'd be a right bitch if you say that . . . ' I tried to take that home and there haven't been nearly as many arguments.

Laughter also helped her gain some distance and relax.

Roger said after the first group: I'm more able **to step back** from things.

The voices people hear which impel them to obey commands are underdistanced: there is no space between a voice hearer and their voices: therapy must enable a space to open so the person can *step back* and develop their observer ego, rather than be overwhelmed.

Gloria: (speaking about using two chairs and the space between them to represent opposite poles of a situation) Somehow it enables you **to create space mentally** to allow you to visualise opposing points of view and come to a decision about the situation.

The development of an observer ego enables people to reflect on experiences rather than being controlled by them: for example **Pat** created a wise woman friend who advised her to take **three steps back,** not to get involved (between her husband and his mother) and let others sort themselves out: **It goes back to seeing myself through other people's eyes** (i.e. from the distance and perspective of the other).

Distance enables people to put things into perspective:

Jimmy: It's good to be able to express how you feel, because if you're spinning out of control and you've got no direction in your life (you're confused); then (through dramatherapy) you've got this ability to **put things in perspective for your self** later because it gets it out of your system.

This space for reflection can save lives from impulsive action:

Dave: I have been depressed/suicidal but *it's not been I must do this imme-*
diately. I feel we worked on this a lot: it's benefited me.

Dramatherapy offers the opportunity to work at a distance, through metaphor, story, play. Gradually the person can move closer to reality. Of her dramatherapy work with abused children Bannister (2000: 105) states: 'This gradual move from metaphor to reality protected the children from being overwhelmed by re-enactments of traumatic scenes.'

Being able to play then, is to play with distance: negotiating relationships through activity and metaphor, expressing the self and encountering the other at a safe distance. The child does this with the transitional object and their relation-ship to their carer: dramatherapy and psychodrama provide an opportunity to play again. Slade (1980: 35) saw that children 'build and rebuild Self by Play.' The therapist must therefore become a playmate: facilitating play with distance without being over-intrusive to aid the person in rebuilding their fragile self. The distance is negotiated: at times the client will want greater or lesser degrees of distance and the therapist must be able to moderate and manage the distance of the relationship to what is appropriate to the client's need at that time. The therapeutic aim is not simply to achieve middle distance but to discover, as we did as babies through 'peek-a-boo', that it is possible to play with distance (Scheff, 1979). This play with distance creates the space between therapist and client: space for the growth and expansion of the self. Such play enables us to discover that we can feel, think, move, achieve control, let go of control, choose, negotiate, change, lose and find self and other.

Dramatherapy and psychodrama methods can provide a metaphoric, containing whelm to provide sufficient distance so the person is not overwhelmed by the wave of psychosis. Buoyed up by the creative act the person is empowered. The metaphoric distance protects the vulnerable person; the creative play strengthens the ego; the degree of distance is varied until the person is strong enough or wishes to be more direct, to move closer to self and other.

Chapter 8

Individual dramatherapy
Cheryll

In this chapter I offer a single case example in which I explore the use of specific creative methods that enabled a client to reveal and re-create herself. All the sessions were one-hour long. We worked together for 156 sessions over three and a half years.

Introducing Cheryll

Cheryll was 40 when I met her (though she looked much younger and sometimes behaved in childlike ways). As a child she had been depressed and withdrawn, unable to function at school with a specific learning difficulty in maths. She wrote:

> Life for me was difficult. I dealt unknowingly with early depression . . . being
> reserved, set apart . . . never bonding with any one at all. I felt like the stray
> ugly duckling . . . left out of all social activity.

She had first seen a psychiatrist at the age of 13. At 21 she was depressed following the difficult, painful birth of her only child during which she hallucinated: she later gave this child up to the care of her parents. During this period she struggled with extreme isolation, poverty, deprivation and neglect. She was diagnosed as schizophrenic. She had accepted her diagnosis of schizophrenia with despairing resignation yet also had aspirations of recovery when psychiatry appeared to offer none. She said: There is no future, no cure. I'm always going to feel poorly. I sometimes feel normal, it's delicious; want to feel happier.

By the age of 24 she was hearing voices. She occasionally acted out in violent ways, smashing things, attacking medical staff. She was regarded by the service caring for her as 'difficult'. She complained of headaches and brief fainting spells. She dissociated, saying that sometimes an evil personality took over. She also had a baby self and a child self: she heard six voices including a gentle female voice aged about 30 and a callous, controlling male (who seemed at least partly to be modelled on Jed, a previous sadistic partner). She described her voices as vicious, subhuman (a voice had once ordered her to kill a cat) but also as soothing. The male voices were especially controlling and oppressive. She felt oppressed by her voices; however, when lonely she had summoned a voice, hoping it would be friendly. One of them, whom she named Fiddlededee, soothed her when she was feeling powerless. When she was hearing voices she withdrew from contact with others and had inner dialogues with the voices. They reminded her to do things and controlled her choice of food, clothes and home decor. Over the course of therapy she talked about and showed me different selves. I did wonder whether she was in fact suffering from dissociative identity disorder but did not feel it was my role to challenge her diagnosis: my job was to work with her as a therapist. She described herself as a diamond, with its different facets being different personalities that sometimes caused confusion. She also told a psychiatrist that she didn't have a personality and would like one. She said she had a twin self (whom she called Paula) who had too many feelings and was overwhelming; this twin self seemed the polar opposite of her usual self: the twin had too many feelings whereas **Cheryll** characterised herself as having no feelings. She showed me, in a dance, the process of transforming from one self to another: an anguished non-verbal struggle. I began to get to know her other selves/voices: Thing, Seek (short for Secrecy), Fiddlededee, Wolf. She said: I've never spoken with anyone about them. She showed me these over time, revealing them gradually through mask work and toy theatre. She said I would never know all the facets of her personality. Although the work was often challenging I found her always interesting – a puzzle that never entirely lost its mystery.

Assessment sessions

In an early session we used Guatemalan worry dolls (miniature figures in a small round container). These enabled **Cheryll** to talk about the birth of her son: how she had hallucinated due to the pain and hated the baby, wishing the doctors would kill 'it'. Now she pushed the doll representing her son away to protect him from being embarrassed by his mother. (During the subsequent therapy I witnessed the changing relationship between **Cheryll** and her son, culminating in his wedding: a happy family event.) Other Guatemalan worry dolls were roles, personalities, babies who were safe together. The following week, reflecting on this work, she disclosed she had had two abortions. When we drew her family tree (genosociogram: see Schutzenberger, 1998) we discovered her mother had lost a female child a year before she gave birth to **Cheryll**: mother hardly ever mentioned this girl. There is considerable evidence that depressed, grieving mothers are unable to bond with a 'replacement' child (see also Casson 2000b).

Piecing together the fragments of the story

As the work proceeded I sought to find appropriate creative methods to help **Cheryll** symbolise her difficulties. As she had talked of fragments I offered her the tangram (a Chinese puzzle with different shaped pieces that can be fitted together in any order to make patterns): she used this to speak of her strengths and the struggle to bring the pieces together in various ways. She wanted to reject her vulnerability and made strength, a diamond others could not see or appreciate, central. She was then able to show me her disintegrated self, speaking of splits in her personality, of other selves. She used the tangram to develop a story of boxes containing many things, some of which were lost: jewels, maps and disgusting things. A merchant gave away his box to avoid conflict. He gathered up the fragments of old smashed boxes and put a ribbon round an ugly box. The fragments could be contained and integrated in a story. Later, after 88 sessions of therapy she was able to talk of her experience of fragmentation and of putting herself back together. She wrote: I feel like a smashed diamond but piecing me together is . . . hard work . . . to get each piece of me properly into its own place . . . I feel sort of fragmented not human at all and I've forgotten what feeling human is . . .

Babushkas

As the therapy proceeded we went on to use Babushka dolls, which are also containers (Illustration 5). Playing with the dolls stimulated **Cheryll**: inside the adult she found the child. She said the outside of the armoured figure hid a beautiful inner self: the outside shut its door against the world so people could not see in. She was fearful that my shell will fall away and leave me vulnerable to the way I feel physically, emotionally . . . In the collection of Babushka dolls was a world sphere containing other spheres, within which the central sphere was painted with an uruborus snake: this recalled memories of her childhood in a tropical country. The snake image recurred: one day she wore a T shirt with a snake skin pattern. She described the snake as sensitive, aware of vibrations,

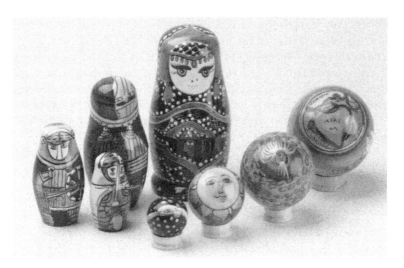

Illustration 5 The Black Russian doll, the armoured figure and world

able to taste the air: not human but alive. Years earlier her hospital notes had recorded her sensation that she had a cold snake inside her which buzzed and made her walk around. Later this had become a bee or a fly buzzing. She wrote a poem about a fly with its multifaceted eyes as an image of herself. She spoke of having lost her human identity: of not being able to feel, being blank and referred to the time with Jed when she felt she'd lost her self. She wrote: I am no longer a human being: the truth you should know is that the dream of a snake can become you and you see your body the body of a snake . . . underneath the headless snake is a human being called me . . .

Her therapy gradually enabled her to feel, express thoughts and feelings and reclaim her humanity. This was due at least as much to the warm, containing relationship with me as any technique.

> **Cheryll** wrote: The Russian Dolls are **delicious**, the Black one with **onion** ring etching and a door on his **tummy** roused me so too did the little blue ball with the gold spots that I didn't at first identify with connecting the balls and the black doll till in my favourite place the night, in the twilight dream I saw **two forests** one of **serenity and enchantment** and strong golden hugh (hue) reflecting off velvety soils and grass . . . the other . . . one was **a reality forest** . . . then through the **stomach** of my dream on a smokey blackened doll I saw perversity nice faces became evil **smells** and corruption lurked . . .

Food and feelings

The images here are full of meaning: the olfactory senses relate to her need for nurture. Her mother, depressed when **Cheryll** was born, was unable to nurture her: indeed her breast milk was not palatable for baby **Cheryll**. Mother bottle fed her. **Cheryll** remembered her mother forcing mashed egg on her until she was sick, disgusted by the *smell*. Mother and child did not bond well. She described herself as a thin child who was not nourished/loved, who grew to feel separate, different and rejected. Years later with Jed, her psychopathic boyfriend, she survived sadistic physical humiliation, sexual abuse and rape. **Cheryll** withdrew into fantasy (the enchanted 'forest of dreams') from such a harsh reality (the 'reality forest' which she also called the 'forest of perversion'). **Cheryll** told me she had worked as a hospital operating theatre assistant and been involved in the disposal of aborted foetuses. She brought in some bones and bit them, inviting me to suck out the marrow and spit, be sick. She brought mussels to eat, biting them aggressively, then disclosed that when she killed the budgie she had bitten it. It seemed she was trying to disgust me (and so either test whether I would reject her or see if I could express disgust) and showing me her sadism as she tried to digest things she had done in the past. **Cheryll** was sick, vomiting the raw liver after the session in which she ate it in front of me. The next week we talked about what disgusted her, what she could not stomach. She spoke of child abuse and when her son was taken off her by her parents (who brought him up because

Cheryll could not parent him). She brought in a perfume called Poison. She spoke of olfactory hallucinations of dirty, unpleasant smells. She spoke of accepting her voices' *taste* in choosing clothes and decor for her home. I offered sensory stimuli to encourage her creativity. We explored perfumes, tastes, colours (including finger paints), textures (including cloth and clay). This sensory play, named by Jennings *et al.* (1994: 97) 'embodiment play', offered **Cheryll** a developmental recapitulation (see also Cattanach, 1994: 28–40). Slowly **Cheryll** began to bring more palatable food: fruit, milk, honey. She began to accept my interventions (the 'food' I had to offer her) and use her therapy creatively. She later referred to her therapy as delicious. **Cheryll**, speaking about a Tiger puppet, said that its aggression had abated because it was well fed and had got what it needed. All these bizarre actions then can be seen as metaphoric, symbolic communications that were meaningful rather than mad.

Anger

In eating raw liver and a cactus in front of me, Cheryll said she was showing me how anger could enable her to overcome disgust or block pain. Internalised anger, unexpressed, can lead not only to depression but also to splitting of the person: the anger thus becomes symbolised, encapsulated in one part of the self. This then can become a source of voices:

> **Cheryll**: (writing in her journal. Paula is the name she gave to her alter ego.) When I feel anger, it's extreme – *I can't speak* . . . I have felt very violent holding so much that I sweated *I then split into two people* I saw a responsible person at the wheel of a car too fast and big and angry, always alert and on my guard feeling as vicious as an alsatian dog . . . I saw my anger in time as abnormal, people saw a quiet person *I split my character took on two meanings* the person in the back relaxed and looking on at my anger and the anger itself and other person controlling it at a terrifying intolerable degree . . . I don't know why I'm angry but I am very tired too . . . but it won't go into my special diary written by Paula, however Cheryll say you are special you know why because you sit amongst Jed and all the others you *warm* them up with your human love and your innocence, we *pokefire* at them in our own cold ways . . . I don't want to shut my eyes to them they are still open with past fears and when they have gone I may shut mine and you will be gone and and I will become innocent and Jed is mad and my eyes will close, Paula will come and I don't want her to because I can be mad and she can't . . . what *irritates* me more is that Jed is in the room . . .

Jed was **Cheryll**'s sadistic, psychopathic partner who physically, sexually and emotionally abused and humiliated her. He died before he could murder her and she felt haunted by him. The above, apparently 'mad' writing has meaning, half-concealed, that reveals the anger she could not feel or openly express to Jed lest he attack her. She connected the mute rage she felt towards him (he'd once said he wanted to sexually abuse her son) with her mute rage as a child. She had learned to block pain and fear, to dissociate, when she was with him in order to survive. She self-harmed: here a match struck *furious* and fast on a colourless face it drew its *fire* on my arm but left no pain . . .

I have written elsewhere on the symbolism of fire, abuse and anger (Casson, 1998a). **Cheryll** survived Jed by not feeling, discovering she could dissociate from pain. She wrote: sometimes I am very sensitive, other times I *cut off* from the pain. She learned to numb herself, even to enjoy the pain. It became a source of strength to know she could survive. She demonstrated this to me one day by biting the cactus. One way of coping with overwhelming feelings is not to feel, to cut off feelings. She said: If I got back to normality I would have normal feelings but now I cut off from feelings and people. She talked of her fear that the blocks that kept her at a distance and protected her, might go and she would then be overwhelmed and collapse into feelings. She was afraid of her anger emerging when she was ill: that it would be out of control and dangerous. My aggression is all bad, nasty: it can't speak. If it could speak it might be possible to control or express it in safe ways. She used sessions to express her anger and destructiveness without harm to either of us.

Mask work

Using a mask helped **Cheryll** disclose the circumstances when she killed a cat, relating the mask of a wolf to one of her voices. She spoke of a white wolf with a stag's body, a spiritual figure of power. One voice she said was a dog: god, spelt backwards. Of her anger she had said she was feeling as vicious as an alsatian dog. Over the months and years of the therapy and the analysis of her imagery I gradually came to understand some of the meanings within her cryptic communications. We went on to make masks: **Cheryll**'s first was plain white, expressive of her fear, of being frozen. She wrote: take a look behind the mask and you would find that the only real meaning life has for me is to die, I see a flat abysmal world full of human frailties and suffering. Drawing a mask she was able to symbolise her experience through form and colour: showing the holes in her head (lost memories) and using the colour of forgetting (green) she drew little people on the mask: these became thoughts in her brain. She then created another mask of singing and loving. She laughed: she wanted to be happy. The creative work lifted her mood. In a following session she drew another mask, its face split, a hand reaching out over fragments, weeping: she stated her tears were not far away.

Make-up

At the next session I offered her the opportunity to move from mask to make-up: the latter being a less distanced technique as the make-up is on the body, whereas the mask can be held off the body. **Cheryll** used make-up to create two faces on a white base: a polar bear and a puppet. The polar bear was an isolate in lonely, cold places. The puppet was powerless, manic and controlled by an unknown puppeteer. She spoke about whether Seek (one of her voices) would make her leave home (just as Jed had made her walk the streets at night in winter). She reflected that part of her was depressed (the polar bear – a white creature who lived at one of the poles of a bipolar world, able to survive out in the cold), part manic (the puppet) and that different aspects of herself had different feelings. When she had washed off the make-up I gave her a string puppet so that she became the puppeteer (returning before the end of the session to more distanced play). She later wrote about the puppet as an image of her stuckness, the strings wrapped around her, mute.

Control

The unknown puppeteer controlling the stuck puppet introduces the theme of control. Dramatherapy and psychodrama aim to give the person more sense of control. Taking control might mean a change in personality as well as in behaviour:

Cheryll: Part of the year the voices disappeared altogether. I was relieved and liked that but then other things started happening – I seemed to take a loud/dominant role – the voices made me meek.

Cheryll at the start of her therapy felt unable to say 'No' to her mother. Mother was invasive, critical and controlling. **Cheryll** could not bear to be with her long. She had said 'No' to Jed twice and been violently punished. He had raped her at knife point. Jed had taken total control of **Cheryll**: he had starved her, deprived her of sleep, exhibited her naked to his friends, publicly humiliated her, physically and sexually abused her. She still felt haunted/possessed by him and heard his voice. She said her voice Seek was a controller. This voice had appeared contemporaneously with Jed with whom it was in alliance but in control: a part of herself that 'allowed', observed and 'controlled' Jed, giving her a sense of things being in control when in fact Jed was in control. She feared him coming back and taking over: of losing herself again. Jed took control by suddenly hitting her, shocking her and taking her breath away.

Through her therapy **Cheryll** struggled with issues of power and control, attempting, and sometimes managing, to control me. At times I had to model saying 'No' to her attempts to abuse me (when she asked me to share some raw liver) or please me (when offering inappropriate gifts such as a set of knives). She expected that I would reject her and tested me, asking whether I was bored, whether I liked her: so often had she been rejected that she expected me to do so. Therapy then must give the person experiences of being in control, negotiating power, having choices and responsibility. For example **Cheryll** enjoyed having control of the lighting in the room, changing the brightness of the coloured spot lights to match her mood, at a time when others (parents and boyfriend) were taking control. Eventually she was able to re-assert control of her life.

Costume and colour symbolism

When I first met **Cheryll** I was struck by her dress: a yellow caftan with stags and entoptic forms which I recognised from prehistoric, shamanic cave paintings. She was playfully eccentric in her costumes, deliberately not conforming to 'normal' societal expectations or fitting in with her 'normal' parents, though when they visited her she wore plain clothes to avoid their criticism. I've *cut myself off* from normal people, don't want to be judged . . . My parents still see me as a child: I've had to dress down/formal for them: they'll take me over when they're there. They disowned me . . . She described her parents as controlling and invasive: they criticised her dress, food, home and read her diary. **Cheryll**'s parents came to visit her, bringing their dirty laundry to exploit her washing machine. She felt overwhelmed by their demands and decided to withdraw and listen instead to her voices. During the period of therapy she began to separate from her parents emotionally, placing limits on their contact with her and their invasive visits.

Cheryll came to therapy every week in a different costume, sometimes theatrical, sometimes ordinary. She brought a ballet dress, a pink ball gown, a man's suit, a 'sexy' leather dress; she told me that the voices sometimes told her what to wear and that she was reproducing hallucinatory figures: by wearing their costumes she was trying to gain their meaning. Although the hallucinations were brief she had an intense feeling of meaning. One day she asked me if I wanted to see her split in two. She went in another room and changed into a man's suit. She showed me a male figure, strong, dependable and caring, basing this role/aspect of herself on a previous partner, Reg, who had died. Thus she expressed her grief and incorporated these aspects into herself.

Gradually I understood she had a system of colour symbolism: green = forgetting; brown = father (dull absence); red = love (a colour Jed didn't like); pink = child/babyhood and the colour of 'Secrecy' (a voice); orange the colour that connected them all. (This colour symbolism had first become apparent when we worked with buttons and Cheryll explained the meanings of the colours of the buttons she chose.) She brought in her pram beads: primary coloured spheres on elastic that stretched across the pram, 'to protect her'. The different colours also seemed to symbolise different aspects of herself. The pram beads could be seen as a transitional object in the space between herself and the other, the world.

In an early session she brought pictures of babies, including one inside a red melon. She then chose to create a red room using the coloured spot lights and sat on the floor in her red dress. Red in her colour symbolism meant love. She was creating a safe space within which she could go back to begin again. She dreamed of me wearing a red shirt and a passive woman who accepted what was offered without objection. As red was the colour of love, of passion, I noted the times it occurred as when she brought raw liver, a red rose, and wondered about the possibility of seduction and abuse. Over several weeks **Cheryll**'s behaviour was seductive: she wore a see-through blouse, a leather dress, changed her clothes in a session, brought photographs of herself in the nude. I refused to look at these and maintained appropriate professional boundaries, inviting her (when she wanted to change costume) to use an adjacent room. My ability to maintain appropriate boundaries enabled her subsequently to talk about the abuse she had suffered at the hands of Jed.

Slowly we found a way forward: in one session we restaged her first birthday party:

> **Cheryll**: (writing in her journal) Thankyou for the pink cloth. (we had used pink cloth to set the scene for the birthday party) . . . my party is in my dreams (I! dream) Party girl dreams . . . a dress of any description and my birthday girl socks with the picture of the lit candle on them, the party less child grew up . . . som-how birthdays for me never were parties, deep inside I felt a **solitude I hadn't relationships with children that could support a party** . . . The unusual thing about being a little girl was about having babies one day yourself, here I was different, **my baby would want me to notice and play and feel good and understood**, but these arn't in the imaginings of myself as a child my thoughts were brutal corrupt and perverse I wanted to be crap all to my baby when it was born and green words would come through my ugly childlike lips when I was alone, I don't remember them being out loud.

Unable to give to a child what she had not received herself she had been envious of (green words which could not be voiced out loud), even hateful (be crap) to the child. She needed her own experience of nurture before she could give such to another. And so back to pink Thanks for my birthday pressy John (a symbolic toy box I gave her in the session) dreams so full up of pink I smiled broadly in them and my first birthday party I felt a part of my own dream I liked it I'm still liking it, my first birthday . . . We had repaired something through this birthday party. **Cheryll** chose pink again when, during a sensory play session with colours and textures, she wrapped herself in pink cloth, put on the red and white spot lights to create a pink room and relaxed. (In some police stations experimental cells painted pink have been found to calm violent offenders, the specific wavelength of the colour affecting the brain wave patterns to calm the prisoner.) In a later session she wore red: she was bright, warm, expressive and read her poem about happiness.

Happiness

The smell of heather and un-polluted air . . .
The tide rushing in waves foaming between your toes cleaning
your feet and the soft warm sand sifting softly over your

fingers and under foot.
Indeed the colour pink, fair, bright, warm and true, sweet
like a candy floss and hot too like hot ice that burns
your fingers in the deep depths of winter, many pink
merry faces, but come away from my fire my pink . . .
Happiness can be found in taste the succulence of a honey dew
melon or your favourite chocolate truffles . . .
but deeper lies the mental pain the cruelty of existence but when in
deep below the surface
you may be surprised to find the opening of a large
fresh red delicate poppy, to bring a warm beaming
smile to your lips, not forgotten a smile on a face.
1998 was a happy year.

Creative therapy is not just about problems but about discovering strengths and the pleasure of creativity. Out of pain and pleasure **Cheryll** began to create poetry.

Theatre

Cheryll had wanted to be in school plays as a child but was never chosen: dramatherapy offered her an opportunity to play, perform, be witnessed. She spoke about *A Midsummer Night's Dream*. I offered her a toy theatre, a reproduction of Shakespeare's Globe Theatre (Illustration 6). The toy theatre reminded **Cheryll** of puppets: of when she, as a child, had been unable to play.

This play had many meanings for her: the forest, fairies, the lost lovers, the conflict with parents. She asked: Why would Oberon mix up the lovers in the forest: why be cruel and confuse reality and dream? Reading the text (she had a remarkable ability to sight read Shakespeare) provided her, a very distracted and fragmented person, with a containing structure. Reading aloud has been found to reduce voices (Watkins, 1998: 208; Slade and Bentall, 1988: 189). Reading together we were playing together: I was a playmate. She was no longer the lonely child but had a companion and was able to be the star of the show. She enjoyed playing Puck and being mischievous. In the toy theatre she picked out figures from the 'play within the play', of Pyramus and Thisbe, the *wall* and the lion. These seemed metaphoric of her anger and the way she protected or blocked her feelings. After Jed's death she said: I've been unpenetratable since then, *a wall*, I have the ability to cut myself off from life. She said she was *walled off* from reality. Others did not see or know a part of herself that she hid (the voice she called 'Secrecy').

She showed me how she could go into a safe place at will: dissociating and entering a space *walled off* from the world (which she called a psychotic state. She stated that this disturbed others but was OK for her). Reading the text of *A Midsummer Night's Dream* prompted her to talk about the possibility and

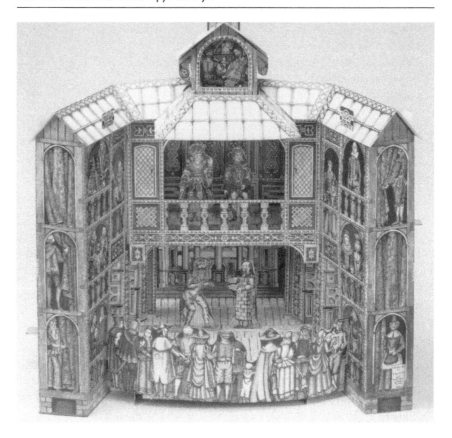

Illustration 6 Toy theatre: *A Midsummer Night's Dream*

difficulty of emotional bonding between mother and child, of her own relationships with her mother and her son. The lack of attachment bonds with them had impoverished her emotional life so that she did not feel a person and her masochistic bond with the sadistic Jed had resulted in emotional abuse and dissociation.

She created a scene with three fairies who were her voices:

- A wide eyed depersonalised fairy, only half-human, angry, jealous.
- A fairy who ate a magic mushroom and went green (the colour of forgetting in her system of colour symbolism) and lost herself. By eating the red berry (the colour of love) she found herself again.
- A glittering fairy with strong delicate wings: a beauty that others could not see. She was not alone but dancing with others.

The following session she talked of three lost siblings (one of whom died less than a year before her birth, the other two were miscarriages) and her mother's mental illness. She brought in Spencer's *Fairy Queen*. She wrote, If ever a book understood me this one does and quoted:

> For all as soone as life did me admit
> into this world, and shewed heavens light,
> From mothers pap I taken was unfit
> And streight delivered to a fairy
> > (Spencer (1910: 55) *Fairy Queen*,
> > > Canto IX, iii)

Cheryll read the passage of the Red Cross Knight and the Filthy Dragon who devoured her babies. We used toy theatre to play out the encounter of the dragon, the knight and a dwarf (baby). It was possible to play with fantasy safely and creatively: to express this disturbing material at a safe distance. She was now able to talk about disturbing experiences and reflect on them. The following week we created a play in which the star of the show felt joy and satisfaction at the fulfilment of her dreams. In this role she enjoyed the audience's pleasure at her performance. **Cheryll** then tore the scenery up to express her envy at this star. Her younger brother had been born within a year of her and she had had to give up her place in the pram and walk. She said: I always felt rejection. **Cheryll** was passive as a way of surviving her mother's rejection and hostility. She spoke of being a lonely child, unable to play.

Destructive and creative play

The creative work then had facilitated significant disclosures. It also allowed her to play out aggressive, angry feelings. She imagined hurting others (indeed she had attacked staff in the past). She was allowing me to know of her sadistic care-less attitude, contrasting this with accounts of her compassion for others (suicidal friends and people with learning disabilities whom she had befriended and was helping). Slowly an integration of these split-off, opposite aspects of her self occurred. She was able to reveal both her functional, sane, compassionate, creative self and her dysfunctional, insane, destructive self. In the dramatherapy it was possible for her to express these aggressive impulses in a safe way without harming anyone. I reflected that a baby needed her aggression to encounter the world (to reach out, grab, bite, meet the other) but if baby was met with aggression, as when mother physically abused her (see p. 138–9) she would withdraw and experience aggression as bad. Her own aggression might then be internalised and turned against the self. The withdrawn, depressed child (of a depressed mother) would be unable to relate or process anger. One of my aims therefore was to turn the anger outwards in creative play. In one session **Cheryll** enjoyed demolishing a house I built from toy bricks. She enjoyed teasing me, playfully expressing hostility. She played with a soft toy devil. In therapy she was able to tell me of her 'bad' side, her anger, her murderousness which she feared would be released when she was ill. In dramatherapy she could play out evil fantasies in a safe way, as Slade (1980: 73–74, 109) said of his work with children: drama enabled them to play 'out evil in a legal framework'. Play can be cathartic and destructive, enabling the expression of angry feelings. **Cheryll** tore up a dress, tore up the scenery of the toy theatre, cut off a doll's hair. She then told me Jed had cut off her hair. Some of her play was hostile: a way of expressing her aggression to me. She broke up a doll: telling me she had hidden the contraceptive pill in a doll when she was 13 so her parents wouldn't know, (thus this destructive act was creative: she was revealing a fragment of her story).

Another example of such cathartic, destructive play was when another woman tore up a telephone directory to express her rage at her abuser's telephone calls. She threw the pieces into the air and saw how they fluttered like butterflies; her rage transformed into exuberant delight. The destructive act was transformed into a creative image: passion becoming soul. The possessive power of the abuser (victims often describe feeling haunted by their abuser) must be destroyed before the person's free will can be released. The self is recreated through play. The butterfly has been a symbol of the psyche (soul) for over 2,000 years. The fairy is in effect a human butterfly. Roman fresco and mosaic images of Psyche show her wearing butterfly wings.

Mother and child

Cheryll didn't feel loved as a child. The atmosphere at home was full of shouting and hostility. Her mother physically abused her when she was a baby. **Cheryll** wrote in a poem:

> What hides itself behind the maternal veil,
> Through violence all innocence shattered,
> No difference between night and day,
> No watch no time no sleep
> Through fear . . .
> Pictures scattered in pieces fragments only the past left.
> I now a picture of glass on unpenetrable glass with eyes void
> of emotion . . .
> I am no longer a human . . .
> and you live on knowing something about
> life that with no-one you can share because no-one would
> understand the blackest diamond of all is innocent as a lamb.

Cheryll's mother was depressed following the death of her previous child. **Cheryll** spontaneously role reversed with her mother in one session and I interviewed her as mother. She disclosed that she had always had difficulty relating to her child. She had been grieving and anxious throughout the pregnancy and when **Cheryll** had been born had rejected her: she was subsequently cold and withdrawn from the child. During this role reversal **Cheryll** was clear, cogent and in touch as never before. In the following session she wept, grieving the death of the child her mother lost before she was born and her own unmet needs as a baby. She then remembered, at age 3–4, being shut in a cupboard and mother frightening her that there were ghosts. She was in a complete panic, banging on the cupboard door, fearing no one would hear her.

It may be that **Cheryll**'s mother's lack of empathy for her as a child was most damaging: in working with a psychotic client the therapist's capacity for empathy is challenged. I hypothesised that when **Cheryll** was born she was not seen or appreciated: her mother was unable to respond to her. **Cheryll** dreamed of herself as a child, withdrawing from shouting and feeling bored and not cared for. She felt the womb had been a safe place.

This pattern was repeated with **Cheryll**'s own son: after a difficult birth **Cheryll** had been unable to bond with him. Gradually over the period of the therapy **Cheryll** developed her relationship with her son until she was able to attend his wedding.

The countertransference

I define countertransference as the feelings the therapist has about the client and the work. These will be composed of a mixture of the therapist's own material and the impact of the client on the therapist: what the client projects into/onto the therapist. I have at times found the countertransference, when working with people who hear voices and have psychotic experiences, overwhelming and needed supervision to understand what was happening.

Snow (1996: 230) stated that the 'therapist will need to contain chaotic and often painful countertransference. I believe that anyone who has spent a good deal of time working with psychotic individuals will recognise the pangs of what Lewis (1993, 17) calls somatic countertransference' (see also Ellwood, 1995: 78; Eigen, 1993: 136, 177, 193, 201).

At times the countertransference seemed liable to destroy the relationship. I felt warm towards and interested in **Cheryll**, yet repeatedly I felt sleepy during her sessions: so much so that at times I had to bite my tongue hard to keep alert. I was not bored, as she feared: I did not feel rejecting of her yet I would suddenly find myself drifting off to sleep. Was there something I did not want to hear? Was I escaping because I could not comprehend what she was saying or from the disturbing effect of her fragmentary communication? Was I hypnotised by her voice? Was I avoiding contact with her (or she with me)? The other side of fascination is the powerlessness of trance. I took this to supervision and we wondered if I was being propelled into the unconscious for some reason (see also Lewis, 1993: 13). I struggled to stay awake. Then in one session **Cheryll** disclosed that her mother had broken her arm when she was a baby. Suddenly I understood: a baby would have no possibility of escape or way of comprehending such experience. The only option would be to withdraw into the unconscious from such danger: to go to sleep. After a subsequent session instead of writing clinical notes I found myself writing a poem as if I was in the role of mother. After consulting my supervisor I read this poem to **Cheryll**. For the first time in her therapy she wept. Through the countertransferential communication I had been able to process the feelings that did not make sense and return some meaning to **Cheryll** in a form that she could accept.

However processing such unconscious material is not without its challenges and costs. After a session in which she spoke of when Jed had raped her at knife point, threatening to cut off her head, and how she had then regressed to being a baby, I wrote in my journal:

> After seeing Cheryll I have a real sense of the toxicity of this work. Horror, disgust, confusion, powerlessness: that I hardly know what's real/unreal, where to go, what to do. Anxiety floats and hardly is there relief afterwards as I feel hopeless, helpless: the undigested affect she cannot stomach that I must metabolise for my own well being. I need to go out, walk, be grounded in the calm of nature: to see the simple order of things, of external reality, recognisable and predictable after the confusion of our encounter. As I confronted her she became clearer and I wonder if she uses me to get clarity just as I get confusion from her.

There were many times when I did not understand, when I felt baffled, frightened, '*out of my depth*' (and therefore fearful of being *overwhelmed*). As well as my professional skills I needed to draw on my personal strengths to sustain me.

> The therapist's ability to contain and endure this primitive fear is of great importance in the psychotherapy of someone suffering from schizophrenia.
> (Thomas, 1997: 68)

It was at times like this that the supervision sustained me: as I felt *held* so I could hold on, *holding* the person in therapy (see Mollon, 1996: 154). Such holding provides a container that counters the possibility of being overwhelmed.

The child within

In my therapy room I have teddies and other soft toys. A kangaroo with a baby in its pouch reminded **Cheryll** of her childhood and was also a metaphor for her relationship with her mother, with her son and with her own vulnerable self. Therapy can facilitate the healing re-emergence of 'the child within'. As a child **Cheryll** had desperately wanted to grow up. She described her mother as being unable to play with her as a child. Now she wanted to regress to be a child again, to enjoy being little and play in her therapy sessions. Dramatherapy and psychodrama offer playful opportunities to recapitulate developmental stages that have been blocked or delayed by abusive experiences (see Bannister, 2000:

102). Other participants in my research reported that at times they experienced involuntary regressions to childhood. These were not necessarily due to therapy:

Gloria: I feel as though I've regressed back to childhood, where I barely function and find it difficult to cope alone.

Diane: I still feel very young, emotionally.

Several people echoed **Diane**, stating they felt very young.

When **Jill** went into hospital it reminded her of when she had been put into care as a child: I felt like I was in care in that building . . . it felt like I was being locked up.

In dreams, fantasies and delusions the image of a dead baby or child occurred. One person had a delusion that their father had confessed to being a child murderer. **Diane** said one of her voices was Myra Hindley: vindictive, cruel, revengeful.

Cheryll talked of aborted foetuses, a dead sibling, a dead bird, a dead cat (which she was told to kill by a voice). She sometimes felt dead. Due to Jed's brutality she did not feel human. She said he had killed her: now she was dead. In this state she felt very powerful, not caring for herself or others: fearless. The voices joked about her wanting to be human. She wrote: So long as I can say I am not human it makes things seem better . . . the living dead needn't have feelings . . .

Dillon also wrote: I don't feel human.

Roger said: I felt dead inside.

Anton sometimes felt dead, not feeling, not connected, free. Another man who had been the victim of a serious assault said he felt he had died. **Harry** as a child enjoyed playing the role of a dying, wounded cowboy. He felt haunted by ghosts. He sometimes felt like a zombie: withdrawing from contact with others, not thinking, not feeling (see Chapter 11). Neuroleptic medication may also contribute to such emotional indifference (Healy, 1993: 33).

Cheryll dreamed that my anger split a baby into millions of bloody pieces ripped from my womb . . .

Dave also recounted a dream:

> Janet pushing pram with baby totally enclosed in covering. I pull back a small flap to let the child breathe and Janet complains the baby will be cold. I find a large white bag in the street with blood on its fringes and discover it contains a dead baby, the others walk off unconcerned . . . In some way I feel my childhood died at an early age and my parents too when they divorced. Perhaps the child reappeared looking for its parents in psychosis . . .

I have previously connected this type of experience with abuse:

> I regard sexual abuse as soul rape or soul murder, and many abuse survivors speak of themselves as having died as a child or experience themselves as containing a dead child, a frozen inner self, buried.
>
> (Casson, 1997–1998: issue 64: 59)

The healing drama (Bannister, 1997) enables the inner child to re-emerge through play. Speaking of dramatherapy **Jimmy** said: You feel as if you can be born again . . . It's like being a kid again . . .

Jenny confirmed this: We played . . . you got in touch with the kid in you.

Harry: (speaking of physical warm-up exercises and games in therapy) playing football, throwing the ball to each other: that was quite fun, brings the child out of you. It was all right.

Anton enjoyed playing in therapy: it's as if I have to go back to an earlier stage, to beginning and learn to play again. I had the impression that **Anton** had been interrupted when playing as a child by a critical/invasive other and so was unable to concentrate, to play. He told me he wanted to learn to concentrate/focus. He spoke of his mentally ill mother's negativity towards him, her blame and criticism and his father's hostility. Slade (1980: 28) showed how the absorption of play enabled the child to develop the ability to concentrate.

Play with children

Possibly as a result of being able to be playful in therapy, several people reported their ability to play with children outside therapy improved.

Cheryll said mother had not been able to play with her and consequently she had been unable to play or have friends as a child. After playing with the toy theatre **Cheryll** reported that she was more able to communicate with her niece, telling her about the theatre: She loved it. I therefore enjoyed her company – it was not in silence . . .

Harry also had this experience: I can play with my kids better whereas . . . I used to keep the kids distant, didn't want to know, hated them actually, it was so sad . . . **Harry**, in effect, had learned to play during his individual therapy sessions (see Chapter 11).

Pat also found her ability to relate to her children had improved: And I think the kids have been better. I'm not as ratty. As she was able to play more in dramatherapy so she was able to play more with the children at home. As she found an outlet for her anger she relaxed more and so was more able to respond to her children. As she received attention she was able to give attention: I'm much more outgoing with the kids. I take my time to listen whereas before . . . I'd tell them to go away . . . I feel stronger.

In my view the potential preventative mental health benefit of this work for the children of voice hearers is incalculable.

Structuring chaos

I did not impose these various creative methods on **Cheryll** but listened to her to discover what method would be appropriate. She had, for example, mentioned *A Midsummer Night's Dream* several times over the weeks before I offered her the toy theatre and the text. The play already had multiple meanings for her: she'd even called herself Hypolita after her first marriage. I was seeking appropriate creative stimulus and metaphoric containers: she specifically asked for more such structure after sessions when talking alone did not seem helpful to her. Theatre then provided a containing structure (see Chapter 9).

Many sessions were chaotic: **Cheryll** had difficulty concentrating and would move from one image to another, from reading to playing, from talking about memories, fantasies, recent events, to dancing. Though it was often baffling to move with her through this chaos, slowly sessions became more coherent as she learned to use the time. Sometimes it was as if she was showing me the fragments of her self and slowly gathering these jigsaw puzzle pieces and putting them together to form a more or less complex picture of her whole self. What this organised and coherent account, written after years of analysis of the material, may not give the reader is a sense of my own experience of confusion, even bewilderment at the chaos of fractured material that **Cheryll** presented. It was sometimes months, even years, before I understood some of her cryptic communications.

Working towards closure

In bringing any period of therapy to a successful closure the final sessions must be planned and time taken to reflect on the therapy and bring matters to a close. In one of the final sessions we worked with the image of doors (exits): I offered **Cheryll** a collection of photographs of doors and she enjoyed choosing different images to represent different feelings. An abandoned, ruined castle (which had been built to protect those within from hostile attacks) symbolised her attempts to wall herself off in the face of hostility. Other doors were images of happiness, of safe boundaried places where people could live. As we approached the boundary of therapy **Cheryll** was more able to establish safe boundaries for herself in her relationships with her family and arranged her own house move from a block of flats where she was stressed by the environment and vulnerable to scapegoating/hostility, to a housing association which was safer and more pleasantly situated. She also began to separate from the mental health services, choosing to find meaningful activities and roles in the community, thus recovering her sense of agency and control of her life. Of dramatherapy she said: It's active, fun, motivating – when you're down or have low self-esteem it's uplifting and **brings you out of your shell**. If you're in your shell it's OK, it brings you out. It's good not to be a cabbage.

She also was able to grieve more and to appreciate the humanness and vulnerability of others, including mental health workers she knew were off sick with stress. She gradually became more compassionate to others. She wanted to talk with rather than at people and established a new and caring relationship with a man who proposed marriage: Cheryll accepted an engagement. One day when I said the sessions were coming to a close she left feeling '*severed*': she associated this with a previous time of extreme loneliness in her life. She felt particularly depressed that day. The loss of therapy seems to have had at least a short-term deleterious effect. At the end of her first period of 44 sessions of therapy (which had been all I could offer her in the research) she wrote: Losing John Casson is something I'm not sorting out, this is a situation I'm trapped with, because before I knew him I was not a human being . . . I want John to know he gave me a life, I breathed in his company. She was then able to assert herself with her social worker, who supported the continuation of her therapy with me. At the end of the second period of 112 sessions, she wrote:

> I feel like a human being. I'm a person . . . You were there John, you mattered to me more than anything ever did in my whole entire life. For 3½ years I sought your room hardly letting you speak for myself. I felt I was starting from the beginning all those years lost could suddenly in my own un balanced mind be surfaced and given life and that is what I did in my time with you, for it was no time at all and the hour flew by too fast. You gave me dreams which made sense, previous dreams although significant were unnatural, haunting and displaced. Your room dreams and memories were new and I liked this, and will cherish those memories. I became a person again.

She felt respected and stimulated. She gradually became more creative than destructive during sessions and in her life outside, making things, embroidering, knitting, dancing, painting, writing poetry, making Christmas cards, jam, cake, wine. She was able to establish a new, loving relationship and was experimenting with new roles, attending college, caring for others, doing voluntary work. After therapy was over she courageously achieved one of her ambitions, showing the world, she told me, that people with major mental illnesses could recover and make a contribution to society. After therapy her diagnosis was changed from schizophrenia to personality disorder.

In answer to the research assistant's question, 'What did you find helpful in dramatherapy?' **Cheryll** said: I've enjoyed *being me* more . . . Being able to feel and *be myself* without being pulled up. I tend to judge myself.

Cheryll had stated at her 18th session: I enjoy coming here. The voices are quieter: they are curious about what I do and interested so they listen. They sometimes speak . . . After the 44th session she said that the therapy had been very helpful: though she still heard voices she said they had become soft, not harsh, not making threats. Part of the year the voices disappeared altogether. I was relieved . . . She said she was changing a lot. I don't know me. I've enjoyed being me more. At the 54th session she said that being in therapy had helped her stay in her own home (as opposed to going into a hostel). At the 67th session she said:

you give me motivation, give me interest . . . that she had been able to stay out of hospital and give up suicide as an option. She lost four friends, fellow psychiatric patients, in three months, through suicide and spent time in her sessions grieving them and expressing her own suicidal thoughts. She said that dramatherapy had helped her survive. After 70 sessions **Cheryll** was becoming clearer: not hinting at things but saying straight out *I killed a cat* . . . *I hate* . . . *I am angry*. As she was more able to feel and tolerate emotion so she had less need to overdistance herself and hide in craziness or act out in dangerous, anti-social ways: she became more coherent, more integrated. At the 104th session she said: *I've found me, I'm myself again.*

Chapter 9

The theatre model of the self

Drama's Vitallest Expression is the Common Day . . .

It were infinite enacted
In the Human Heart –
Only Theatre recorded
Owner cannot shut –

(Dickinson, 1975: 363)

In 1863 Emily Dickinson envisaged a theatre within the human heart. Her metaphor implies we can be the actors, audience and owner of this inner theatre. I now explore the history of this idea and its potential as a model that can inform therapeutic practice.

Theatres of memory

In the sixteenth and seventeenth centuries Hermetic Neoplatonist philosophers developed theatres of memory. These theatres used images, myths and visualisations. The architecture was symbolic and full of meaning. Guilio Camillo (who at the time was regarded as one of the most famous men of the sixteenth century) had read the Hermetic texts, including the *Asclepius* (an ancient Egyptian-Greek medical text attributed to the God of healing, see p. 148) and his theatre was based on classical models (Yates, 1966: 156). In Venice (1532) and Paris (1534, it was still standing in 1558) Camillo designed and built memory theatres which incorporated a comprehensive symbolic system to enable people to remember large amounts of material: the theatre contained, according to Camillo, 'all that the mind can conceive and all that is hidden in the soul' (Yates, 1966: 158). It 'represented a new Renaissance plan of the psyche'. The theatre reflected 'the divine macrocosm in the microcosm of his divine *mens*' (Yates, 1966: 172). The theatre not only contained, but also provided the distance for the observer to appreciate the whole, a perspective that 'gives us true wisdom' (Camillo, quoted by Spence, 1985: 20).

In seventeenth-century England John Willis (1618) and Thomas Fludd (1619) also developed theatres of memory. Whereas Camillo actually built his theatres,

Willis and Fludd invited people to visualise the memory theatre in their imagi-nation. Fludd's was influenced by the design of Shakespeare's Globe Theatre (Yates, 1966: 342–367).

It was in the Globe that Shakespeare himself played the role of the ghost in Hamlet. The ghost demands to be remembered and Hamlet uses the play within the play to prompt Claudius' guilty memory, because of his experience that:

> guilty creature sitting at a play,
> Have by the very cunning of the scene
> Been struck so to the soul, that presently
> They have proclaimed their malefactions.
> (*Hamlet*, Act II, Sc. 2)

Cox (1992: 141) reported on the way Shakespeare's plays prompted memory in the special hospitals for offender patients: one said of watching *Hamlet* in Broadmoor, 'the knife scene reminded me of an incident when I threatened my ex-girlfriend, and it brought home to me the fear she felt.'

Another patient told the actor:

> When you picked up that skull it really got to me; hit me in the stomach; I've killed a person and I've done a lot of work on how the relatives must feel . . . but it never crossed my mind until now that there is a corpse some-where of the person I killed. I have never thought about the corpse before.
> (Cox, 1992: 148–149)

Theatre then stimulates memory: *Living Memory* is a theatre that performs exclusively to elderly people. Paul Sneddon, the director, said: 'The work is a stimulus to long-term memory. It also enables people to establish their own identity, which has often been taken away from them . . . It's also a good way of people getting to know each other. They feel they have some common ground' (*Guardian*, 8 June 1993; Casson, 1997c).

Dramatherapy, psychodrama and playback theatre can be seen as theatres of memory wherein past scenes are revisited for healing purposes. Harrow (1952: 154) quoted a patient as saying that one result of psychodrama was: 'My memory has been revived. I remember lots of things now.' I have found similarly that drama can stimulate memory. For example in a psychodrama **Harry** replayed a scene from his youth and said: It brought a good piece of memory back!

Roger said of dramatherapy: the group brought back memories.

A woman at a playback theatre performance said: 'I was absolutely amazed at the instant improvisation. It made good therapy too, because to see what was, for me, a traumatic event re-enacted, helped me to exorcise the ghosts that still haunt me' (Casson, 1998b: 16). In the theatre of memory ghostly images from the past may return to haunt our dreams.

The theatre of dreams

Healing through dreams is of course an ancient practice. At the beginning of the Christian era people suffering from ill health went to Asclepius' temple: they slept there, hoping for a healing dream in which Asclepius would appear to diagnose and treat their ailment. Their dreams were interpreted the next morning by the priests and healing actions prescribed.

In 1803, Reil, who proposed therapeutic theatres in psychiatric hospitals (see Chapter 4), connected the phenomenon of dissociated personalities with normal dreams:

> The actors appear, the roles are distributed; of these, the dreamer takes only one that he connects with his own personality. All the other actors are to him as foreign as strangers, although they and all their actions are the creation of the dreamer's own fantasy. One hears of people speaking in foreign languages, admires the talent of a great orator, is astounded by the profound wisdom of a teacher who explains to us things of which we do not remember ever having heard.
>
> (Ellenberger, 1994: 146–147)

It was this inner theatre Reil proposed to externalise on a therapeutic stage. Fechner (*c*.1850)

> found the difference between the waking state and the sleeping state was not mainly a difference in the intensity of a certain mental function. It was as if the same mental activities were displayed alternatively on different theatre stages or scenes (a remark that was the starting point of Freud's topographical concept of the mind).
>
> (Ellenberger, 1994: 313)

Evreinoff (1927: 54–55) quoted Freud: 'The most abstract thought is dramatised in the dream without the participation of our conscious self . . . it becomes the aim of the dream to provide the connecting links and to make thus possible the presentation of a unified dramatic whole.'

Evreinoff comments:

> The famous psychologist has here given us a lucid and penetrating picture of the very essence of our subconscious self, and has proved that this self is pre-eminently dramatic and theatrical in its mysterious activity. Is this strange author of dreams so masterfully described by him not a real playwright and stage manager? The dream is a drama of our invention. It is the monodramatic theatre in which one sees oneself in an imaginary reality.
>
> (Evreinoff, 1927: 55)

This statement echoes Moreno's concept of surplus reality and psychodrama. Jung (1974: 52) stated: 'a dream is a theatre in which the dreamer is himself the scene, the player, the prompter, the producer, the author, the public, and the critic.'

Landy (1986: 157) also used this metaphor: 'the dreamworld can be seen as a stage containing sets, props, costumes, colors, and characters.' Jennings agreed: 'we dream in dramatic form. Our dreams are like miniature private theatres where we are either actor or observer' (Jennings and Minde, 1995: 23).

Dramatherapy and psychodrama can be seen as dreaming while awake: a kind of lucid dreaming in which the dreamer is in control and can alter the dream at will (see Casson, 1999b). This is in contrast to psychosis which can be seen as being trapped in a waking nightmare, unable to tell the difference between dream and reality, nor in control of one's fantasy or real, external life (Jennings, 1998: 119). Esquirol (1832) characterised people who hallucinate as 'dreamers while they are awake' (Slade and Bentall, 1988: 8).

The psychoanalytic theatre

Freud based psychoanalysis on the interpretation of dreams and free association. Anna O., Breuer's famous patient at the end of the nineteenth century, who played such an important role in the beginning of psychoanalysis, referred to her free associations during therapy as her 'private theatre' (Jennings and Minde, 1995: 23). Despite Freud's denial of the value of action in therapy he often referred to theatre, using Oedipus as a central myth. McDougall has written psychoanalytic texts on *Theatres of the Mind* (1986) and *Theatres of the Body* (1989). The analyst is the audience for the drama on the couch. Freud however also realised there was another hidden audience member:

> Even in a state so far removed from the reality of the external world as one of hallucinatory confusion, one learns from patients after their recovery that at the time in some corner of their mind (as they put it) there was a normal person hidden, who like a detached spectator, watched the hubbub of illusion go past him.
>
> (Eigen, 1993: 10)

The theatre for oneself

Evreinoff, prophet of theatre as therapy (see Chapter 5), had published his *The Theatre for Oneself* in 1915–1917 in Russia (Casson, 1999a). This was a private theatre, part visualisation, part role play, in which players could imagine, either in the privacy of their own home, in the street or indeed anywhere, other identities and scenarios than those they normally played in life.

> People will play themselves, and for themselves, needing neither actors nor spectators . . . Every artist of 'the theatre for oneself' must be his own

playwright. It is exactly in the free improvisation that lies one of the greatest attractions of this institution.

(Evreinoff, 1927: 256, 195)

This is akin to Moreno's concept of psychodrama and surplus reality (though Moreno's method included an audience). Such solipsistic activity is not without its dangers and in terms of therapy such play is perhaps best carried out in the container of the therapeutic space with the supportive witness of the therapist. Dramatherapy and psychodrama are the heirs to Evreinoff's idea.

Moreno's theatre of the self

Moreno proposed an interpersonal model of the self in his interrelated social, cultural and role atoms (Casson, 2001b). These show that the self is not confined to the body but extends out into the environment and especially into our relationships. These relationships are affected by role and culture. The survival and enrichment of the self depends on the number and quality of these relationships. Moreno's atoms are valuable tools in assessment and treatment. The atoms are described by plotting symbols of interpersonal and intrapsychic relationships within three concentric circles: the inner circle being the place for the most intimate relationships, the outer circles being for progressively more distant relationships. The area beyond the third circle is for those relationships that are in the past or deceased (see Figure 1).

Moreno's design for his therapeutic theatre was likewise three concentric circles: a mandala (see Figure 2, overleaf).

The pattern of the mandala occurs in the circle of the therapy group and is often created in a psychodrama group: a circle and a centre. Such a ritual structure is an archetype of wholeness, relating the parts to the whole, the individual to the group. Jung (1972: 240) saw the mandala as a symbol of the self.

Jennings' theatre model of the mind

Jennings (1996) proposed a theatre model of the mind. She argued that the

> infant is born already dramatised and that the dramatic relationship has been established in utero. Notice how pregnant women talk to their unborn children and answer on their behalf. The child becomes a confidant and friend as well as a little monster when overactive, keeping its mother awake. The dramatised relationship continues after birth and is gradually modified as the child increases in autonomy.

(Jennings, 1996: 206)

In Jennings' view the child develops through cycles of activity enabling him/her to know and gain control of the *body*, play *projectively* with objects in the world

SOCIAL ATOM

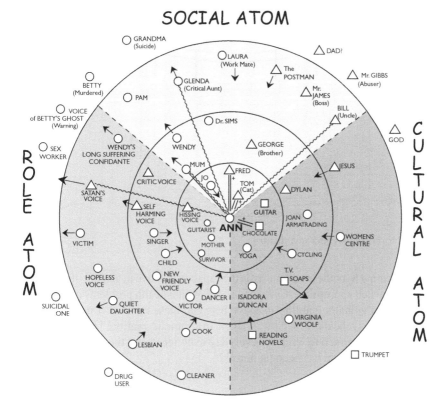

Normally shown individually in three separate concentric circle diagrams these atoms are presented simultaneously here to allow comparison. Ann is fictional. Voices are plotted as roles.

Notation Key:

    ～～ = angry/hostile/negative relationships
    ≈≈ = ambivalent relationship
    ± = positive relationship
    → = arrow pointed inwards = attraction and/or wish to draw closer
    ← = arrow pointed outwards = rejection and/or need for distance

Figure 1 The social/cultural/role atom

and to assume *roles*. Her developmental paradigm of *embodiment-projection-role* (EPR) provides dramatherapists with a schema for their work. She also noticed that in this process

> the child becomes increasingly able to distinguish between everyday reality
> and dramatic reality (otherwise referred to as the reality of play or the reality
> of the imagination). Without dramatic reality we would not be able to imagine
> how something could be in the future. The dramatic imagination is essential

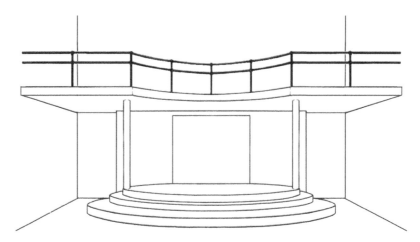

Figure 2 Moreno's psychodrama theatre

for forming hypotheses. Maturity is the capacity to move in and out of dramatic reality when appropriate. Certain kinds of mental health problems can be seen as an individual's inability to move between these realities. I maintain that when in psychosis, a person is stuck in dramatic reality. The distinction between the concrete world of everyday experience and the symbolic world of the imagination has become blurred.

(Jennings, 1996: 206–207)

Jennings' model has clear implications for clinical work; to enable clients to move in and out of differing realities, develop flexibility and the observer (audience) ego: to play and so recapitulate developmental processes for healing purposes. If reality can have multiple aspects, perhaps the self in response has multiple facets?

Landy's role model of the self

Landy questioned the idea of a unitary self:

In a nuclear age, all things once considered indivisible are now splittable. Not only have we split the atom, but also families through divorce and abandonment . . . nations through holy and civil wars . . . In splitting the self, one enters a new mythological system – one that is not only polytheistic, but also paradoxical . . . the self is dead, at least in its monolithic version.

(Landy, 1993: 21–22)

Landy wondered about a self without a centre: 'Peel away the layers of the onion and there is nothing there.' An empty stage? He proposed a role model of the self. He referred back to James (1890/1950):

From this there results what practically is a division of the man into several selves; and this may be a discordant splitting, as where one is afraid to let one set of his acquaintances know him as he is elsewhere; or it may be a perfectly harmonious division of labour, as where one tender to his children is stern to the soldiers or prisoners under his control.

(Landy, 1993: 20–21)

Hillman (1983) agreed and suggested that therapy aim not for integration of the personality but for an acceptance of our multiplicity:

Personality is imaginatively conceived as a living and peopled drama in which the subject 'I' takes part but is neither the sole author, nor director, nor always the main character. Sometimes he or she is not even on the stage.

(Hillman, 1983: 53)

The roles we play, the scripts we play by, the stories we re-enact, our style of acting, display our character, our public persona (mask): the way others experience us as a person. But there may be other parts of the self that are hidden behind the mask or backstage. As **Cheryll** said: Behind the scenes are voices.

The theatre model of the self that I now propose contains this multiplicity.

The theatre model of the self

Hyppolite Taine (1828–1893), a French philosopher, compared the mind to a theatre (Baars, 1997: 52). In 1937 Murphy titled his article about psychodrama: 'The Mind is a Stage'. He described how Moreno invited people to play fantasy roles to rebalance their personality, develop their spontaneous creativity and experience catharsis. Mitchell (1987: 275) also used this image of 'the stage of our minds'.

Ryle (1990: 149) criticised the Cartesian dogma of the mind–body split and the 'ghost in the machine' doctrine to explain mental life. He used the metaphor of the mind as a theatre in which consciousness and introspection discovered scenes. Dennett (1991) investigating the mind–brain problem developed 'the idea of a Cartesian "theatre", located in the pineal gland, the point at which the mind and body interact, in which the mind sits like an audience observing that which the senses portray of the external world' (Thomas, 1997: 165). Baars (1997: 7) also used a theatre metaphor to describe the brain, declaring that 'all our unified models of mental functioning today are theatre metaphors.' Greenfield (2002) basing her ideas on Baars and referring back to Camillo's theatre of memory, picked up this metaphor:

the theatre provides an appealing framework for describing brain function. The stage, for example, is small and limited, just like a moment of conscious experience. We can press the comparison further: behind the stage, the

> conscious experience, is a vast area of offstage activities, both past and present, that sets the context that will give the momentary experience a particular quality . . . The attention needed at any one moment can be likened to a spotlight.
>
> (Greenfield, 2002: 26)

There is then a continuum between brain, mind and self, rather like that between backstage, stage and the theatre as a whole.

The theatre model does not posit a singular, but rather a multifaceted self.

> According to G. H. Mead (1934) and William James (1890) . . . the self is comprised of an 'I' and a 'me'. The 'I' is an objective, generalised set of permanent attributes, and the 'me' is a subjective, more specific set of behaviours determined by social circumstances.
>
> (Landy, 1993: 20)

Moreno's seminal work *Who Shall Survive*, in which he explored his role theory, was published the same year (1934) as Mead's role theory in *Mind, Self and Society*. Moreno and Lacan both posited a mirror stage of development (Casson, 1998b). In a mirror the 'I' observes 'me' (I observe myself); I am audience of my own performance; the subject 'I' and the object 'me': 'I' instructs 'me' (I tell myself what to do, direct myself). Eigen (1993: 237) stated: 'The mirror or imaginary I (ego, moi) lives as an actor (performer) with an eye to the audience, the other . . . As both actor and audience, the ego is other to itself.' Moreover, as Mead (1934: 142) put it, 'We divide ourselves up in all sorts of different selves with reference to our acquaintances . . . There are all sorts of different selves answering to different social relations.' James (1890/1950, vol. 1: 24) took a similar view: 'a man has as many social selves as there are individuals who recognise him and carry an image of him in their mind.' This accords with Moreno's social atom. 'I' and 'me' are but two aspects of self and identity: both connected to ego. Freud posited the ego, superego and id; Jung the archetypes. The theatre model can accommodate all these 'I's and 'me's, roles, subpersonalities, subselves and more (see also Rowan, 1991, 1993). We are multiple rather than singular creatures. In 1894 Janet stated that there were 'crowds of things which operate within ourselves without our will' (Ellenberger, 1994: 370).

Armstrong-Perlman (1995: 94) used the theatre metaphor in describing how a child internalises bad object relations: 'Internalisation and splitting do not after all eliminate the bad aspects of the real object . . . They just transfer them to an internal theatre.' Winn (1994) also used the theatre metaphor for the intrapsychic world:

> If we recognise that in each of us there are a number of sub-personalities or different facets, then our inner world can be thought of as a stage on which various conflicts, arguments and dialogues are carried out.
>
> (Winn, 1994: 85)

Radmall (1995) suggested that the self can be regarded as a stage: the space that expands as more roles are played upon it.

> The inner stage of a client may be equated with the concept of the self. It may be an appropriate metaphor for self, as self appears to be not so much a single entity but rather an arena wherein interaction between different components takes place.
>
> (Radmall, 1995: 14)

The stage is a place where roles are played. Moreno (1993: 47) stated that: 'Roles do not emerge from the self, but the self may emerge from roles.'

Roles and relationships from the real external world of the other become aspects of the self, internalised and acted out upon an inner stage as we mentally rehearse scenes. Parts of self may be encapsulated and dramatised in voices and in dreams. Parts of self may also, through projective identification, be acted out on the interpersonal stage, when we put others into role as significant parts of ourselves, transferring to the other what is intolerable to ourselves. Seth-Smith (1997: 98) described the image in art therapy as a container for such material. The image or role in drama can likewise be a container, enabling the person to temporarily display or inhabit aspects of the self that might otherwise be split off. We may also project onto others ideal or unfulfilled aspect of ourselves: in psychodrama these aspects of ourselves can be taken on by auxiliaries and witnessed within the theatre of the self. Thus the theatre model enables either a reintegration of disowned parts of the self, or for these disowned aspects to be held at a safe distance, acknowledged, witnessed and contained.

The theatre then can be a metaphor for the self: by self I mean the whole human being (mind, body, spirit), by theatre I mean a theatre building or space. The space may be an internal space or a space between people. The theatre model of the self acknowledges that we perform in relation to the other. An empty theatre is a pretty depressing place: we need a witnessing audience even if it is only another part of ourselves, the observer ego. When there is no audience the theatre dies. This is in accord with Moreno's recognition that poverty in the social atom is an indicator of a danger to survival, and is a reason for bringing isolated people together: to offer them the support and validation of an audience. The theatre model of the self provides us with an image of the human being as both private and public. In psychosis the theatre is often too private, leaving the person in an impoverished, isolated world, lacking an audience. The therapist then may be the first member of the audience who can tolerate the strange world that the psychotic person has endeavoured to keep private for fear of rejection or judgement. Theatre with its surreal, magical elements, is an appropriate container for what others may reject as crazy. How might we understand what occurs in this theatre?

The explicit and the implicit drama

The theatre model allows for paradoxes, deus ex machina surprises: it does not reduce human beings to pathology but allows them their full glory and wealth: a mixture of fantasy and reality. It illuminates two dramas: the *explicit* drama and the *implicit* drama. The explicit drama is the one declared on the bill boards outside: I am in the role of . . . this performance is about . . . The implicit drama is the one behind the scenes that the audience may not see. Charlie Chaplin's explicit dramas were hugely popular but it does not take much to see through to the implicit dramas about the abandoned child whose mother was mentally ill: the cheery laughter is suffused with a tragic grief, the child in need of rescue and relief. His films are not thereby reduced: the explicit dramas were successful and meaningful. There were also multiple implicit dramas: his relationships with young actresses, his financial success, his artistic creativity and power, his social and political satires.

In dramatherapy and psychodrama the explicit drama carries the implicit therapeutic drama, just as metaphor carries meaning (see Chapter 7). For example in a psychodrama the protagonist was tense, could not breathe freely and felt he was wearing a metal shirt that kept him restrained. I role reversed him with the shirt. I asked a member of the group to take the protagonist's role and had the protagonist stand behind this person and embrace him as the shirt, tightly holding the auxiliary's chest. The beauty of such a role reversal is that it both reproduces the experience the protagonist speaks of, externalising it so that it can be worked with, exaggerating and intensifying it so it can be experienced more fully and at the same time produces exactly what the protagonist said he was not able to do – namely get close to some one. The *explicit* drama here is that he was being a metal shirt; the *implicit* drama is that he was embracing another group member. After he had spoken as the shirt and clarified the nature, purpose and script of such body armour, I role reversed the protagonist back into his own role to experience such tension and containment. The implicit drama however continued, now the protagonist was being hugged by another person. Having the body armour externalised and played by another person the protagonist could now be vulnerable, relax and let go of tension and be held, contained by another. The *explicit* metaphor carries the *implicit* therapeutic process. The theatrical metaphor of the symbolic costume contained the emotional material at sufficient distance to be worked through. Had I asked the protagonist to allow himself to be hugged or invited him to hug other men he would not have been able to do so. Here the container was a costume. In another drama the container was a cage in which there was a monstrous demon: the protagonist's rage and violence. To set the scene I invited the protagonist to role reverse with the cage, to own the container and reveal the purpose, nature and history of this structure. Thus playing the role of an item in the scenery may provide the person with the necessary distance and opportunity for catharsis, as when a protagonist role reversed with the gas fire in her abusers' house and promptly blew up (Casson, 1998a: 77)! The explicit drama may seem crazy but the implicit drama, during which the isolated client is joining and playing with the group and the therapist, carries the person out of isolation into relationship.

The theatre model in therapeutic practice

How is this theatre metaphor useful to therapists? The metaphor enriches: some will have poor theatres but, like Grotowski (1968), produce powerful, meaningful theatre. The theatre model can inform the clinical decisions of the dramatherapist: does the person need to change roles, is s/he role bound? Is there a need for a change of scenery? What costume is s/he wearing? If s/he were to be director of this scene how would s/he change it? At any one time the theatre model might suggest appropriate ways of working. Breathing may relax and ground the person in the here and now. Movement in the space offers the opportunity to express and release tension. Working with props enables projective, expressive work and empowers, extending movement and stimulating creativity. Toy theatre enhances the observer ego. If you play the victim role too often what other role might be helpful: what is it like to be the rescuer or a villain? How can we change the story? What does the critic say? What script could the writer now create: do I, as my own playwright, rely on outdated scripts written by previous generations or compose my own lines?

A person who is flooded by psychotic experiences needs clear boundaries, sufficient distance and a container for what would otherwise be overwhelming. The theatre model provides such a container.

The method

The method may use visualisation, drawing, commercially available or specially created toy theatres, movement and role enactment. While what follows is a scheme, any part of the model may be introduced according to a client's need at a particular time.

Visualising the theatre architecture

Theatre has a stage and the public are let in to see the show (*theatron* being Greek for 'a place of seeing'). There is also a backstage area into which only some are allowed. There are spaces under and up above the stage where few, if any, are permitted. The model then incorporates various limits and permeable boundaries. There are boundaries between on stage and off stage, the actor and the audience. The body of the theatre can be large and magnificent or poor and neglected. The show in the former may be dull and boring and in the latter poetic and full of spirit. The front of house may be gilded, the backstage dilapidated. The building however has a history and architects who more or less planned it. The culture and our ancestors were involved in the design and development.

A useful question then might be, 'What is the history, what are the traditions of this theatre?'

Invite the client to relax, possibly conducting a guided relaxation when the person is comfortable lying down or alternatively breathing and moving about in the space. Invite them to imagine/visualise a theatre: what sort of space is this? Is it an outdoor theatre or a building you go into? Look at the structure, the spaces: as you enter what do you notice?

Note: significant material can emerge from considering the place, architecture, state of the theatre, facade, the posters and name of the theatre, the foyer, box office, front of house, even before we enter the auditorium. Once inside we look at the audience space, the stage or explore the backstage. A plan or drawing of the theatre can elicit further material. A physical model can be built either in miniature or with furniture in the room.

What are the roles?

Every part of the theatre has different roles implicit in it. The person can be the actor, director, front of house manager, ticket and programme seller, dresser, prompt, critic, playwright or designer. The lighting technician may cast light upon the stage or throw all into darkness. Creating and playing these roles offers opportunities for self exploration, expression and expansion. Who then is coming to the theatre: who is the audience for the play? Chantal was a shy woman with learning disabilities. She chose to be the ice-cream seller when the group performed their show: this role enabled her to interact with the audience.

What is the stage curtain like?

Bringing the focus now onto the stage the therapist invites the client to choose the colour of the curtain and decide whether to open it. In effect the person is in charge of when this revelatory act occurs. What do the actors behind the curtain feel before it is raised? What is the stage manager doing?

What is the scenery in this first act?

Once the curtain is raised the therapist asks what the scenery shows. This may be drawn or painted in the miniature theatre. I have already suggested role reversing with the scenery or embodying metaphors inherent in the scenery (Casson, 1998a: 75). Does the client want to change the scenery? What colour is the lighting? Is the stage empty? What is the stage set, props, objects, furniture? What is missing? What is the next scene?

Conrad visualised an empty stage with a set of a cold, lonely city. On stage a figure struggled up an incline down which rubbish poured, hoping for happiness at the top. The actor enjoyed the physical struggle and then went to the greenroom, backstage, to relax. Thinking about this image he realised that happiness was always somewhere else when he was young: that his childhood in two different countries meant that, when unhappy, he looked back nostalgically to the other country. He also realised he needed time to relax rather than struggle all the time.

Who is on stage?

Now we look, from the audience space, at who is on stage. Are there puppets, masked actors, characters in costume? How are they behaving? This is in effect a projective technique that may eventually lead to the client embodying the projected roles. For example in exploring the aftermath of an abortion Claire imagined seeing the scene on a film screen. This gave her the necessary distance from the event to feel safe and not be overwhelmed by her distress. She later stepped into the action in the role of an advocate for women undergoing this procedure and confronted the doctor for his insensitivity, asserting her needs and expressing her anger.

What is the action?

What story is told? What is the script? What do the actors do? We may now actually improvise scenes, using, if in individual therapy Johnson's (1992) Transformations, Landy's (1993) Role method or Mitchell's (1996) Ritual of Individual Therapy.

The theatre of the self includes working with the body: actors use their bodies to express character, emotion and through non-verbal communication convey meaning (Cox, 1978a; Pisk, 1990). The body is a container of the tensions that, as Reich (1980) recognised, express the psychological life history of the person or symbolise the defence structure created by the person to contain and manage their pain. Dramatherapists and psychodramatists work with the body encouraging breathing, movement, expression, play. The body is clothed in a costume that may express significant material. Carol was somewhat stuck: for three sessions we had gone over her fears about going back to work. I had wondered if she needed me to hear a deep reservoir of fear that had been unexpressed over many years, dating back to when she was an abandoned and abused child. I wondered where she might find a source of power. I noticed she was wearing a leopard skin patterned blouse and asked her, 'If there were a leopard in the office what would it do to the boss?'

'Go for his balls and shake him,' Carol replied, laughing. We continued this fantasy as Carol embodied the leopard and accessed more of her anger at the pain she had been caused by those with power over her in the past. Later we visualised the leopard under her desk at work as a source of female ferocity which, when threatened, could remind her of her power. She went back to work, empowered by this image.

In group therapy we may discuss scenes emerging in people's imaginations, choose to enact one or create a compilation (see Chapters 10 and 12). The group enactment implicitly involves the social skills of sharing, co-operation, give and take. If this is a rehearsal what does the director say s/he wants to change? If this is a performance what happens?

What is going on backstage?

Who is the dresser? What gossip is there in the greenroom? What make-up is the actor applying? Is there a theatre cat or a ghost? Who brings flowers to the stage door? What are the 'voices off' saying?

Gloria felt she was backstage with an audience out there waiting: she had withdrawn from the world and she needed to get back on stage. We explored ways that she could master her feelings rather than be overwhelmed by them. We used (1) being aware of the feeling, (2) breathing, (3) expressing it by talking, (4) colour and imagery: visualisations of a theatre and of painting. These revealed her fear of dark spaces, voids, loss of self and feelings 'blackmailing her' – hiding in the darkness – fearful of being seen. When a male figure came into the spotlight he was powerful and spoke his truth, faced reality. **Gloria** benefited from these creative visualisations. They empowered her and enabled her to disclose further material about the rape, at a safe distance.

What cannot be shown on stage may haunt the theatre so that, as in *Six Characters in Search of an Author* (Pirandello, 1994) the apparent confusion on stage speaks of an invisible, offstage, trauma.

After the performance

Who is in the audience? What does the audience feel, think, say in the interval? What changes do they want? What does the critic say/write? What is the head-line of the critic's notice? Reflecting on the experience it may be useful to identify who has the power in the theatre. Nick could not cope with the strong emotion in the group. He withdrew to the audience chairs and was able from there to tolerate being present while feelings were expressed. Later he spoke of his own feelings.

Closure

To end the session we go back to the theatre: we may rehearse the curtain calls, then finally bring down the curtain and leave the auditorium. At the end of a long-term group this theatre ritual enabled the members to celebrate what they had achieved and gave each person a moment in the spotlight.

As people leave the theatre what do they feel? What do they think as they emerge into the light of day? Reflecting on the experience is a normal and essential part of a visit to the theatre. The therapist then invites the person to speak of the next day, the week ahead, their real responsibilities, possible activities, ways the person can cope and enjoy, care for themselves during the week before the next session. This transition from dramatic reality to everyday, social reality is important before the person leaves the session.

Adapting the theatre model

It may be objected that for many people the theatre is not a relevant cultural form. The theatre model is a template metaphor. It is possible to adapt this idea to other cultural forms such as film (see the example of Claire on p. 159), to computers (which offer an infinite series of levels and virtual realities: Edwards (1993) has already shown the possibility of using a computer metaphor) and TV. Each of these offer a container with multiple roles and realities. Video can also be used as a containing method which provides a group with a mirror and an observing ego (see Chapter 10; Pettiti, 1989). The model must be fitted to the client's needs, not the client to the model: it may be useful in just one session or may form the basis of a period of work. It may be used in individual or group work.

Application to therapeutic work with people who hear voices

The theatre model of the self provides the therapist with a normalising model that can contain psychotic experiences without having to regard these as manifestations of 'illness'. The Morenean model of madness (see Chapter 3; Moreno and Moreno, 1984) sees madness as a manifestation of inadequately channelled spontaneity and creativity and promotes the acting out of delusions and hallucinations in order to satisfy act hungers, gain insight, experience catharsis and connect the protagonist with a social reality suitably adapted to his/her needs. The theatre model of the self is in harmony with this and normalises voices and visions as part of human and theatrical experience for millennia. The theatre model accepts that devils and spirits will appear, offstage voices be heard and surreal scenes be impressive even if their meaning is not apparent. Perry (1974) pointed out that many people struggling with psychotic experiences actually feel they are participating in some form of drama or ritual performance. One benefit of a therapeutic method which uses a theatre metaphor is that 'off stage' figures such as 'deities on Alpha Centauri' can be brought on stage or at least within the therapy room, represented and contained instead of being split off. Voices and psychotic experiences can be acknowledged and worked with, contained by the theatre metaphor or literally contained in a toy theatre, mask or puppet. They may then be held at sufficient distance to be observed, and if not comprehended at least related to and contained.

The theatre model of the self incorporates ideas of distance, boundaries and role. The audience (when an intrapsychic role, the observer ego; when interpersonal, other people) is at a safe distance. The model provides dramatherapists and psychodramatists with a containing metaphor for the work, combining embodiment, projection and role play in an intrapsychic and interpersonal space which expands the sense of self and empowers the person.

Chapter 10

Group dramatherapy

While some people who hear voices will choose individual therapy for the feeling of safety, nurture and privacy it offers, group therapy can be empowering and helpful. Furthermore, Ellwood warns:

> One-to-one therapy could be seen as potentially dangerous for a very damaged person, for whom the most threatening thing in the world would be to relate to one other human being, who would represent the dreaded other into whom all their worst fears and most hated aspects of themselves would be projected. Thus one-to-one therapy would be likely to bring out all their resistances in a very extreme way, which could result in the therapy being broken off and destroyed.

> (Ellwood, 1995: 5)

In group therapy such intensity is diluted to more manageable levels as different people carry different projections for the person struggling with psychotic experiences. Group therapy may also be more real and offer shared compassion and nurture from other voice hearers.

Dave: enjoyed being in a group of oddballs – marvellous characters, enjoyed the humour and relationships . . . There is a lot to be said positively for group therapy (even though it can be publicly painful) which I didn't realise at first when I was fixed with the idea only 1 to 1 sessions were helpful.

However, it may also be a place where hostility is expressed. For some who have withdrawn from social contact group therapy may seem too threatening and they can use a period of individual therapy to establish a safe, nurturing relationship with the therapist which later enables them to make positive relationships with others in a group. In my research, participants were more likely to attend individual therapy than group therapy (which seems to belie Ellwood's concern) and a period of individual therapy helped participants prepare for group work. People must be offered a choice.

Preparation for group

In the penultimate individual assessment session before joining a group we might use Guatemalan worry dolls, chairs or other objects to represent the other unknown members of the group the client is about to join. This will enable an exploration of the fears and fantasies the person might have about the group, what they might project onto the unknown, prospective members. The client may then role reverse with one of these group members and say how they feel: thus the client realises that the others may also be fearful and not hostile. Questions can be answered and necessary information provided to reduce exaggerated fears.

Group size

It seems that a group of six is an optimal size; however, given non-attendance it may be wise to have a group of eight so that there will be between four and eight attending: useful work can be done in a small group as **Sheila** reveals:

> I used to be in a group . . . but it was a big group and I found it difficult to talk in: this group is only four of us, it was six to start with, and I find it easier to talk in. In the other group we were asked questions and asked to bring our views forward but I always felt a bit worthless. I used to get upset when I came away because I used to think, 'Well I didn't get anything out of that group today.'

From this statement it seems that structured, playful activities facilitate group cohesion and functioning more than discussion alone. However, when a group drops to below four it can be disappointing, even demoralising, for those who do attend. People may need support to get to a group: maximising attendance is therapeutic not only for the individual who has difficulty attending but also for other members of the group.

Creating a safe space

In the first session I invite people to create a safe, personal space in the room using chairs, cloth, sticks, cushions and other equipment. This is further to enable them to 'own' the space. Many professional spaces are 'owned' by the professionals: clients enter these spaces and sit where they are indicated: they may not be given a choice. A dramatherapist is able to offer the person the opportunity to sit on the floor, on cushions, or under a table if they prefer: to have their own space. For people to choose where to sit, to get up and walk around, to lie on the floor, to move chairs, to take up space, is empowering: this gives people a greater sense of control of the environment, a sense of agency rather than passivity. **Dave** said that creating his own space was particularly helpful. **Jimmy** reflected that creating the safe space made it safe to play:

we made a private space in the room, decorated it towards the way we felt. It was helpful because it was nice to see what other people did. It showed what sort of people we were. I really enjoyed that . . . It's safe to do it there. Everything is behind closed doors, there's safety there: it's a bit like exposing oneself as a fool, but it's safe to do so . . .

The audience chairs

To ensure a feeling of safety in therapy sessions I place two rows of chairs across a corner or at one side of the room (I also use this technique in individual work with people who dissociate). These I name the 'audience chairs'. I explain that as this is drama we need an audience and if sometimes people don't want to take part in things or need to withdraw, they can sit in these chairs. If they sit in the front row they are indicating they need to sit out but are willing for group members to engage with them and draw them back into the session. If they sit on the back row it means that they want to be left alone. In this case only I, as therapist, might visit them and check out how they are feeling. Other group members will respect this withdrawal and wait until the person chooses to rejoin the group. On several occasions using the audience chairs has enabled people to stay in the room rather than leave because they felt overwhelmed.

Anton: I withdrew (to the audience chairs) *to protect myself from you. I had a rush of thoughts, things going too fast. That was helpful to withdraw to the audience chairs and be in control.*

Even when group members did not use these chairs they found the fact they were available helpful.

Sheila: *The chairs were put in one corner: where we could just observe if we wanted to do or if we sat further back we were left alone. We had that choice, which I found quite helpful. I didn't actually do that: I didn't have the courage to do it, but I knew it was there. It was always there in the back of my mind that if I wanted to escape I could do from whatever were going on . . .*

From this place the observer ego is still engaged and the person need not flee or dissociate. I have written elsewhere of how people can gain therapeutic benefit from being in the audience (Casson, 1997c). The audience chairs enable people to distance themselves, if they need to, from the group. During an early group session we can all sit in these chairs to imagine what 'the play' will be like, thus inhabiting the audience space. Such control, through which people can own the space and achieve the distance they need, results in the space becoming safe and the therapy not being overwhelming: people have some power and choice. The audience chairs represent a safe place and symbolise the right to say 'No/Stop' or withdraw. When someone uses the audience space I praise them and eventually, when they are ready, I ask what they witnessed from that place.

Group agreement

Group members negotiate their own agreements in the first three sessions: usually agreements include commitments to respecting each other's confidentiality and to no violence to another member of the group. These agreements can be made into a contract, signed by all and each member given their own copy.

Group dramatherapy method: theory into practice

In describing my practice I will use Jennings' (1990) developmental model of dramatherapy of embodiment, projection and role.

Working with/through the body: embodiment play

Empowerment cannot only be a mental concept but must be experienced in the body: power and control must be felt in the body and expressed through physical behaviour. For people who are survivors of abuse and who have psychotic experiences this issue of control is often experienced in the body: a sense of someone/something having control of the body. Dramatherapy, in using physical activities, can foster a greater sense of physical self-control.

To achieve a greater sense of control in the body, in the here and now, it is useful to practise breathing, walking, running, rolling, jumping, movement and mirroring exercises, Tai Chi, dance, physical games, playing with a parachute or other objects such as sticks. Many activities can be used as warm-ups for the group. Warm-ups can stimulate the body, promote relaxation, interaction and thereby relationships, develop spontaneity and creativity. In groups we have used trust walks; practised relaxation; given each other back massages; played catch with balls and bean bags; created a web of string (by one person throwing the ball to another across the circle while retaining the end of the string) to show the connections between people; created rituals; worked with props and objects such as hoops, cloth, ribbon sticks. These activities stimulate, engaging people in co-operative action and promote breathing, fun, relaxation.

After control of action in space and role play, embodiment play was judged the next most helpful aspect of dramatherapy according to the research participants. Dramatherapy acknowledges the connections between mind and body and engages the whole person in action. Jones considered:

> the body as a means to express, discover and develop the self . . . The body is often described as the primary means by which communication occurs between *self and other*. This is through gesture, expression and voice.
>
> (Jones, 1996: 152, added emphasis)

Working with the body will therefore consolidate the sense of self.

Dillon: Medication makes it more difficult to express self – you become more cerebral – a talking head . . . It's useful that dramatherapy involves movement of the body.

Movement increases breathing, reduces tension, promotes relaxation and clearer thinking. Through physical action the emotional energy held in the body's muscular tension can be released and people gain a sense of power and control.

Jimmy: The group I enjoyed simply because it alleviated the tension within my body which is a source of anxiety: it relaxed me.

Watkins (1998: 210) differentiated between voices resultant from a high level of arousal, when the voice hearer may benefit from physical activities that promote calm and relaxation, and a low level of arousal, when the voice can be reduced by physical exercise. Giving people a choice as to which physical activity matches their need is therefore important and the audience chairs give permission for someone to withdraw from an activity that is not appropriate.

Physical action can enable people safely to express their hostility to the world: the men's group enjoyed kicking the world (an inflatable globe); kicking and hitting, with padded sticks, cushions, boxes, soft balls.

Tom (kicking ball): Lets your tensions out . . .

Dillon (beating a pile of cushions with a stick): I feel cleaner, got rid of some of the rubbish and can see/think clearer.

Active relaxation

Some survivors of abuse cannot relax when lying down: they can however find gentle movement relaxing. Tai Chi, the Chinese slow motion movement and breathing exercise and martial art, provides a structured discipline and practice that can channel aggressive feelings away from violence towards a sense of power in co-operation with others. **Roger** enjoyed teaching **Ben** martial arts moves, sharing his experience. Tai Chi is especially safe and gentle yet it can also be vigorous. Elements of Tai Chi can be adapted to different levels of ability. **Ben** complained that the voices sometimes made his body ache: he was fearful that the physical sensations would cause damage to his body. He complained of the effect of medication on his body. He said that he benefited from using Tai Chi. **Tom** said: It's very calming.

Breathing has been essential to enable people to relax, reduce panic and anxiety and to be able to voice, to express themselves. At times of trauma people may stop breathing; holding the breath may be a result of shock and also an attempt to survive, resulting in a survivor holding tensions in the body. For **Tina** and others there was a vicious circle of anxiety, inability to breathe, asthma, tension, loss of confidence about going out, isolation, low mood, anxiety. Difficulty breathing also translates into difficulty speaking which may be a trigger for voices.

Tina: My asthma brings me right down: she's (doctor) put my anti-depressants up. Breathing exercises help my mental state as well . . .

Speaking of the breathing exercises in dramatherapy **Sheila** confirmed this: I found that really good because when I was having . . . a lot of asthma attacks . . . it really did help me.

Physical problems

Many psychiatric patients complain that when they suffer from a physical illness they are not taken seriously, that it is presumed that their symptoms are psychosomatic or 'all in the mind' (see Roberts and Holmes, 1999: 21). Such physical problems and the resultant negative feelings about their body can lead to increased isolation and hence exacerbate voices. For example, increased weight can be due to medication side-effects and lack of exercise. Such increase in weight coupled with a decrease in physical activity can lead to shallower breathing, increased anxiety, decreased self-esteem (in a culture that prizes thinness and fitness) and withdrawal from society, increased isolation and voices. Motivated by his attendance at the group **Roger** began to take more care of his physical condition:

Roger: (after the first group) I want to become physically fit . . . I've cut down on comfort eating. Since joining the group I've eaten less chocolate. (after the second group) I've lost weight, over three stone . . . feel good.

Dramatherapy, as reported in Chapter 5, can promote physical well-being. For example, Andersen-Warren (1996: 111) reported lessened psychomotor retardation in participants in a therapeutic theatre group who had a diagnosis of a psychotic illness.

Song

As indicated in Chapters 5 and 6, an essential area of embodiment and empowerment is encouraging the use of the voice. Singing lifts mood and has other health benefits. When she used to sing **Pat** had less asthma. Singing can also be a socially cohesive source of pleasure. We composed group songs: each person contributing a line, improvising. Below are two such songs.

Men's group song

It doesn't make you less of a man if you cry.
Laughter hides my fears.
Playing football for Oldham town.
Listening to music and dance,
Watching TV in a trance.
A tot a day keeps the doctor away.
Sing a song, sing it simple, sing out strong!

Group 2's love song

When I first met you,
You were like a star:
So I know who you really are.
You're mine! You're mine!
It's like walking on sunshine.

The themes of these songs show group members' interest in feelings, identity, encounter, relationship, attachment, belonging, love, fun and joy.

Leah: We . . . made up a love song . . . I really enjoyed it today . . . singing and playing instruments made me happy . . . I sing to myself, I get happy: it helps.

Tom: a good song makes me happy . . . all my problems go away . . . I don't notice the voices . . . I associate certain songs with certain times . . . (when) I was happy. (i.e. before his breakdown.) I like singing a lot. (Was that helpful, singing in the group?) Yeah 'cause I like to give people a good impression of myself, put a good image across. I love ABBA, just singing along . . . it strikes a chord with other people, 'Oh I know that song.' . . . I've always liked music and I think it's very helpful. When I was hearing the voices I used to switch the radio on. Humming does relax you. I've tried it before . . . Music can make you happy. I sometimes reminisce about things . . . We have sung some songs in the group, mentioned music we like. We've played instruments . . . It was enjoyable . . . (Singing) was quite good as everyone joined in.

For **Tom** therefore music and singing raised his self-esteem, brought happy memories, improved his mood, involved him with others, relaxed him and reduced his voices. Humming has been found to be helpful to voice hearers (Watkins, 1998: 208). **Ben** said that sometimes singing helped him cope with the voices. Singing also helped **Sheila** block intrusive voices. We also played musical instruments, improvising with keyboard, drums and percussion.

Sheila: We did a music sessions . . . I found it really good . . . because we were all involved, it was fun, we all had a laugh, changing instruments, I was trying to keep up . . . I was trying the castanets. I was laughing more at myself because I was making mistakes . . . that was really good fun. (See section on Fun, p. 212–7.)

Some people who hear voices find listening to music helpful: it may be that the stimulus of the right brain (where music is processed) enhances mood (which is predominantly modulated in the right brain) and displaces/diminishes the activity of the speech area of the left brain, stilling the voices (Casson, 1998c). **Dillon** said that his voices were reduced by music.

Jimmy: Music helps: distracts me, helps me forget about the voices.

Sheila: The other day I put a tape on, put my stereo on try to shut them (voices) out which helped a lot because Roger's bought me a couple of tapes and he's got me a relaxation tape as well. So I've been putting the tape on when I've started hearing things. That's helped a lot. That's what I was frightened about the other week because they were saying, 'You're not worthy,' it just got on top of me. I put some music on . . . put my headphones on.

Pat also found music over her headphones helpful.

Drumming can release energy and relieve tension. The stimulus of rhythm can produce altered states of consciousness: 'rhythmic shamanic drumming produced a drum beat frequency in the theta wave EEG frequency (4–7 cycles/second) the brainwave range associated with dreams, hypnotic imagery and trance' (Drury, 1989: 39). This is also the range of creative thought (Casson, 1997–1998). For over 20,000 years shamans have used drumming for healing purposes.

Dave wrote in his journal: Had stimulating/creative session in John's group with percussion instruments. I think I could develop their use much further. Relaxation/stress management and awareness . . .

Pat: I enjoyed doing the instruments that was good: I was in a right mood that day. I just bashed them drums to hell . . . A release of tension . . .

Jimmy: We had a chance to play musical instruments. Instead of taking it out on something we would try and make a rhythm of life, banging the drums.

Drumming can be a safe way to express aggressive feelings. It may be that hostile voices encapsulate aggressive feelings and when these can be more directly expressed there is a reduction in such voices. I therefore give permission for people to shout and use of the whole range of their voices: the aim being to empower them to own their expressive, vocal power.

Leah enjoyed shouting her lines in drama: it took it out of me.

Anton: I shouted at them (voices) and they diminished. I felt better.

Many people did not swear, for cultural and religious reasons, so it was distressing to them that the voices swore. When appropriate I gave permission and encouragement to people to swear, to release anger and aggression.

Simon: I swear at them (the voices) when I get annoyed: it relieves the stress . . . I've never been a terribly aggressive person; when the voices got to me I found a short outburst relieved the tension. I've started to swear: it relieves some of the frustration/exasperation.

Talk

Voicing one's opinion, speaking up for oneself is asserting identity. Talking therefore in a group enables people to relate to others and express themselves. Verbal warm-ups encourage people who are not confident, to speak: such as passing an object around; name games; word games (The Good News, The Bad News); simple 'check-ins' when people say how they are feeling or what they need that day. Group therapy is an antidote to isolation and offers people an opportunity to talk, communicate and relate to others:

Tom: I enjoy it because it gives me a chance to say things which I wouldn't get the opportunity to say to anyone else. That's what the groups are there for . . . We're actually talk about the voices, whereas if I was at home with my Mum I might shy away from talking about the voices through fearing that they'll come back again. But talking about them directly that puts them in a normal, everyday thing . . . Makes them normal.

Sheila: I've discussed things in the group that I wouldn't have done six months or a year ago. I've talked about my feelings which I would have kept inside, so I'm more confident in the group to discuss my problems. I'm more confident . . .

Speaking up for oneself may mean saying 'No': as stated in Chapters 5 and 6 this is an important element of people being empowered.

Leah: We did an exercise about decisions, how to say, 'No' that helped. I've felt stronger as a person: I could say 'No' to people if I wanted to.

Roger: I'm more able to say 'No'. He was more able to stand up for himself, more self-respecting and others, including relatives, were more respectful of him. He refused to join the family for Christmas (thereby achieving the distance he needed at that time). Having rehearsed it in therapy some people were able to take this skill into their lives. This practise in saying 'No' to others may also enable someone to say 'No' to a voice. **Roger**, after the second group he said he was more able to say 'No' to ideas and could block out voices:

Funnily enough . . . when I thought about going over the balcony I thought to myself, 'Why am I thinking this? that's a negative thought. I'm not doing.' I thought to myself, 'No chance.' I feel more confident I can block them out . . . They're the same old stick in the mud voices: 'Do such a thing, do this and do that.' But I'm saying to myself, 'No chance.'

Furthermore group therapy can facilitate the development of social skills.

Dave: I can talk more openly with other people since being in the research and socialising has helped me when I'm low.

Pat: It's (therapy) like learning again how to talk . . . (What was helpful?) Exploring different ways of talking to people.

Talking in a relationship involves listening: an essential social skill.

Ben: Group work helped me to learn to listen to others.

Leah realised the importance of listening as well as talking in social skills: I learned a lot about making conversations . . .

Ben said that developing communication skills and having fun were the principal therapeutic benefits of the group. Such play and humour facilitates relationships.

Simon: I'm glad I met the people. It was interesting to speak to them . . . We started as a group that didn't communicate well and ended up with, unfortunately close to the end of the group, starting to communicate better.

Projected play

In group therapy we have used visualisation, imagined landscapes and paintings; made maps, drawn mandalas; used photographs and other images on cards; told stories with symbolic objects, containers, toys, doll's house furniture, toy animals, Babushka dolls. We have written poems and short scenarios for plays. Such creative work provides both a container and some distance: it stimulates and enables communication. Visualisation enabled people to share their inner worlds and relate to others:

Sheila (speaking about projected play and visualising): I found that was quite good because it made you realise what the other person was seeing in their mind's eye . . .

Jimmy (recalling a session in which the group made a map and developed the story of a journey): I put a big star on the piece of paper . . . we made a map . . . we're travelling . . . every one had a suggestion . . . it's as if we had a compass, we all had something to offer while we were doing that.

Images stimulate creativity. Storymaking, a projective technique (see Gersie, 1990, 1997), provides the basis for dramatic enactment:

Leah: We looked at some picture cards, picked out three each and made an imaginary story. I liked this exercise. We then acted it out and I was the news presenter which had a lot of thought put in.

Some people find visualisation without any concrete object difficult. It is helpful therefore to provide objects to stimulate projected play and encourage creativity. I have used a collection of containers in individual and group therapy: different objects such as a cage, glass box, post box, toy safe, heart, dustbin and treasure chest:

Sheila: One week John brought some little trinkets and asked us what they were and what they represented to us. I found that fascinating . . . I think (I chose) a little jewellery box . . . at the time I didn't realise it but afterwards I thought, 'Ooh it's like secrets being locked up and you're opening the box and your secrets coming out. That's what I've done in the group: I've opened up. Some of my secrets have come out to people in the group . . . Before I went to the group I wouldn't open up to anyone, I wouldn't tell anyone how I was feeling: if they asked me if I was all right. I'd just say, 'Yes,' or snap at them. Whereas now I'm coming out of myself a bit more: I've got that little bit more confidence than I had . . . We made stories up about them all: what we thought they were from or whatever. Each one of us had a different experience: I think it was very helpful because each one of us did something different.

Playing with text

Another metaphoric container for projected play is a theatre text. We used texts from *Waiting for Godot* (Beckett, 1954: 40–41), *Adult Child/Dead Child* (Dowie, 1987 – see Chapter 4) and *The Mahabharata* (Carriere, 1988: 104–105). I had selected passages that included voices. Working with such existing written material helped group members speak of their own experiences of voices: they also enjoyed rehearsing and speaking their parts. 'The temporary use of scripted roles is also useful in lowering the patient's anxiety' (Johnson, 1981: 56). Dramatherapists work with texts which provide a containing structure (Jenkyns, 1996).

Leah: The play was called **Waiting for Godot**. We rehearsed between us and then in front of the others, it was brilliant doing the play. I actually thought the information (in the) play was a schizophrenic person's symptoms . . . I was happy today 'cause of the role play.

Rehearsing scenes, returning to familiar material conserved in a text, can be reassuring and offers people who struggle with chaotic experiences some safety, predictability and pleasure. However distracted the person is, the text awaits their return: it holds attention, being a constant container for projections (as the text of *A Midsummer Night's Dream* was for **Cheryll**: see Chapter 8). After using these texts group members created their own improvised drama so the texts acted as stimuli for discussion and participants' own creativity. We also used poems and drawings as texts.

One day **Dave** brought Byron's (1970: 94) poem *The Dream* to a session and the group decided to dramatise it.

> A change came o'er the spirit of my dream
> The Wanderer was alone as heretofore,
> The beings which surrounded him were gone
> Or were at war with him; he was a mark
> For blight and desolation, compassed round
> With Hatred and Contention; Pain was mix'd
> In all which was served up to him, until,
> Like to the Pontic Monarch of old days,
> He fed on poisons, and they had no power
> But were a kind of nutriment; he lived
> Through that which had been death to many men,
> And made him friends of mountains: with the stars
> And the quick Spirit of the Universe
> He held his dialogues; and they did teach
> To him the magic of their mysteries;
> To him the book of Night was open'd wide
> And voices from the deep abyss reveal'd
> A marvel and a secret – Be it so.

Each group member chose a role in the poem that interested them. **Roger** played the 'Wanderer in the Abyss' and benefited from laying to rest the spirits of the dead. **Dillon** played the 'Pontic Monarch', built a temple and offered prayers for the exorcism of a ghost. **Ben** said: Even after all that has been lost the temple can be re-built, the seasons turn, the crops grow. He felt hope from this drama. Through the metaphoric container of these roles they were able to work on profound sources of disturbance without plunging into distress. The poem's imagery had 'touched the depth before it stirs the surface' (Bachelard quoted by Cox and Theilgaard, 1987: xiii) The group members enjoyed the drama yet **Roger** was referring to an incident in the Second World War when his father watched his comrades machine gunned to death; **Dillon** had lost family members in the holocaust and in exorcising a ghost was referring also to psychotic experiences; **Ben** was a survivor of a civil war in which temples had been destroyed and thousands had starved. Despite the horrors of the past this creative activity was suffused with hope. **Dave**, who was suicidal and depressed, played the spirit of the mountain: the role lifted his mood. Here the containing structure of the text/metaphor/role, the explicit drama (see Chapter 9), provided the necessary distance to enable therapeutic work, the implicit drama, to be done.

The following week **Ben**'s drawing of a skeleton was the source of a ritual in which **Dave** played the role of 'Yin and Yang' which had lost its balance. He dived into the ocean and transformed into a comet. 'Embodied expression . . . is needed in order for transformation to occur' (Lewis, 1993: 174–176).

Of this session **Dave** said:

> The most helpful thing was transformation: being free to be anything you wanted to be. I died then ran around with white material . . . You said, 'You don't have to die in real life.' I found it useful emotionally and conceptually. The point about things change was made more strongly and personally because it was on an emotional level with people – it was something I knew but it was made stronger. You don't have to die physically in order to change but you do die in some way. (He wrote in his journal): Today in dramatherapy we enacted our own 'creation – mythology' and as a result my obsession/need to talk about death has been alleviated. In particular it's been made aware to me that without darkness/death/evil/ends there can be no lightness/birth/good and beginnings a balance is needed this balance constantly changes and we need to be both executioners and clowns/jugglers in life . . .

Mehl (1988: 133) who developed shamanic healing methods in a modern pain clinic, stated: 'Healing always involves a death and transformation of some part of the person.'

Dave dreamt he was

> a Mesolithic shaman 7000 BC . . . I was . . . being threatened by two tribesmen; smeared with a grey clay slip and carrying spears. They cut large pieces of flesh from my body until I saw my skull on the floor. With a bare foot the skull of myself was crushed into powder with the heel into the soil. I was happy and began dreaming again . . . of a healing ritual, men in ancient clothes, amber, head-dress of metal pieces . . .

This shamanic dream was helpful to **Dave**. It is in accord with shamanic initiation rituals of death, dismemberment and resurrection: the trance experience (see Eliade, 1989: 38). The ritual enactment of dying, going under the sea and being transformed held **Dave** back from acting out his death fantasies in overdoses.

Being someone else: role play

Shamans are masters of transformation, of changing role and changing perspective from the human to the divine, to the animal, to the demonic: they are maskers and shape shifters (Casson, 1997–1998). In dramatherapy and psychodrama people have the freedom to transform themselves, to become the other. Moreno discovered that people are more spontaneous when they play another role. In being able to play other roles, whether real or fantastic, people are able to expand their sense of self, to inhabit more of the theatre of the self (see Chapter 9).

> As mediator between *self and other*, between self and the social world, role embodies qualities of thought, feeling, and behaviour taken on from another and represented in a way prescribed by social convention.
>
> (Landy, 1986: 92, added emphasis)

Moreno wrote:

> Role can be defined as the actual and tangible form the self takes. We thus define the role as the functioning form the individual assumes in the specific situation in which other persons or objects are involved. The symbolic representation of this functioning form, perceived by the individual and others is called the role. The form is created by past experiences and the cultural patterns of the society in which the individual lives . . . Every role is a fusion of private and collective elements.
>
> (Moreno, quoted in Fox, 1987: 62)

Role play therefore brings people into relationship with the other, indeed plays with the relationship of self and other.

Puppets can provide a bridge between projected and role play, providing creative stimulus and some distance.

Jimmy: I could communicate to the others through this glove puppet which was using my imagination . . . I found myself thinking, 'Can I introduce this character to the group which isn't me: it's just a friend I know which is quite nice,' . . . that you could converse with, that could converse with the rest of the group rather than it being you on the spot.

Jimmy found the distance afforded by the use of a puppet helpful in being able to relate playfully to others without feeling pressured.

Playing another role can also give us a sense of liberating distance from our usual self: when we were not being our habitual selves (which may be limiting, especially if in a patient role, to a pathogenic degree) we can be more of our greater, potential self and through such roles we can gain insight, energy, power and a greater sense of self, of identity. Creating another character may enable someone to discover an ability they did not know they had:

For example, the actor playing Lord Bootlace had, through this dignified and controlled man, found what he described as 'a centre of stillness!' This was very precious to him and quite a startling discovery, as he had previously viewed himself as a very agitated and restless person.

(Andersen-Warren, 1996: 120)

We created characters with hats, gloves and cloth for costumes and told their stories.

Jimmy: (I) could be a pirate, a Russian dissident or anything. We get dressed up . . . it's like discovering what goes on in my mind . . . It's good fun. It's safe to do it there . . . I like it (role play). I've got very little at home to interest me . . . it's just me at home so given a chance it's like saying, 'I've got a different persona that I can portray to other people.' The sense of imagination is wonderful. You don't want to be yourself all the time: you can break out and be someone else . . . You're wearing a hat, you can pretend to be someone else . . . it's like having a free licence . . . You feel as if you can be born again . . .

After playing the role of another I return to myself, renewed and expanded.

Jimmy: I got encouragement to be more extrovert – it was nice when some people would sit back and be passive and allow me to do my thing: to be exuberant . . . I was allowed to *be myself* more. Being creative I found that a very soothing experience because I allowed myself to be radical where I'm normally laid back.

The enactments gave people confidence, released tensions. In answer to the question: What have you found helpful? **Theo** replied: The drama, acting things out, taking people off, group discussion . . . I enjoyed it. It gave me more confidence. I sleep better . . .

Video

In the group I ran (1985–1993) for people with severe social anxiety (most were diagnosed as schizophrenic) we created comedy videos (Casson, 1986). One of these was *The Space Odyssey of Dr Watt*. The group devised the story and script, made puppets, sets, the sound track and edited the film. We filmed in the dramatherapy studio and on location (a park where there were large dinosaur models). Dr Watt's spaceship was more or less controlled by two computers. These machines spoke to the Doctor, giving him information, orders, warnings and gobbledegook. The Doctor talked back to the computers as he struggled to control his spaceship, encountered aliens, visited hostile worlds and returned safely home with three dinosaur eggs from another world. It was only after we had finished the film that I realised the computers were a metaphorical representation of the voice-hearing experience; that the journey from the family home to outer space and the eventual return to the family, was a metaphor for psychotic illness; that the hostile environments of other planets, aliens and erupting volcano symbolised the terrors of their experiences. All these were held at a safe distance by the metaphoric container of the film which was a reality process: playing together we worked out how to make a film, had fun and over two years accumulated enough material to make a satisfying comedy of which the group were justly proud.

Mike initially regarded himself as entirely uncreative and avoided eye contact. He had an interest in photography and so he became the camera man. I noticed, as we watched the film he made of our activities each week, how he looked at people through the camera lens. As he developed in confidence he began fleetingly to have eye contact with others. His confidence grew in wider social settings. The camera had given Mike the distance he initially needed in social relations, as Powley (1981–1982: 48) stated: 'One of the advantages of experiencing through a camera is that we do not have to engage life directly.'

The group decided that there should be a showing for their families and friends and so the journey ended with a return to the staff room which had originally been the living room of Dr Watt's family where now their own family members gathered to enjoy the film. The impact on the group members' self-esteem of this public showing was positive. The family of the man who played Dr Watt now saw him not only as a disabled schizophrenic but also as a comic actor and the star of a film.

Reflections of working with video

Powley (1981–1982: 51) pointed out that the video image is the world in miniature: 'it's so small! So much in our control, at the press of a button. What power we have over experience!' (See also Pettiti, 1989: 7.) Thus video can be empowering for people who may not have power over their voices or psychotic experiences. Mike's preference for being the cameraman must alert us to the possibility that some may not want to be filmed, preferring the safety of a backstage role: people must have a choice. Some perpetrators of sexual abuse film their victims. Before any camera is introduced into the group feelings about filming and ethical concerns about the group's confidentiality must be addressed: again group members must be empowered to say 'No' and even when the camera is accepted into the group I explicitly give permission to any group member to call for it to be switched off and filming stopped. When the camera is introduced useful work can be done before it is switched on with an exploration of what the camera might see, what people want to say to the camera and with group members role reversing with the camera. Pettiti (1989), who used video successfully to develop confidence and work through issues in adolescent groups, explored the psychological functions of the camera as a transitional, externalising object: the camera stood in for significant others from the patient's life. The video also stimulated creativity, playfulness and disclosure. The camera is a recording witness (see also Landy, 1996: 22).

Group work in hospital with more disturbed patients

All the group work cited above was carried out in day centres with people who were able to live in the community. I have also worked with acutely mentally distressed patients in hospital. With a team of therapists (occupational therapists, nurses and a psychiatric physiotherapist) I provided a twice weekly ward-based 'recovery group' from 1991 to 1993. This was specifically for people struggling with psychotic experiences. Basing our work on dramatherapy theory and practice and Yalom's (1983) *Inpatient Group Psychotherapy*, we provided a structured, supportive group where the focus was on the here and now. As well as providing stimulus we also provided predictable structure: always beginning and ending the group with a simple, recognisable ritual. When all group members were present the therapist began the session with the following introduction (based on Yalom, 1983: 287):

> I am . . . and these are my co-workers . . . Welcome to the Recovery Group which meets twice a week on Tuesday mornings at 11.00 and Thursday afternoon at 4.00. The group lasts forty-five minutes. We try to remind you a few minutes before the meeting so you can come to this room. Our aims are to enjoy being together, learn to relax with each other, trust each other, and learn to concentrate; to listen to each other, share things that are important to us, overcome shyness and have some fun. We've planned some tasks today and there'll be time before we finish to review the group activities and how you feel about them.

In the last five minutes we asked group members to remember, preferably in order, the activities we had done together and in remembering share how they felt about these: what they disliked and what they enjoyed. This enabled the therapists to assess how members had perceived the activities. This was also an opportunity to ask for suggestions and help us plan for future group meetings.

This containing structure held very anxious people: the structured exercises and games enabled them to take part. We always established people's presence and identity in the room by asking them to state their names, say hello and participate in a name game or introductory activity, bringing them into contact with each other, achieving a sense of arrival. From this beginning we moved into exercises of awareness of here and now reality: noticing and focusing on sensory experience, providing stimuli for seeing, hearing, touch, taste, smell. From these we could develop into a sequence of

> I notice . . . I feel . . . I imagine . . .

This might lead into storymaking and drama.

We conducted embodiment warm-ups and exercises: promoting physical relaxation, breathing, voice, movement and mime. We used structured pair work including trust walks and mirroring to promote interaction and conversation. We conducted whole group movement exercises, including back massages, hugs, games with elastic, softball, percussion. We used objects to stimulate projected play. Occasionally it was possible to conduct a brief psychodrama (see Chapter 12). More usually we used drama to promote spontaneous interaction between people in the here and now. From group members' statements we might explore a theme through simple drama activities or introduce a situation for improvisation:

The vet's waiting room

Each group member imagines they have a pet. (The therapist encourages variety by saying that anything goes – including bats, crocodiles, elephants.) They meet in a vet's waiting room and talk about their pets' ailments. A variation on this is that the person may role reverse with their pet and then the pets talk about their owners.

Reflections on structuring

For highly anxious and disturbed patients a structured group provides a safer environment than an unstructured group. Given the social anxiety, lack of social skills, paranoia and the possibility that vulnerable patients may feel overwhelmed, it is important to build into the practice of group dramatherapy some safeguards: to balance the risk with familiar ritual and safe structure that can contain anxiety. For example at the start of the group we might use a familiar ritual of passing a small globe round the group so that each person can in turn speak about their world.

Occasionally a group will tolerate a space, filling it with discussion, sharing or silence. As group members gather in the room such a space will occur: the therapist may well pick up concerns or themes in the snatches of conversations that occur and be able to follow these up in the group. A long silence will not be helpful and therapists must be willing to model appropriate responses to suggested exercises. Group members' ideas must be picked up and expanded whenever possible: e.g. during a movement exercise if a member moves differently the therapist can invite the whole group to copy the movement, paying attention to how 'Phil' is moving. The group is about noticing and being noticed and about making connections in action, relationships, thinking and bringing meaning out of chaos. The organising skills of the therapist are therefore to support the members of the group to make sense of the time spent together and to positively connate all contributions, even when they are negative so that members feel they are respected as autonomous human beings. For example:

Therapist: Jane, you've told us how low you're feeling and that you thought the dance exercise was silly. Thank you for telling us how you feel and for expressing your opinion.

(NB: Of course this must be said without any hint of condescension or sarcasm!)

Group dramatherapy can empower, enabling people to relate and play with others, grow in confidence, expand their role repertoire and have fun. **Dave** said that the dramatherapy group is an important means of developing well being (and) for this reason I believe should be offered long term to people with not only voices but also other mental illnesses.

In Chapter 13 I will report more broadly on the benefits of the method as expressed by the research participants.

Chapter 11

Individual psychodrama

Harry

Although psychodrama is usually considered a group therapy, Moreno's first use of drama as a therapeutic intervention was in individual work: at some time between 1908 and 1912 he worked with Elisabeth Bergner, a troubled child. At first he worked individually with her, encouraging her spontaneity and creativity through poetry and dramatic play, later inviting her to join a children's theatre group (Marineau, 1989: 35–38). She was to become one of the most famous actresses of the German stage in the twentieth century and acknowledged Moreno's role in developing her creativity. This is what Moreno himself says on a recently rediscovered audio tape:

> Psychodrama can be done also on an individual basis. You cannot do group psychotherapy except in a group – that is what the word means. You can do psychodrama a deux. You can do psychodrama just like you do psycho-analysis. Instead of being on a couch you are on a stage in action, in a series of actions. You can do group psychodrama and individual psychodrama. Psychodrama is really more inclusive than group psychotherapy.
>
> (Moreno, 1965)

I have written elsewhere about individual psychodrama (Casson, 1997a) and will focus here on an individual case study to describe the practice of psychodrama with an individual who hears voices.

Introducing Harry

Harry was 34 when he was referred to me by his social worker, who was concerned that he might be violent. **Harry** was also frightened: he withdrew from people because of his hatred and his fear that he would lose control and kill someone: his son was in care because he had beaten him and he also feared he might 'touch' his daughter. As a child **Harry** had been beaten by his own father, a perpetrator who was eventually sent to prison for sexually abusing **Harry**'s daughter and his siblings. **Harry** felt rage but also said he loved his father. He found communication difficult: I've never found it easy to express emotions. He withdrew into silence, spending hours drawing abstract patterns, mandalas, which he called 'doodle art', in a trance-like state: he found this calming. He heard the voices of his son; of a middle-aged man who told him to attack his son or cut/kill himself (sometimes he did cut, on other occasions he dissociated, as he had done when his father had beaten him: I get into a trance); a loud, scary voice that called his name; a mumbling crowd, whispering and confusing. The voices started after his mother's death. The family fell apart: she was holding it together. He had been unable to grieve her death and wished to be with her. He had also seen/felt a ghostly presence on several occasions: an eight foot tall woman: dark eyes, white skin, long hair, black dress: she looked like Satan. This was more frightening than the voices. **Harry** also heard an evil voice he named Satan: a destructive part of him he did not want to own.

The voices annoyed him and occurred often when he himself was feeling angry. He acknowledged the voices as being in his head and had the insight that they voiced the distress he was unable to voice. He had put his own violence behind him but felt a growing pressure: he 'switched off', dissociated, to escape from angry feelings and went into a trance state. He had difficulty sleeping, was suicidal, depressed. His diagnosis was 'vulnerable personality secondary to childhood abuse.'

Due to adolescent petty crime he had been sent to a 'boarding school' and been physically abused, humiliated and bullied. He was also victimised by his elder brothers. He felt he had to do as others said and obey the voices. He was unable to assert himself in relationships. He chose individual therapy because of his social phobia, shame and fear of attacking someone. The description of his therapy that follows is necessarily simplified for clarity. We did revisit themes and I have telescoped time and psychodramas to illustrate key processes, theory and practice. All the sessions were one-hour long.

Spontaneity training: permission to play

In an assessment session **Harry** imagined and then role reversed with a friend, who was an advocate, able to stand up for his child self. The friend insisted that children could play instead of fight and have fun instead of being aggressive. We began therefore with spontaneity training in which I gave him permission to play, explore the room, rediscover and expand his creativity.

Exploring the room

A psychodrama often begins with walking about the room. I encouraged **Harry** to explore the room and take some ownership of the therapeutic space. **Harry** wanted a light-filled room: he opened curtains and put on extra lights. Having this control made him feel safer.

Harry: I hate any room that was too dark: it helped me feel more confident, secure.

His father had not allowed **Harry** to have a light on in his bedroom at night and used to come into the dark room and beat him with a black belt.

I encouraged **Harry** to look in the cupboards, not only so that he could own the space and the resources for creative work but also so that he felt nothing need be kept hidden. This reminded him of father's angry injunction not to look in cupboards.

Harry: I started getting a bit paranoid. I didn't like going into cupboards and wardrobes that are not mine; I kept back a bit . . . I couldn't get things; John had to get things out . . . At home I was restricted or anywhere else, whereas John said, 'Explore the room.' . . . at the time I would not go in cupboards . . . because I was always told not to by my father . . . now I'm more relaxed; life is full of curiosities.

Harry internalised my permission to explore and recovered his childhood curiosity which father had prohibited. From the objects he found in the cupboard he created images:

I was building things, I made a clown (out of objects) on the floor . . . I didn't like it; it didn't look right to me. So I built in the middle of the room this three-dimensional doodle art. I really liked that; we used ribbon, cushions, that chime thing . . . It's something I'd never done before . . . of all the drawings I done, they were flat but this was three-dimensional: I enjoyed that.

The negative voice told him to spoil this creation but **Harry** refused. He felt empowered.

Preparing for safe action: breathing

In the first sessions **Harry** was volatile and potentially violent. I knew that before any cathartic work on his rage could be safely done I needed, for both our sakes and the safety of others, to do some preventative work to enable him to control his explosive temper. I explained to him the value of taking 'time out' (walking out of the room) when he felt he might lose control. He never did this in therapy but used the technique at home. Key to him having some control were the breathing exercises we practised together.

Harry: We've worked on my temper as well. The breathing exercise comes into that. When you get into really stressed moments walk out or wait until later and try to talk it out . . . And I've done that a few times and that has worked, but it doesn't always work but I have got the gist of it: it can be controlled . . . When I first went to John I was tense: he noticed I wasn't breathing. Now when I get in a real flutter I do that (breathe) . . . and it's useful

*... **breathing helped ... so I can talk fluently ...*** release the energy but *not violently: not hitting doors ... Even when I get in a stress situation I can take the breathing exercises, calm down, go through it slowly ... I don't feel confused.*

Becoming more aware of his breathing enabled **Harry** to think, giving him the mental space to be more in control of his reactions, have more choices, be more able to speak and assert himself. We visualised large advertising hoardings with huge letters saying STOP, THINK, BREATHE. He practised this at home and it helped him cope.

Harry: *think, breathe, sometimes I walk up and down in the kitchen to get a bit of the stress out of me ... I've got to say to myself, 'Relax, take it easy, take deep breaths, and just think before ... '*

Safe anger energises and empowers

We then sought safe ways to channel his angry energy. **Harry** immediately noticed the world ball in the room:

Harry: *We started out with a world, a big blown up world, we were just basically pissing about, kicking it, it was all right ...* It's all right to kick back at the world ... There was a drum kit in the room and I gave him permission to play with it: *I started playing the drums then; that was pretty interesting, I enjoyed that. It was just too loud, I gave it up. He got this chime thing* (cymbal) *it weren't loud and I was pounding on that: I liked the sound. I've got tapes with that kind of sound on it: it's therapeutic for me, it relaxes me. It is different* (playing rather than just listening) *but if you've got an imagination for music like I have, you can blend it all together.*

He enjoyed discovering that he could allow his aggression out in controlled, creative ways. We also rehearsed how he could manage his anger. We used Tai Chi (he had previous experience of martial arts) to help him breathe and feel a sense of grounded self-mastery.

Harry: *I did martial arts myself years ago: It's a good way of getting some of the stress out of you rather than hitting a wall ... Now I'm a lot more calmer ... John taught me to shake limbs, breathe, relax. When I started doing that at home it did help ... it helps to clear your mind, relax.*

Psychodrama 1

The first psychodrama was about his relationship with his wife. He was jealous of her relationship with his son. The threatening voice told him to argue with his wife, be obnoxious, aggressive to her. This could be seen as symbolic of the difficulties in their relationship. Unable to communicate his feelings to her, he withdrew and translated his rage into 'doodle art' so that she felt frustrated, angry, hurt. Their marriage was on the verge of collapse. In this first psychodrama I played the double role, as an empathic witness and support, helping him speak of his feelings. He wept.

Harry: I went through a really bad patch, my family were splitting up and I went there and the whole of that hour I just cried. He was there; he gave me the guidance, the comfort . . . because I never get this off any of my side of the family, or anybody else come to think of it. It made me cry more and made me want to get all this energy out. He was there, just talking to me . . . he found little ways, he was there, listening . . . when that hour was over even though I was still depressed I'd got a lot off my chest.

In a later session he was able to role reverse with his wife and have psychodramatic conversations with her, gaining insight and empathy for her position. Following these rehearsals he was more able to talk with her at home.

Harry: I'm able to talk to Sue a bit better whereas one time we hardly talked at all. I can talk better to Sue. I'm able to speak a bit more how I think and feel to any other person . . . It's a lot stronger – my relationship (with my wife) than it was six month ago . . .

Once when suicidal he created his own funeral scene and in Sue's role as grieving widow s/he said that she loved him, that his life had been wasted and he deserved better. S/he blamed his family, especially his father and said he missed his mother. S/he said he had a heart of gold and a head full of shit. Through this psychodrama he was able face death, to grieve his mother, express fears and realise that his wife, despite their quarrels and difficulties, did love him, value him and would miss him. After this psychodrama his suicidal feelings abated. (On the safe practice of psychodramatically enacting suicide see Appendix 5.)

Psychodrama 2

The second psychodrama was about his relationship with his son, Tim. Communicating with Tim was also difficult as the boy was deaf and despite being able to sign, **Harry** was often frustrated and unable to control Tim's behaviour. He said he hated Tim and as **Harry** had been violent to him, Tim was taken into care. When Tim was due to return home **Harry** felt stressed and heard voices telling him to harm himself.

Harry: Due to the fact we were just getting my son back: I wasn't too keen on that. I didn't want anything to happen like it used to do: that was playing on me a lot. (The voice said,) 'Hurt yourself, stab your self . . . ' I had to have three stitches . . . give myself pain so I could forget everything . . .

We began the psychodrama by representing Tim with a large teddy bear. **Harry** held the bear lovingly and poured out his passionate concern for the boy: he was angry with the system for failing to educate him and he made connections with his own boyhood experiences of being bullied. He punched cushions and hit a drum to express his rage. **Harry** then said he heard a voice which he identified as his son's. I asked him to role reverse with this voice. He growled aggressively. I interviewed him as the voice/son. As the voice he said, 'I love you Dad.' I returned **Harry** to his own role and repeated the words the voice had said. It was a moment of transformation: from that time onwards the relationship with his son began to improve. Indeed the voice saying, 'I love you Dad,' returned later in his therapy: this disturbed **Harry** as his son was not able to speak in such an articulate way but he acknowledged that it was true: his son did love him and he loved his son. This further illustrates how voices may express feelings that cannot otherwise be directly expressed. Their relationship continued to improve until Tim came home permanently.

By role reversing with a voice a person can express feelings, gain insight, control and a sense of ownership of such ego-alien intrapsychic material. *Role reversals with voices should however be brief*: the aim is not to potentiate the voice but to enable the person to move between voice and self and gain some mastery. While it can be helpful to have an auxiliary play the role of a voice in group therapy (see Chapter 12) it is perhaps unwise for the therapist to play this role in individual therapy. I repeated the words of **Harry**'s voice but from my own role. It may be possible to briefly double the empty chair representing the voice but for a therapist to become the voice might well be disturbing and confusing. Zerka Moreno (1978: 163) warned that the therapist playing such roles could result in role confusion for therapist and patient. It is possible to use a trained auxiliary to assist in individual therapy and play such a role.

Psychodrama 3: role training

I have earlier written of the importance of empowering people who hear voices to say 'No' (Chapters 5, 6 and 10). Dramatherapy and psychodrama offer opportunities for rehearsing behaviours: through such rehearsals people are able to become more assertive. **Harry** had been chronically unable to assert himself in relationships or say 'No' to others' demands. We began the next psychodrama by **Harry** playing the role of his brother Bill who regularly pressured **Harry** to join him in his drinking. I then played Bill's role, basing my performance on **Harry**'s. In his own role he capitulated to Bill's pressure to drink. I invited him to role reverse with Bill again and played **Harry**'s role, mirroring his passive behaviour. The mirror technique provides distance (which may be a source of humour) and strengthens the observer ego (Casson, 1998c). Of this mirror **Harry** said: It was quite funny: when he was taking me off . . . it was quite interesting: to see yourself amused me. I didn't take it that seriously. It weren't offensive. He weren't taking the mick.

In his role I then modelled him asserting himself, saying 'No' to Bill. Having provided this model I invited **Harry** to play his own role again. **Harry** rehearsed calmly saying 'No' to Bill.

> I've got a bad thing of just saying what I say and not think about it first. Sitting on the chair and he'll (J.C.) be someone else, like my brother . . . and he'll talk to me . . . 'I'm coming round for a drink, a beer.' Well me I used to say, 'Yeah.' Then he'll (J.C.) say, 'Let's try and practice saying, 'No' 'cause you're living on yes, yes, yes, let them have what they want, make them happy: it doesn't work.' So he'd repeat the question again and I said, 'No,' dead snappy like, 'No.' Then he'd say, 'Relax, take deep breaths, when you say it, it's not going to go over to him as a hostile thing' . . . so I said, 'No you can't drink here. It's messing up the family. It's encouraging me to drink, and I don't want to drink. And it's just not good.' Now after that when I went home that day my brother came across, he'd already bought the beers and came into the house. I looked at him, breathed deeply, (and said to myself) 'Oh shit . . . Calm down.' He handed me a can and I said, 'No thanks.' He said, 'Go on, go on,' because he's very persuasive, he tries to get it in my hand. I said, 'No, you're right Bill, thanks for offering but No. Drink it yourself if you like . . . ' 'Why don't you want a drink?' 'I don't want a drink. When I want a drink I'll let you know.' At least I kept there. I refused it point blank: that's another way he's helped me. I've got confidence . . . It's very helpful to say, 'No.' Very helpful indeed. Before I met John I would do things despite that I really hated it. When my brother comes round with a couple of cans I can say, 'No, I don't want that.' John made me realise you can say, 'No.'

Harry was also able to say 'No' to me. Asked what he had found helpful in the psychodramas he said: being able to say, 'No' . . . Sometimes you asked me to do things and it was too much . . . I had to say, 'No.'

In further psychodramas **Harry** rehearsed overcoming his social phobia, coping with meeting professionals and asserting himself.

Harry: I went in once and said, 'My confidence is pretty low, I go all red, withdrawn, I'd rather sit in a corner than go and talk to someone.' We worked on it and now I'm able to talk to people . . . I've got confidence . . . My son's been in care . . . I had to go to this meeting, being one to one is hard work but being with 15 people is over the top. When Sue (**wife**) said, 'Would you like to come to this meeting?' I said 'No' at first. She said, 'Well I need you there to help me and support me.' I thought OK then, it's for the family. Do It. So I went to this meeting, I didn't say much I must admit.

I went. I did as much as I could . . . He worked on my feelings, helped me feel less panicky, less irritated, guided me through that.

We also rehearsed a meeting with his consultant psychiatrist. Such rehearsals can empower people in relationships and develop their social skills.

Harry: Now I am more assertive. At one time I weren't violent, I was bad tempered, shot my mouth off. Now I talk, I say to them, 'I'd rather talk about this . . . rather than argue about this because we're not going to get anywhere fighting so if you want to sit down and talk about it fine, if you don't go out.'

Harry was able to generalise his new-found ability to talk: to practise outside the therapy session, to speak to others.

I'm thinking: I feel more confident. That's how the therapy has worked: cos now they don't have control of me; I don't have control of them (partner, relatives, friends) because I don't want control of them, just me, that's good enough for me. They still think they have control over me . . . It helped to bring my way of thinking out, it's made me less aggressive, have some kind of control over what I do, what I think of my life, to deal with certain situations regarding people.

In these rehearsals **Harry** role reversed with the other, gaining insight:

Harry: Acting different people I found it quite hard but at the same time I found it quite amusing. It helps you to learn about the other person. You get a more broader idea of how people are working. (Changing from one role to another) makes you understand better about yourself and the other individual.

Psychodrama 4: intrapsychic roles

The fourth psychodrama was about **Harry**'s relationship with different parts of himself. Moreno (1939) termed this 'auto-tele' and plotted these parts of self, as intrapsychic roles, on role-relationship diagrams. He explained that as well as considering the patient's relationships to significant others (the feeling relationship between people he termed 'tele', plotted in the 'social atom', see Chapter 9) it was necessary to understand the patient's relationship with himself.

As an infant grows he does not only experience other people but also experiences himself . . . Gradually he develops a picture of himself. This picture of himself may differ considerably from the picture others have of him but it becomes considerably significant for him as life goes on. The gap between him as he is and acts and between the picture he has of himself is growing. Finally it appears as if he had, besides his real ego, an outside ego which he gradually extrojects. Between the ego and his extrojection a peculiar feeling relationship develops which may be called the 'auto-tele'.

(Moreno, 1939: 4)

Voices may then be seen as such 'extrojected' parts of the self or intrapsychic roles encapsulating aspects of self. Leudar and Thomas (2000) have suggested a dialogical model of voices as inner speech. Speaking to oneself is a normal activity. The dialogue suggests there are different aspects of self: I and me, parts of self which may be integrated, split off and/or extrojected as unacceptable to the ego: roles, in effect, that are offstage, 'voices off' in the theatre of the self (see Chapter 9). Psychodrama facilitates such self talk. **Harry** used objects and chairs to represent these different parts of himself. Thus there emerged the following roles:

Victim, Child, Persecutor, Judge, Rescuer, Protector, Observer, Carer, Sick Patient (carrying shame), Dissociator, Escaper, Quiet one, Desperate one, Furious one, Mad one.

This list does not exhaust the roles **Harry** played but are those named in the following psychodrama. Describing this 'psychodramatic splitting' of himself into various roles to a research assistant **Harry** said:

> I sit down, we've got a few chairs: I've to be another person, well me but in another way, split the personality up a bit . . . We worked on certain feelings: I've got four chairs: in one chair I've got depressed mood, in another chair I've got a really mad mood, and so on and so on, from one chair to the next. It helped, it was tiring work but it is effective . . .

The judge role emerged when **Harry** expressed a fear that I would judge him if he disclosed a shameful secret from his past. This role was first projected out onto me as therapist. By placing an empty chair to hold the role I was able to place this part of his self in the space between us and then invited **Harry** to show me the role as he perceived it, thus ensuring he temporarily owned the projected role. As we examined this role, the judge was further subdivided between a critical, condemning figure and a compassionate figure of justice. As the compassionate judge he recalled the circumstances of **Harry**'s upbringing and responding to the question of shame felt by the patient role, declared, 'He was not all to blame.' The judge, as justice, returned the adult responsibility for what had happened when **Harry** was a child to where it truly belonged: to his father.

Coleman (1998) stated: A psychodramatic trial . . . requires you to look at *all* the evidence. That allows you to *take power*, through playing different roles.

Such 'psychodramatic splitting' clarifies the nature of intrapsychic roles and can reveal when a role has become contaminated by feelings that belong elsewhere. **Harry**'s persecutory super-ego combined an introjected abuser role, shame, rage and loathing for the powerlessness of his child self. He said he hated his child self for being manipulated and not realising what his father was doing. (By directing the rage and hatred at himself **Harry** in effect protected his father from these feelings: due to his father's violence it was impossible for him to express these feelings when younger.) When **Harry** was a child there was no adequate protector, carer or advocate. He had learned persecution and internalised that. There was no rescuer: the only escape was dissociation. He was a passionate carer for others and tried to rescue vulnerable animals; he dreamt of rescuing his family from a whirlwind: he needed to learn to care for himself.

Clayton (1994: 131) showed how roles can be arranged in clusters and so analysed into those that are progressive and functional; fragmentary and dysfunctional; coping and survival strategies. We can constellate **Harry**'s roles into clusters as follows:

- *Progressive and functional*
  Rescuer, Protector, Carer, Compassionate Judge, Observer.
- *Fragmentary and dysfunctional*
  Child, Victim, Sick Patient, Desperate one, Mad one, Furious one, Persecutor, Critical, Condemning Judge.
- *Coping and survival strategies*
  Escaper, Dissociator, Quiet one.

In working through such intrapsychic roles in psychodrama the aim is to observe what was adequate, overdeveloped, underdeveloped, conflicted and absent (Clayton, 1994: 142) and then maximise the progressive and functional: to promote the growth of a healthier role system. For example, not being yet ready to disclose the shameful secret he carried, **Harry** protected himself from premature disclosure by playing in a fantasy, escapist psychodrama. This enabled him to recapture good memories, develop hope for the future, strengthen himself in the face of his current depression and the challenge ahead. The week after he created a drama about Noah saving the animals from the flood, expressing his passionate anger at human destructiveness. Thus his ethical anger was being expressed as he developed the role of advocate for the oppressed: a role entirely absent from his childhood experience (he had first created the role of an advocate for his child self in an assessment session, see p. 183). In these dramas he was rescuing his capacity to play, protecting himself and finding safe ways to escape (which had been impossible when young, except through dissociation), to express anger and rescue those vulnerable to destruction. Given his hatred of his son, which I now recognised was the projection of his hatred for his powerless child self, I felt it was essential he develop the role of compassionate judge. After expressing his rage (see p. 193) I therefore invited **Harry** to play the role of the compassionate judge and as such he told himself that he had been an innocent child, his father had been responsible and that he could forgive his child self. He then remembered trying to protect his sister from his father and being physically punished for doing so. Thus he was able to rescue the image of himself as a child from his abuser's view and decontaminate it: enabling him to re-establish a healthier, functional 'auto-tele' with his own playfulness and ultimately re-establish himself in relation to his own children as an adequate father (see p. 194). The child role could then be moved from the dysfunctional to the functional category of roles.

Of this work **Harry** said:

> I had to play three or four different people: that was exhausting cause one minute I'd got three me, four me, in different chairs, personalities, that was extremely hard work, sometimes I got a bit depressed about it. Worn out . . . I was a bit baffled by it but when I got home I could use some of that . . .

This post-session confusion is not necessarily a negative outcome: as the intrapsychic furniture is rearranged there will be a period of confusion as the new self organisation is integrated. This reorganisation was further facilitated by the use of the Five Story Self Structure, which is, in effect, a miniature psychodrama theatre (see Chapter 6). This provided necessary distance for **Harry** to acknowledge different parts of himself including an evil, murderous part, (previously projected onto the Satan voice and the vampire ghost), and set them in relation to his whole self including his positive spiritual aspirations, thus integrating the bad with the good. The Five Story Self Structure is in effect a mandala when viewed from above. This explains its integrative power. **Harry** said of the Structure that it was

> quite amazing actually. I didn't realise how at the bottom I'd got three or four bad things in my life and I didn't realise how severe they were and how good I was at the top because everything at the top were stars and an angel and I've got more good things than bad things really. I figured that if my things are only this small and bad and I've got so much good then I've got so much going for me. So it's just learning to live with the bad things and carrying on going up.

A technical note on the empty chair

In individual therapy, due to the lack of people to play different roles there is more reason to use the empty chair technique, so that significant others, voices or parts of the self can be represented. However, not all clients can use an empty chair. **Jill** did not like using an empty chair:

> It's hard . . . Talking to someone who's not there, pretending someone's there in the room. I can do it in my head but not openly . . . I feel silly, upset, agitated . . . I didn't like talking to an *empty* chair. She spoke of creating music during a session as taking away some of the *emptiness* and complained that in previous experiences of therapy long silences had been unhelpful: You didn't let big *gaps* happen . . . where . . . we just sat there and *nothing* said

*or did anything . . . I can do that and just trap off (dissociate) . . . Of sculpting she said: We did that with animals: it were using something you knew what, **instead of using empty chairs**, something you could see . . .*

From this I wondered if the *empty* chair represented too much emptiness, a lack of someone being available in her life when she needed their presence. Concrete objects (buttons, toy animals) facilitated her ability to play projectively, providing a richer symbol than an empty chair.

A further consideration is whether the empty chair is too large: if a client imagines an abuser or voice in the chair there is a danger that in a regressed child or powerless state they may perceive the abuser or the voice as larger, more powerful than them. An alternative strategy then is to miniaturise the psychodrama, using objects, dolls, puppets, toy theatre or the Five Story Self Structure. An empty (doll's house) toy chair a couple of inches high can contain a voice and so the person themselves be much more powerful and in control.

Psychodrama 5: expressing rage

Having done the above work on his intrapsychic roles, realising that the 'sick patient' felt deep shame and owning his internal condemning judge, **Harry** disclosed the secret he carried: that following observing his father sexually abusing his sister, **Harry**, aged 11, had also sexually abused her. In a psychodrama he talked to his sister, expressing his grief, guilt, regret and hurt. He then returned responsibility to his father. He felt rage at his father for sexually abusing his sister, brother, daughter and girlfriend. He was frightened of his father but also said he loved him so was unable to express this anger. He dissociated to escape from these angry feelings. I offered him a life-sized figure on which to express this rage. This dummy had been made specifically for working with survivors of abuse (Casson, 1990). It was made from foam, cloth and paper. Its purpose was to enable people to safely express murderous rage by being able to attack a figure they could associate with an abuser. I explained that the dummy was for his use and that he did not have to worry if he damaged it. For safety the figure is best placed on a mat and surrounded with cushions.

Harry: Punching that doll was quite a good help really. When I saw that doll it was just a case that I saw my Dad and our Robert (brother) and Keiran (friend): I saw all these people in one go. At first I hesitated because I don't want to go there but I thought, 'Sod it I've got to get this out: I'd rather take it out on this than a proper human being. It would be more safer for everybody,' but my head went: I did blank out when I was hitting the doll I must admit cos I can't remember much of hitting the doll but when I'd finished it was a massive weight coming right off your chest and off your head. It was out. I knew what I'd hit was going to damage nothing else. So I felt a big relief from it. I enjoyed that . . . took a lot of aggression out of me. It was helpful

> because all the hurt I'd had in the past and all the people that'd hurt me; doing that was a good relief: to actually hit something because I'm not a violent person. It takes a lot to get the aggression out of me. I busted its face and everything. It took so much out of me and I sat on the step and I was shaking and crying and it took all that energy. I felt free, Oh I felt free, no problem. Free of my Dad, free of all the bits of problems that my brothers and family had given me. Free totally. It was great, fantastic, couldn't have timed it better.

He ended this cathartic session relieved and smiling, recalling a happy, triumphant memory of clowning in a circus when his creativity had been witnessed and applauded by a large audience.

Psychodrama 6: the good enough father

I had noticed that **Harry** rarely mentioned his daughter, Stella, during the sessions and as he had started his therapy fearful that he would 'touch' her, I was concerned that he consider his daughter's needs before the end of his sessions. Following his disclosure about his relationship with his sister, his grief and the expression of rage at his father, his fears about his relationship with his daughter evaporated: he had in effect separated from his father and could fulfil the father role for his children in a safe and caring way. Half-way through his therapy he began recognising Stella's needs as a girl on the verge of womanhood. Eventually he role reversed with her and told himself that she loved him and that she missed him when he 'switched off' as a coping mechanism when he found things difficult. Following this session **Harry** talked to Stella, apologised to her and re-established his relationship with her.

At his follow-up interview **Harry** reported:

> my daughter at the moment she's trying to learn me numbers in German. We have such a laugh . . . and when she goes to bed I kiss her . . . it's natural now it doesn't feel ugly. I'm being me now. Tremendous. We have a good time now . . . I used to keep the kids distant, didn't want to know, hated them actually, it was so sad . . . It made me think what I was losing. I didn't want to leave it till it was too late. So now I'm making up for a lot of lost time. It's very important to get on with your kids, understand them. If Stella's miserable I go to her and (say), 'You want to talk about anything?' She's getting it off her chest . . . we play . . . laugh . . .

His relationship with his son had also improved: he was able to play football with my son, I talk to him, best I can. **Harry**, in effect, had learned to play during the sessions:

> I can play with my kids better whereas I wouldn't do practically anything but

now I can play with my kids: do what they do, be a right jerk if you have to be,
but it gets a lot of aggression out of you and at the same time it's fun.

Closure

In the final sessions **Harry** returned to his fear that he might be violent. He created
the role of a wise friend and said, 'You're OK – you won't kill: you love life.'
His ability to play compassionate, wise, friendly roles was in stark contrast to his
earlier self-hatred. He had created and thus integrated a positive self-role. He was
able to grieve the end of his therapy, though he complained that a year (forty-four
sessions) was not long enough. His sense of humour had emerged. He was calmer
and more playful. Despite the difficulties in the family the marriage had survived
and his relationships with his children were much improved. He had not been
violent during the period of the therapy and had ceased self-harming. He also
reported that the voices had cut down dramatically; now and again, very rarely
I hear my name being called but it doesn't bother me. At his follow-up interview
a month later he stated: I've not heard any voices since.

Harry's views on his therapy

Half-way through the forty-four sessions **Harry** reported:

> The voices are hardly there now . . . it goes to John and my social worker
> in their own ways they've talked to me and listened to me . . . I'm thinking
> now was it just my own imagination I heard them voices, was it just me
> . . . I know through the time I've been with John something has happened,
> that's stopped me, it hasn't stopped me completely, it has stopped me
> to a large degree, of hearing these voices. Whatever happened I can't really
> explain that. Gradually through the months since I've been with John it's slowly
> gone.

Psychodrama helped **Harry**, who had previously coped by withdrawing from
painful experiences (in an attempt to escape), to face up to things: I recognised
the problem in front of me better and clearer: it's easier to face it than run away
from it . . .

In summary psychodrama psychotherapy resulted in a reduction of **Harry**'s
voices, his potential for violence to others, his self-harming behaviour and suicidal
feelings; it led to an increase in his self-esteem and interpersonal confidence;
improved his social skills, his ability to relate to others and communicate his
feelings; enabled him to think more clearly; gave him a sense that he could control
his anger; expanded his sense of himself, integrating aspect of himself he had
previously split off and projected into voices and visual hallucinations; enabled
him to relax and become more spontaneous, creative, playful; gave him hope for
the future.

Harry told me that psychodrama/therapy had helped me a lot: gave me more self-esteem, helped me collect my thoughts better . . . The therapy that I was doing with you was helping me to relax . . .

Harry told the research assistant that therapy had

> made me less aggressive, have some kind of control over what I do, what I think of my life, to deal with certain situations regarding people . . . I've had so much emotion and so much crap in my head for years and he's helped release a lot of that. I can walk into the streets now head high and not having to look down . . . I'm not as stressed, tense as I used to be . . . Confidence, boost in waking up to reality. I feel happier in myself. I don't feel depressed. If anything does get me down it's for a very short time. I can get out of it and get on with what I'm doing. I don't feel confused. Even when I get in a stress situation I can take the breathing exercises, calm down, go through it slowly . . . Sometimes I've come out of there and a whole lot of pressures come off me so I'm walking free headed. Clearing my mind. Every time I come out of there my head's getting a little clearer.

In his final follow-up research interview **Harry** stated that: The therapy helped . . . (me) be more spontaneous . . . I'm being me now.

Chapter 12

Group psychodrama

Psychodrama has been used with groups of people struggling with psychotic experiences and hallucinations since the 1930s (see Chapter 5). In this chapter I describe my practice. I also present research participants' opinions and relevant theory focusing in particular on the techniques of doubling, mirroring, role reversal, the use of auxiliaries to play roles in a protagonist's drama, concretising, spontaneity and creativity. **Roger** said of psychodrama: I find it very helpful because you can act out your own problems and you can help other people as well at the same time.

Psychodrama and sociodrama enabled group members to explore the voice-hearing experience; to develop coping strategies; to re-enact dreams/nightmares and take control of these intrapsychic dramas; to review and rehearse family scenes or scenes with professionals where protagonists wanted to assert themselves. The method empowers. Psychodrama enabled participants to come closer to significant material, or through the mirror technique, step back and observe themselves. There were many issues people brought to therapy: unfinished business, unresolved traumas, grief, relationship difficulties. Psychodrama offered the opportunity to work through these issues.

Warm-up

Essential to effective living is the ability to warm-up to tasks and roles: to enable us to be appropriately spontaneous. Warm-up may be less necessary in groups of people who are 'self-starters', who have motivation and experience themselves as having the locus of control within themselves. Conversely, for those who have low motivation or who have had experiences where the control was in the hands of another (whether that be an abuser, a voice or a professional) more warm-up activities and spontaneity training will be helpful. Structured group warm-ups to promote cohesion and trust are also more necessary for people who have difficulty relating to others. In addition vulnerable clients may be unable to move directly into personal work and need to work at some distance from their issues. It is therefore useful with people who hear voices and who have psychotic experiences, to work first through structured, supportive exercises such as are outlined in the earlier group dramatherapy chapter (10). As a warm-up to more personal psychodrama, drama on a group theme using hypothetical situations, sociodrama, may enable the group members to work together, become used to creative action methods and still address personal concerns at one remove (see below pp. 198–201 for sociodramas on voices and dreams).

Warm-up operates over time, so that activities one week can stimulate disclosures and work in subsequent group meetings. One day in the men's group we used a colourful parachute, wafting it up and down. This brought the group together in a co-operative activity, was stimulating and fun. **Theo** however found it overwhelming and feared the group were about to attack him. It led in following weeks to his disclosure of being bullied and his psychodrama about that experience (see p. 207). The creative play with the parachute had been a 'warm-up' for his subsequent psychodrama.

Psychodramatising voices

In reply to the question 'What was most helpful?' **Tom** said: It had to be when we acted out the voices.

In one group we worked sociodramatically on the experience of hearing voices: with a hypothetical voice hearer, rather than any one person being the protagonist in the drama. Indeed to further distance themselves from the voice hearing, victim role, the group decided that they would all play the role of voices and I would be the voice hearer. The group members enjoyed playing voices and persecuting me in the role of the voice hearer. **Simon** enjoyed being sadistic and conspiratorial. He said: John did that for us: I described it and he acted it out . . . We did act out some of what I was hearing . . . (He stood on a chair to play the role of a voice), one's coming from higher up. I think that was a bit helpful: it helped explain or describe what was happening. Following this role play **Simon** was more able to stand up for himself. The destructive aggression of voices can be seen as internalised anger directed against the ego because the person fears that if directed externally it would be catastrophically destructive. **Simon** characterised one of his voices as a dangerous psychopath in prison, who gave him 'mental GBH'. **Simon**, a mild-mannered man, encapsulated his own potential destructiveness in this intrapsychic character, thus protecting himself and others from the consequences of the emergence of such feelings and behaviours. In creative play such feelings can be safely expressed. **Theo** and **Pat** also became more aggressive when playing the role of a voice and felt some release of tension as a result. **Simon** noticed a reduction in the aggressiveness of his voice following the above enactment when he played the role of the voice. Using the theory of the explicit and implicit drama (see Chapter 9) I reflect that the explicit drama of the above sociodrama was that the group were exploring the voice-hearing experience; the implicit drama was that they wanted me as therapist to empathise with them, to know what their experience was like and also have power over me, even to be sadistic towards and take control from me as therapist: they were achieving group solidarity and playing together, taking power into their own hands. (It would however be advisable to have a professional auxiliary or co-therapist play such a role: there is some risk in a sole therapist playing such a victim role.) As he developed dramatherapy Slade (1995: 82) observed and supported children's cathartic play in drama sessions whereby they 'spit out' evil and emotions that might otherwise be acted out in illegal or destructive ways. In the theatre a destructive act, such as murder, can be transformed into a creative act, an expressive and safe opportunity to explore our potential for evil. In the above sociodrama the participants were able to express at one remove, through a fiction, sadism and hostility.

In psychodrama voice hearers can talk to their voices played by other people, negotiate, dialogue, rearrange/re-script their inner drama by externalising it. The relationships between the voices and the voice hearer can be sculpted (arranged in symbolic order in space) using other group members or objects, empowering the person to examine the power hierarchies and dynamics of their inner world and explore the possible meanings and identities of the voices. I have suggested that a voice may encapsulate feelings and experiences that cannot otherwise be safely expressed and so playing the role of one of the voices may be potentially overwhelming. For this reason *role reversal with voices should be brief.* When returned to his/her own role the voice hearer may be able to have a dialogue with the voice, answer back and negotiate with the help of another group member playing the role of the voice. It can further be useful then to move the protagonist out into the mirror position to observe the interaction between someone playing his/her role and the auxiliary playing the voice, to gain distance: this can strengthen the observer ego. From the distance of the mirror the protagonist may give themselves instructions on coping or again enter the drama: thus taking greater control and discovering he/she can move between roles and express feelings. The auxiliary can also benefit: playing the role of someone else's voice may be a warm-up to working on their own voice experiences (see sections on the mirror and auxiliary work below).

Such psychodramatic play is healing as it combines both reality and fantasy in the service of the whole person. It brings people together to share their experience and support each other, thus enabling them to break out of pathogenic isolation (see Chapter 2).

Dream psychodrama

Tom: Dreams affect me a lot, at the moment more than voices really . . .

Just as voice hearers may be unable to control their voices so we usually cannot control dreams. Psychodrama offers the opportunity to redream while awake and therefore be in control: to change the dream. This gives people an experience of empowerment instead of powerlessness.

Ben: Sleeping is my weakest point. He was upset by dreams in which he felt physically assaulted by an ***overwhelming*** force.

Several members of a group spoke about their dreams and nightmares but no one individual was prepared to explore a dream: it was too early in the life of the group and members were fearful. I suggested then we create a group dream that combined elements of their experience. The group enjoyed creating this hypothetical dream yet it was clear that they were using their own experience in doing so.

Leah wrote in her journal: Today we talked about dreams . . . mine was about my dad and . . . (when) I was as a child. I hate dreaming about it cause I went through a rough time . . . We also made an image of a dream and acted it out. I was the person who had to run and escape from fear of another person. I think we all enjoyed the role play . . .

In this group dream **Leah** was able to escape, which she had not been able to do when her father had tied her down for a beating.

This sociodrama acted as a warm-up for **Sheila** and the following week she became protagonist in a psychodrama.

Sheila: I had a problem of getting into bed because of nightmares and did a role play about it. I think it's because my Mum died: when she was ill she was in my bed when she was dying, and it must have stuck in my memory and it's just surfaced now . . . That helped a great deal . . . Leah was my Mum, Tom was playing me . . . I think realising the problem was probably down to my mother's death helped because I didn't know what was really causing these dreams and nightmares. It made me come to terms that she's not here anymore and that she is watching over me . . . The hardest part was seeing my Mum in bed again, in my memory, because that's all I remember at the end was her in bed. It was that that upset me really . . . I felt really guilty about it because I was thinking, 'I wish she would die,' because I don't like seeing her the way she is . . . (The psychodrama) was like a flash back to what I was actually going through so it helped because I wasn't having to imagine it: it was actually being role played. I got quite upset, because of the memories. I bottle things up about it anyway. I couldn't carry on: which John understood and we stopped doing it . . . a few days later I settled down a lot in the bedroom and I turned the light on and I thought about things we discussed in the group and that brought me round to feeling more comfortable. I was overcoming the feeling in a few days . . . I've thought less negative thoughts about my mum as well since I've been going to the group. I'm talking to her again. I know she can't hear me. But I'm not getting upset as much as I was before . . .

Roger spoke about a recurring nightmare in which he was unable to rescue a family pet from a fire. We re-enacted the nightmare and then gave him the power to change it, satisfying the act hunger which he had been powerless to fulfil in his paralysed dream role. He could see the dog, whimpering on the other side of a wall of flame. As the fire he identified himself with father's sadistic laughter. **Dave** in the role of the dog said, 'It's not your fault I died.' **Roger** in his own role then confronted his father and told him, 'You have no power now.' He rescued the dog and felt at peace. The following week he reported that the nightmare had not recurred. Goldman and Morrison (1984) also reported success in psychodramatically reworking nightmares:

> the individual enacts the nightmare as it is dreamed and then re-enacts it in a new and more positive way. We have had success in re-training recurring nightmares of Vietnam veterans who previously were unable to divest themselves of the horrors of their wartime experiences.
>
> (Goldman and Morrison, 1984: 25)

I have already likened psychosis to being trapped in a waking nightmare (see Chapter 9). Jung (1960) equated schizophrenia with a conscious dream state. Just as dramatherapists and psychodramatists can work with dream material (Z. Moreno, 1966; Casson, 1999b) so they can work with psychotic images and delusional ideas to achieve a new resolution and empower a previously powerless person.

The psychodrama of an obsessional rumination

Some years ago I had worked with Julia, in a creative dramatherapy group. Diagnosed as paranoid schizophrenic she was suicidal and often asked the question, 'Can God forgive the Devil?' She seemed to identify with the role of the Devil and believed she was irredeemably bad. In the dramatherapy group she played the role of a comic but rather disturbed father and I knew her difficulties went back to her childhood and her relationship with her mentally ill father. However such was her vulnerability and my inexperience that I did not feel it was possible to address this directly at that time and we continued to work creatively at a safe distance. Julia however went on obsessively asking her question: 'Can God forgive the Devil?'

She went into hospital where I was running the in-patient dramatherapy group described in Chapter 10. One day she asked the question again in the group and I felt it was time to psychodramatise this dilemma. I also thought that as she was in hospital she was safely supported and contained by the environment should the work provoke a psychotic reaction. In the group was Nora, another schizophrenic patient, who was a friend of Julia and who was willing to help her explore the question. I invited Nora then to play the role of God (being somewhat manic that day she was happy to do so). Julia in the role of the Devil knelt down and asked, 'Can you forgive me?' I role reversed Julia and Nora and now as the devil Nora asked the question, 'Can you forgive me?' Julia as God replied, 'Of course I can forgive you.' Raising the devil from her kneeling position she hugged her. I role reversed them again so that Julia received this forgiveness and a hug from God. Julia's need to ask this question and her suicidal ideas were thus abated and she was soon able to leave hospital.

This simple drama, looked at through the lens of the explicit/implicit drama theory (see Chapter 9) was effective because it did not plunge Julia back into the hopeless past where she was not able to receive what she needed from her disturbed father. It kept her in the here and now and had a future orientation. Her obsessional rumination was treated as a metaphor and played through to a satisfying conclusion. The explicit drama was between God and the Devil. In the explicit drama Julia was not a powerless child but played powerful roles and was able to get her needs met. The vulnerable ego's fear of the persecutory super-ego was resolved. The implicit drama was of interpersonal warmth and acceptance, forgiveness of herself, the integration of split polarities and friendship. The fragmentary roles were briefly held: Julia was able to inhabit both God and the Devil and return to herself. Bannister's analysis further elucidates this drama: emotionally or sexually abused children, she writes, cannot regard their abusive parent, upon whom they rely for their survival, as 'bad'. 'The children cope with this by designating themselves as "bad" and their abusers as "good" . . . This concept, of being evil or "possessed", is impossible to contain most of the time so the child dissociates and fragments the personality' (Bannister, 2002: 4) In psychodrama these fragments can be presented and played with, much as a child plays different roles and thus integrates these potential selves/roles into a larger theatre of the self (see Chapter 9).

Rehearsals: future projection

In individual and group therapy people can rehearse behaviours. These might be as simple as walking, breathing, singing or develop into practising social skills, assertiveness and ways of coping with voices. Moreno and Moreno (1984: 30) recommend future projections to test out the level of spontaneity a person can achieve in the face of events and as a rehearsal of life skills.

Tom wanted help with his difficulty getting to sleep. We set the scene in his bedroom and he lay in bed, petrified by the voice, unable to move or relax: the voice was . . . like a whispering; SHHHHHH . . . This girl (**Leah**) . . . did it for me, enacting it for me, she did the whispering. (Was that good?) Yeah . . . It was actually getting down to the nitty gritty . . . **Leah** actually identified with what I was saying. **Tom** found it helpful that there was someone who could identify with him, share his experience; he was no longer alone with his fears. To help **Tom** get out of this stuck, frozen place and enable him to think about this problem we played the scene in mirror with **Leah** playing **Tom**'s role in bed while **Roger** played the whispering voice.

From the mirror **Tom** advised himself to move, put the light on, switch the radio on, to look out of the window to see the gas works. I invited him to play the role of the gas works. He introduced himself as an old friend: a familiar, reassuring presence which gave **Tom** a positive message that he could cope. I said to **Tom** in his role as the gas works that he was big and powerful and asked him what he wanted to do. **Tom** expressed his frustration by smashing a cardboard box representing the voice. We then put together these coping strategies and rehearsed him breathing, relaxing, reassuring himself, enjoying the radio, the view from his window and settling down to sleep. I also gave him the information that hypnogogic voices are a normal experience and that they would fade as he went to sleep. (We also discovered that **Tom** was drinking coffee at bedtime, then not sleeping and feeling anxious. Caffeine stimulates tinnitus and anxiety.)

Dramatherapy and psychodrama offer opportunities for behavioural rehearsal. Such rehearsals generalise into behaviour outside the therapy: being able to confront someone in the group enabled **Pat** to confront her husband outside the group.

Sheila: what we do in different weeks I try to bring it into every day life, the problems we have to face, try and overcome them . . . She said that she was asserting herself in response to her sister: I'm answering her back now, standing up for myself . . .

Leah found it helpful to rehearse having conversations: we listed topics and practised in pairs: I learned a lot about making conversations . . . outside I thought about what we said and I used that information to help me make conversation. **Leah** felt more confident and she was able to break out of her isolation. Psychodrama facilitates encounter and relationships in the here and now. Rehearsals, which Moreno (1985) termed spontaneity training and role practice, have a future orientation, focus on problems and behaviour, and are empowering. Rehearsals in group therapy involved social skills practice as part of the process: turn taking, helping others, observing, listening.

Auxiliary work

In psychodrama members of the group play auxiliary roles in the protagonist's drama. **Leah** benefited from **Tom**'s psychodrama as she also heard whispering voices. She played both the voice role and the voice hearer role so the psychodrama was, by proxy, her own drama. Voices can be worked with by auxiliaries at a safe distance, bringing what is invisible and so perhaps intractable, into present, visible reality so it can be worked with and the protagonist gain some control. Zerka Moreno (1978: 164–165) writing about the functions of the auxiliary ego in psychodrama with psychotic patients, lists these as follows:

1   To play the role required (whether this be real or imaginary, alive or dead,

past, present, or future, an hallucination or delusion) and to do so as faithfully to the perception of the protagonist as possible.

2   To investigate, through the role play, how the protagonist perceives the relationship between him/herself and this role.

3   To interpret the role, expressing how this person/role may be feeling in relation to the protagonist, even exaggerating if this would clarify essential issues between them.

4   To act as a therapeutic guide to greater intrapsychic and interpersonal harmony or, if this is not possible, to a separation from the other.

5   To function as a bridge to assist the protagonist's return to the social world.

I would add to this list

6   To trust their intuitions arising during the role play and use these until corrected by the protagonist or director.

7   To accept the directions of the protagonist or director.

To fulfil these complex functions seems to call for extensive training and Moreno did work with professional auxiliaries. However he also used fellow patients to play roles and valued their spontaneity and empathic understanding of the protagonist's experience. He also recognised that auxiliaries can gain therapeutic benefit from playing such roles. I worked without trained auxiliaries and can confirm the ability of clients to do a 'good enough' job of playing roles with brief guidance from the protagonist and director. **Sheila** discovered an ability to play roles in psychodrama; she felt empowered, competent, able to help others: I like helping people and when I was asked to help I felt I was being included in the group as a person . . . When it was for other people it was hard to do but it felt good because you were helpful to the other person. (See Yalom (1985: 13) on the therapeutic value of altruism.) On another occasion **Leah** was able to express some of her own rage by hitting a cardboard box when playing an auxiliary role in **Roger**'s psychodrama. In planning a psychodrama service it would be wise to work in a team (see Chapter 14) but professionals must not underestimate (and so disempower) the ability of clients to help each other or benefit from playing auxiliary roles. A trained auxiliary could be useful if no client wanted to play a needed role or when the role might involve regression or potentially traumatic vulnerability.

Doubling

A double is an auxiliary who helps a protagonist express feelings by speaking as if they were that person. The protagonist can then own these feelings or correct the double. For people who cannot feel, or express their feelings, or who have not had a sufficiently empathic advocate or witness in their life, the double is especially helpful (see Foreword). Zerka Moreno (1978: 165) lists the task of the double:

1   To accurately represent invisible dimensions of the protagonist, copying their body language, facial expressions, vocal tone. This includes vocalising inarticulate parts of the self: the double is an intrapsychic role.
2   To express how the protagonist feels about themselves (the autotele, see Chapter 11).
3   To interpret the protagonist to him/herself.
4   To act as a catalyst to bring the various parts of the protagonist to greater integration.
5   To help the protagonist to rejoin the social world after having reached a deeper level of self-revelation and affirmation.

Leah found doubling enabled her to express her feelings instead of being silent. She valued the empathic witness of the double. **Leah** and **Sheila** were able to double for **Roger** who was not aware of his anger (though he was frightened of an angry voice): with the help of these doubles he was able to identify the sources of his anger and express these feelings for himself.

Protagonists can also play their own double role: in her individual therapy **Gloria** had fallen silent, unable to voice her own feelings. I explained the method of the double. After demonstrating this I invited her to be her own double. From this role she disclosed the rape she had not been able to speak of in her own role.

The 'containing double', an adaptation of the method developed by Hudgins *et al.* (2000; see also Kellermann and Hudgins, 2000: 250–251) is helpful in reducing dissociation and can prevent a protagonist being overwhelmed.

Mirror

This psychodrama technique involves the protagonist stepping outside their own drama and watching, as if in a mirror, someone else play their role. The method provides distance, strengthens the observer ego (Casson, 1998b) and offers an opportunity for the protagonist to adjust his/her autotele (their relationship with and view of themselves).

People who have psychotic experiences have difficulty in establishing the boundaries between self and other. They may project out of the self, into the other, aspects of the self and then subconsciously sense that the other is part of the self. To escape this dilemma the person withdraws into isolation, yet the extrojected aspects of the self return to haunt the person. To recover the person must eventually return to the social world and own their projections. Here group therapy proves its value as it provides a safe micro-society. The mirror technique is especially useful in gaining a sense of separate, boundaried self in relation to others. To have a sense of self we must be able to recognise ourselves in a mirror: to be both subject and object to ourselves, an 'I' and a 'me' and to differentiate ourselves from others (see Thomas, 1997: 192). The mirror technique facilitates this development. It offers an opportunity to see the self and, at the same time, others in relation to the self. It validates the person's experience and gives them sufficient distance to think through that experience. It can also remove a protagonist from a potentially overwhelming scene and enable them to gain sufficient distance to work through the problem presented by the mirror, as in **Tom**'s and **Sheila**'s bedroom psychodramas, above. The mirror can thus expand a person's awareness of the self. Speaking of the mirror technique **Sheila** said: Actually seeing yourself really as other people see me . . . I found when people were acting it out for myself I saw a different part of what I was actually experiencing.

Tom found it helped him communicate more with others about himself: I think it was quite amazing: you could prompt them where they were going wrong . . . It got people to know more about you than just if you told them yourself.

Role reversal

In role reversal the protagonist plays the role of the significant other. Through doing so the protagonist may temporarily own aspects of the self they had previously split off and projected into the other or gain greater understanding of the other.

Tom: We did a lot of what you call role reversal . . . It was quite hard. (He thought it was very helpful and) challenging really to see if you could do it, put yourself in someone else's shoes . . .

From the distance of the other the protagonist can then look back at themselves and gain greater understanding of the self, as **Pat** said of role reversal: It goes back to seeing myself through other people's eyes.

Roger described role reversing with another person as looking through the window of another person's soul, was a spiritual feeling, very helpful.

For two weeks after he role reversed with Jesus and gave himself a message of hope and love, 'Stay alive, for God's sake, stick with it,' **Anton** did not hear any voices. He said he found it helpful to step outside himself.

People must however have the right to refuse. **Dave** refused to role reverse with a psychotic friend: he found the idea disturbing as he feared losing touch with reality.

Concretising

In psychodrama abstract, emotional or imaginary elements can be dramatically symbolised by concrete objects or people. People who are already 'concrete' in their thinking can benefit from active ways of symbolising and expressing things.

Gloria valued the role play where you allocate an object to each source and play out each situation – I was in so much pain I couldn't see it – it helped me to see it, I've got several ways: concretising helped see it and sort it out.

Tom, speaking of sculpting, arranging objects or people in role, in symbolic order, found it more helpful to have people playing the roles: It's much better when it's enacted: you have to use your imagination when someone's talking to you but when they're actually showing you it becomes more realistic.

Sheila said that having voices represented by members of the group – not empty chairs – was very helpful. It made it clearer in your mind what was actually going on.

Roger said it was helpful to imagine someone in a chair as his voice: the voices did have different personalities. In response to the question 'Is talking to your voices as if they were sitting in empty chairs helpful or not?' **Dillon** stated: I don't do this often, but when I do, it helps me get an experiential grasp of reality. Knowing that the owner of the voice is non-existent helps cull the incipient paranoia and gives me a sense of control over the unknown.

The answer to the dilemma whether to use an empty chair for a voice, use an object or put an auxiliary into the role may be to give the protagonist the choice, thus enabling them to have control. The time to use an object, not an auxiliary, is when there is a threat of violent feelings being expressed.

Catharsis

Theo was frightened by the billowing of the parachute when the group were playing with it. **Anton** said the parachute lets out anger and frustration. The following week **Theo** expressed his frustration and aggression by kicking the large inflatable globe. **Theo** started his psychodrama on his voices by telling the group that he heard shouts of 'Fuck off' from white vans. **Dillon** enjoyed playing these voices: the role gave him an opportunity to express his own aggression. **Theo** was able to join in with this shouting and laugh at the swearing. He then connected the swearing to his experience of being bullied as an apprentice: I was 17 when Jamieson (a supervisor) used to shout at me. I was skinny: he was fat. Pinned me against wall and swore, 'I'll kick your fucking arse.' (He) hit me with a paint brush. I was **frightened to death** of Jamieson. **Roger** played the role of Jamieson and **Theo** confronted him, telling him he was angry with him for the bullying. **Theo** psychodramatically slapped Jamieson (slapping the air in front of him while a group member clapped and **Roger** reacted as if slapped. There was no actual violence to a person). I then role reversed **Theo** into the Jamieson role and asked him if he was responsible for bullying **Theo**. Jamieson confessed and apologised to **Theo**. I role reversed **Theo** back into his own role and **Roger**, as Jamieson, took responsibility and apologised to **Theo**. This work led to much sharing in the group of their experience of being bullied and the voices as bullies. The following week **Theo** said the psychodrama had empowered him to cope with the voice; he recognised that he heard the voice particularly when feeling vulnerable. **Theo**: When you shouted 'fuck off' in the group it helped. Now he was able to say 'Fuck off' to the voice so that it went away. I answer voices and tell it to go away . . . (I'm) able to use swear words now. The psychodrama on the voice gave him insight and catharsis. He was able to own some of his aggression through kicking the world ball and hitting cushions: he also gave himself permission to swear.

One of **Roger**'s voices told him to throw his coffee mug at the TV set, smashing it. The fear that he would feel compelled to do this blighted his life at home. We enacted the scene. It emerged that he was very angry with his aunt for her controlling behaviour. **Leah** doubled him and enjoyed expressing her own anger through this role. In the role of the voice **Roger** used a length of pipe insulation material and battered a cardboard box.

Roger: It's all been very helpful, especially when we talked about my aunty coming over from Canada and when we acted it out and all the anger what were inside me and when you gave me that piece of piping to hit the cardboard boxes.

This catharsis provides further evidence that voices encapsulate unexpressed emotion.

Coloured lights

At my private practice and in the studios at two mental health centres where I conducted therapy there are coloured spot lights. They are used for drama and relaxation sessions. In other rooms it may be possible to vary the light levels with curtains and using what lighting control is possible: sadly many professional spaces only have brilliant, rather oppressive strip lights. **Gloria** found the possibility of changing the lights useful. She said that it gives you an element of control; also helps to put you at ease. The lights help with mood enhancement . . . Helps in creating an environment in which you are comfortable.

Sheila: The lighting helped: we had coloured lights. It made the room seem bigger . . .

Deane and Hanks (1967) reported on the value of coloured lighting and its use in psychodrama, enabling people to have control, to get in touch with feelings and significant scenes in the past. In dream and deathbed scenes subdued, blue lighting was especially helpful to deepen the feeling quality of the drama. At the end of such a drama bringing the lights up signals a return to the here and now social reality (as opposed to dramatic or surplus reality).

Spontaneity and creativity

Moreno (1983, 1985) based the method of psychodrama on his research into spontaneity and creativity. He defined the former thus:

Spontaneity operates in the present, now and here; it propels the individual towards an adequate response to a new situation or a new response to an old situation.

(Moreno, 1993: 13–14)

Jimmy responded positively to the opportunity to be spontaneous: I just plunge in: spontaneity is the best answer: don't think about it for too long or it will get stale. Spontaneity can take place only in the here and now. It therefore can help people to be in the present moment instead of dissociated. The presentation of new stimuli in dramatherapy and psychodrama can motivate, lift mood and nurture spontaneity and creativity. **Jimmy** appreciated something new and pleasant each time: creative . . . bringing something new into the group which allows the individual to be able to contribute rather than being inhibited. Even allowing the inhibited person in the group to express themselves without putting pressure on them.

Voices occur spontaneously. Sometimes this is in response to stress and at other times to a lack of stimuli or sensory deprivation: the brain creates its own stimulus. Moreno regarded hallucinations and delusions as a creative attempt to resolve intrapsychic and interpersonal difficulties when a more appropriate response was not within the person's repertoire. The aim of psychodrama then is to bring people gradually, through the enactment of their pathological spontaneity, to a more appropriate spontaneity. Moreno (1971, 1985) believed that spontaneity could be trained. Inappropriate, impulsive or pathological spontaneity can lead to unsuccessful, problematic and destructive acts. **Cheryll**, unable to contain her anger any longer, smashed a cup in the hospital ward toilet and was forcibly injected with tranquillising medication. Both patient and staff were unable to act with more appropriate spontaneity. Destructiveness may result from the release of pent up, frustrated energy (in nature an earthquake, in a child a tantrum, in a nation civil war). The structures of dramatherapy and psychodrama offer a '*whelm*' (a boundaried container, see Chapter 7) to channel such energy, preventing it from becoming *overwhelming* or destructive, to achieve healthier results that raise, rather than lower, self-esteem.

Dillon wrote: The state of total creativity is God. God spends half his time destroying.

Moreno would agree with **Dillon**'s first statement: 'God is spontaneity' (Moreno, 1971: xviii); 'in God all spontaneity has become creativity' (Moreno, 1993: 11). Moreno (1993: 11) knew that spontaneity did not necessarily lead to creativity: 'an individual may have a high degree of spontaneity but be entirely uncreative.' Indeed they may be destructive to themselves and others. To protect themselves from being overwhelmed by painful experience people may block out thoughts, feelings, memories and so block their spontaneity and potential growth. Psychodrama aims to enable spontaneity to be fulfilled in creative ways: enabling people to feel, think, remember and rediscover their potential. Moreno (1985: 90, 91, 101) stated that spontaneity creates, energises and unifies the self. 'As spontaneity declines the self shrinks. When spontaneity grows the self expands' (Moreno, 1983: 8).

Spontaneity and creativity can strengthen a person's sense of self, agency and ability to relate to others. In summary psychodrama can enable people to achieve a more successful warm-up, more appropriate spontaneity, more satisfying creativity.

When is psychodrama not helpful?

Psychodrama is a powerful method and can be overwhelming. Given the vulnerability of this client group, it may well be useful to work at greater distance through dramatherapy methods and to offer spontaneity training. People who hear voices have difficulty concentrating and to ensure they are not overwhelmed psychodramas are more likely to be brief vignettes rather than two-hour epics. Moreno (1939: 6) insisted that protagonists had the right to stop dramas: indeed to do so gave them a greater sense of the locus of control being in their own hands. **Sheila** chose to stop her drama when she felt an upsurge of emotion: her grief frightened her. Nevertheless she did benefit from the work as far as it went.

The timing of a psychodrama is also important. **Tina** told a research assistant: We had a drama about my son. He's not speaking to me. Don't ask me why: I don't know. It's very hurtful. I'm hurt. I just mentioned it (in the group. John said:) 'Would you like to do something with this.' I said, 'Yes.' (We then enacted the conversation she planned to have next time she saw him. Did that help?) No, I was anxious for two days afterwards. (**Jimmy** played the role of son and became upset/angry.) It seems like it was **too much** for him . . . At the time it was a bit depressing, not a lot. It set me off. I felt awful, I shouldn't have said anything. I didn't want all that. I don't like conflict: it causes me anxiety.

Jimmy said that role reversing was stressful. When he played **Tina**'s teenage son it reminded him of his own teenage situation. **Jimmy** was aroused by his own material and was unable to hold this auxiliary role appropriately for **Tina**. He had not had sufficient time to learn the psychodrama method. A trained auxiliary would have been better able to play the role needed. My perception is that it was too early in the group to do a psychodrama: it was just the second session. Cox (1978b) has written about the importance of timing in the therapeutic process. However, when **Jimmy** came to the next session he said he'd found the opportunity to express his feelings helpful.

Group psychodrama can be empowering. However, the psychodramatist's enthusiasm for the method may overpower the client and this needs to be continuously checked: namely that the method is at the service of the client, not the client (or the therapist) enthralled by the method. The therapist's skill is in being able to follow the group and the protagonist's needs through an often chaotic, spontaneous process which moves between different realities and to bring the whole to a containing conclusion. There must be sufficient time for the sharing and closure section of the session and group members need to end the session grounded in the here and now social reality, prepared to go out into the world.

Coleman (1998), a voice hearer who had been diagnosed schizophrenic, became a leading figure in the British Hearing Voices Movement. He regarded his experience of psychodrama at an NHS therapeutic community as contributing to his recovery. His opinion was that *Psychodrama should be encouraged between consenting adults. Psychodrama must be non-controlling, based on the person's view of the world, built on the relationship* (with the therapist).

In the next chapter we listen further to the opinions of voice hearers about dramatherapy and psychodrama.

Chapter 13

What is helpful and not helpful in dramatherapy and psychodrama

In this chapter I report on the research participants' opinions about their experience of dramatherapy and psychodrama. The research falls into the fifth category of evidence for particular interventions, under the UK Department of Health (DoH) National Service Framework for Mental Health, namely: '**Type V**: evidence – expert opinion, including the opinion of users and carers' (DoH, 1999: 6).

The research aimed to give the participants a voice: to value their opinions. From these I have been able to develop guidelines for good practice, which are in the final chapter: this chapter then provides the evidence base for those guidelines.

Play and fun

The analysis of the research questionnaire revealed that participants regarded fun as the single most helpful element in dramatherapy and psychodrama. I therefore advocate a view of the therapist as playmate rather than analyst.

> It is in playing and only in playing that the individual child or adult is able to be creative and use the whole personality, and it is only in being creative that the individual discovers the self.
>
> (Winnicott, quoted by Goldschmied, 1987: 52)

The self is re-created through play. Moreno's view (1985: 91, 101) was that the self emerged through, indeed was created by, spontaneity. I have described the psychotic person as having lost their self (see Chapter 3). It is through play, spontaneity and creativity that the self is rediscovered, reclaimed, reborn.

Fun has intrapsychic and interpersonal benefits: it is a potent antidepressant and stimulant; it can be cathartic, providing relief from tension. Laughter allows the expression of hostility in a socially acceptable way; promotes breathing and relaxation; brings pleasure, energy, and eventually a peaceful, harmonious calm. Fun also is motivating: it encourages spontaneity, innovation and is contagious: people playing together 'share a laugh', enjoy companionship. Humour can also distance us: comedy makes an event that would be tragedy if we were closer to it, bearable. Humour plays with distance: sometimes telescoping polarities and making the impossible happen. It liberates us from the gravity of everyday reality. The bathos of humour punctures grandiosity and over-seriousness: thus it counters overdistance, bringing people together in playful relationship. Such levity promotes buoyancy in situations that might otherwise be overwhelming. Sometimes voices tell jokes with the result that people laugh at 'inappropriate' times. Perhaps such intrapsychic humour helps people survive!

Humour and play can be experienced as childish, daft, silly. People may have been shamed during their childhood and told they are silly or daft. As adults they may feel fearful of being foolish in dramatherapy. McLuskie (1983: 21) commenting on dramatherapy in a psychiatric hospital, pointed out that 'the whole energies of a patient are concentrated on the difficult task of presenting as "normal" and to be asked to deviate in any way from this tightly held conformity can seem a real threat.' The dramatherapist must be careful to choose activities that are appropriate so that people are gradually able to play without shame.

'Daft time'

Pat found dramatherapy liberating: I found it helpful, very helpful. I looked forward to Monday when it was coming: I knew it was 'daft time' . . .

Jenny relished being able to let your hair down and mess about . . .

Dave wrote in his journal: It's so good to act silly; to have fun as a child – to really have a laugh in a way I haven't played since a small child feeling intimidated, scared, guilty, responsible and alone . . . It's good to be loud without feeling someone will think I'm an idiot if they overhear and to use imagination in games in a seemingly trivial and childish way but feeling good about it.

People who have been abused or experienced other blocks to their development, may not be able to play. Therapy then must enable them to play without shame.

> Childhood abuse robs people of their childhood. It also steals off with their capacity to enjoy life . . . Many of our patients . . . could not laugh, relax . . . one of our functions was to create an environment within which fun could occur . . . fun . . . is a spontaneous, creative event.
>
> (Bloom, 1997: 170)

Winnicott declared:

> Psychotherapy has to do with two people playing together. The corollary of this is that where playing is not possible then the work of the therapist is directed towards bringing the patient from a state of not being able to play into a state of being able to play.
>
> (Winnicott, 1991: 38)

Jenny: I thought sometimes, 'What is the point of that . . . something like playing with the buttons and the toys: it was a bit childish and a bit silly but having said that when we'd done it and I got into doing it I enjoyed it, making up my own little games . . . At the beginning I thought I'm not doing that . . . Once you got into doing it . . . We played.

Simon: it's based on play: a bit on the silly side. He said the voices didn't like him playing: they judged it as childish.

Of exploring the space **Tom** said: I thought it was a bit daft. It was useful because it broke the ice between us. A lot of what John did was a bit childish, basic things, I could understand it: like playing with dolls . . . I can see now but at the time I thought, 'Ooh it's a bit namby pamby this.'

Conversely **Theo** found that fun and laughter: gets rid of a feeling of being daft – helps relaxation, gets rid of daft thoughts – helps get rid of negative thoughts.

Harry agreed: it gets you out of the boring part of yourself . . .

Fun motivates

Furthermore **Harry** asserted that: Without having fun in therapy you would not go: it would be just boring, depressing. You've got to have fun.

Cheryll agreed: It's active, fun, motivating . . .

The variety of dramatherapy also motivated **Tom**: I'd been to Hearing Voices groups . . . they were similar but I dropped out of them because I just felt we were going over the same ground all the time . . . I got a bit bored with it. It hasn't happened with John because it's always something different.

Laughter as defence

Freud's view of laughter as a defence is borne out by some participants' statements:

> Laughter hides my fears.
> (Men's group song)

In response to fear people may feel hostile. Laughter can express hostility. Smiling at strangers is a paradoxical signal: friendly and defensive, disarming their potential threat by suggesting we too might have teeth! **Anton** said he sometimes laughed too much in a giddy, anxious way: others experienced this as potentially hostile and so he feared they might attack him. Manic laughter can defend against grief and helplessness.

Diane: I've no idea what to do: I just laugh my head off. I just get so high I just start laughing.

Pat and her sister, as children, coped with their mother's bizarre behaviour (due to her manic depressive illness) by laughing. She later felt that laughter was not OK. In therapy she was again able to laugh freely: laughter helped her gain some distance and relax.

Humour and distance

Laughter may help by reducing distance: **Sheila** said laughing is very helpful: it helps breaks down barriers.

In one drama **Dillon**'s vicious killer voice became like Basil Fawlty, strutting and ridiculous. Through bathetic humour **Dillon** was rebalancing the over-seriousness of his grandiosity. Bokun (1986) has suggested humour therapy as an antidote to the over-seriousness of people diagnosed with schizophrenia. Humour brings us down to earth: **Dillon**'s delusional ideas about extraterrestrial deities needed such earthy humour to counterbalance their lofty pretension. Asked to recall a helpful time in the dramatherapy group **Dillon** spoke of the sessions when Dave played a woolly mammoth. I created a woolly mammoth out of an elephant. This hilarious scene was much enjoyed by the group as it involved artificial insemination. **Dave** enjoyed playing the role of the woolly mammoth: he rediscovered his sense of humour. In this comic scene he was reborn: from extinct, frozen, lost creature he re-emerged through a female elephant. This scene had much meaning for **Dave** who felt he had died as a child. **Dillon**, who was normally an isolate, was, in this improvisation, symbolically co-creating with **Dave**, new life and sharing the joke with others.

Laughter may help by increasing distance

In Sri Lanka, over the course of an all-night dramatic healing ritual, horrific demons gradually become ridiculous until the patient of the exorcism laughs at what was originally terrifying and then is able to dismiss them (Casson, 1979).

Speaking of a dramatherapy session **Tom** said:

> We did a particularly good one last week: he (J.C.) said, 'If the voices were happening . . . what good thing could you think of?' And I thought of Clive James because the television show's particularly funny . . . the laughter made a difference towards the scaredness. So I thought, 'I'll think about Clive James see if, or George Kennedy in Airplane . . . or some daft thing,' and it worked for me that . . . particularly Clive James, it's 'cause it's funny and it's normal.

Ben: having fun – we had relaxation, to forget some of the problems.

For someone who is overwhelmed by problems, being able to distance himself from, even to temporarily forget them, might not be anti-therapeutic avoidance. Indeed to discover that he could have fun with others, instead of paranoid hostility, was therapeutic for **Ben**.

The therapeutic value of laughter

Anton: laughter's the best medicine. (He also referred to the woolly mammoth scene.)

Sheila: because we were all involved, it was fun, we all had a laugh . . . I was laughing more at myself . . . that was really good fun . . . (Fun): yes that was really helpful: we had some good laughs in the group.

Moreno wanted to be remembered as the man who brought laughter into psychiatry through psychodrama (Z. Moreno *et al.*, 2000: 24). Dramatherapy can enable people who are chronically miserable to have fun.

Pat: It's good fun. **You get so bogged down with the seriousness** . . . you feel as if you're always moaning and groaning. After a time in therapy **Pat** described her family laughing together: she found that as she was more able to play with her own children, more able to moderate her anger through playful humour, they were more able to engage together rather than retreat into hostile camps.

Of his work with psychiatric patients Bolton (1979: 13) wrote: 'Perhaps one of the most subtle techniques I have had to learn is to relieve tension with laughter.'

Simon: It helps to have some distraction . . . a bit of amusement: my life is full of serious subjects . . . It's difficult for me to laugh when I'm so oppressed . . . It always helps to have a bit of a laugh occasionally: it **raises your spirits** if you've had voices on you for years . . . We had hats: a bit of a laugh: I chose a Railway hat, I used to work for them. We were having a laugh and joke to **lighten things up.**

Jenny: I think if you bring a bit of **light heartedness** it takes off some of the strain. It did for me . . . it relaxes you a bit . . . it can be fun and there's a fun element and there's a serious side . . . it did make it easier. Takes the pressure away from the situation you're talking about.

Jimmy felt lighter: It's a little bit of magic that just works with me . . . I've expressed myself in such a way **it's taken so much off my mind** that I couldn't give a damn how schizophrenic I am . . . The whole of his concept was sound, working with schizophrenia. It drew out different expressions of our illness. Having fun doing it.

Harry: It (fun) took a lot of tension out of you . . . makes you feel better, instead of coming out depressed and moody.

The heaviness of depression is often composed of repressed anger and aggression: the lightness of humour and play can safely release these, be antidepressant and promote *buoyancy* (see Chapter 7). When **Tina** was depressed she lost her sense of humour and fun: through dramatherapy she got that back: I do like to laugh . . . I think laughter is a good medicine . . .

Power and control

Those activities in dramatherapy and psychodrama that resulted in participants having some power and control over the space and action were regarded as generally the most helpful. Among these activities were creating a safe, personal space in the room; setting the scene (using furniture or other objects); arranging objects or people in the space to represent different things (sculpting); exploring the space in the room; being able to change the lighting in the space; walking about the room; being able to conduct a ritual in the space. Given that I was seeing people in professional spaces this made me realise that it is the professional who usually has control over the space: what's in it, who sits where, what behaviours are accepted or discouraged. For people to choose where to sit, to get up and walk around, to lie on the floor, to move chairs, to take up space, was empowering. Such control, through which people could own the space and achieve the interpersonal distance they needed, resulted in the space becoming safe and the therapy not being overwhelming: they had some power and choice. The audience chairs (see Chapter 10) were the first signal that this was possible. The chairs represented a safe place and symbolised the right to say 'No/Stop' or withdraw.

In my experience as a therapist this issue of control is often experienced in the body: a sense of someone/something having control of the body. Dramatherapy and psychodrama, in using physical activities, can foster a greater sense of physical self-control and empowerment.

Leah: we talked about self-control and lack of power in a person. We gave ourselves two characters, one (of) which was the boss and the other the followers . . . We did a role play . . . I liked being in charge and give orders.

Jenny liked playing another character: Because you're not yourself. You just seemed to have a bit more control when you're doing something when you're not yourself: it seems you're able to do whatever you want: there's no comeback on me: there's the freedom to do whatever, say whatever.

In both dramatherapy and psychodrama action methods enabled participants to take power into their own hands:

Jenny: I feel more empowered to cope . . . Now I am, I'm standing up for myself a bit more. I am feeling stronger. (Speaking about the Five Story Self Structure: see Chapter 6) I was in control of what was happening . . . because of seeing John I decided to do other things, doing more things for myself, taking more control of my life and standing up for myself.

Empowerment leads to confidence and a consequent rise in self-esteem and motivation:

Gloria (Have you changed?): I'm a lot more in control of my life . . . it (dramatherapy) helps you to do the healing itself, to be instrumental in helping yourself, empowering rather than just taking medication which makes me anxious because of the high dose: it helped me understand why I was having problems.

Taking control then may mean a change in the personality:

Cheryll: Part of the year the voices disappeared altogether. I was relieved and liked that but then other things started happening – I seemed to take a loud/dominant role – the voices made me meek.

Conversely, **Harry** stated that therapy had made me less aggressive, have some kind of control over what I do, what I think of my life, to deal with certain situations regarding people.

> Persons who felt empowered in therapy spent less time in hospitals, expected a shorter stay in therapy and knew more about their problems.
>
> (Coursey *et al.*, 1995: 283)

Dramatherapy has also offered a safe experience of letting go of control:

Jimmy: in the group: it's OK to be **schizophrenic . . . 'a thing that is out of control'**. We play at being out of control: it's exciting. We're bouncing around the room. It's good to be able to express how you feel, because if you're spinning **out of control** and you've got no direction in your life then you've got this ability to put things in perspective for your self later because it gets it out of your system. I like it . . . it doesn't half give me a break . . . (speaks of the tension of presenting himself as 'normal', in control.) It relieves the tension (to be out of control).

This was also reflected in **Pat**'s relief at being able to have what she called her 'daft time' once a week. (See section on Fun, pp. 212–14.) Such freedom releases and enriches. Speaking of a session when we threw coloured cloth on the floor as if action painting, **Jimmy** said: I was **enriching** my life with the colours . . . I was feeling like there's a *free abandonment of my spirit* there and what it is to be creative. I was *abandonly* throwing cloth into the room . . .

Flexibility and freedom

Speaking of dramatherapy **Pat** said: It's *flexible* and you can mould it.

The flexibility of dramatherapy and psychodrama can promote greater flexibility in participants. Previous research by Grainger (1990) showed that one of the benefits of dramatherapy was to enable people to become more flexible. Speaking of his individual and group dramatherapy therapy **Dillon** stated: I'm more *flexible* – I was getting too rigid.

Dave wrote in his journal: The great thing about these groups John is that you are *free* to be what you want: – An adult, a child, thoughtful, flippant, sad, happy, you have *freedom* gained from shared and directed trust to be anything . . . I'm actually feeling stronger and more confident by expressing my feelings and insecurities in this controlled/metamorphic group situation.

Showing rather than telling

For some less verbally articulate people physical action and movement helped them express themselves more, to *show* rather than *tell* how they felt:

Diane said that dramatherapy was

helpful in the sense that I've had someone to sound off to, to be able to talk, to *show someone*, and express to someone how I feel . . . *I felt I could show you how I feel* . . . even if I didn't want to say it, I could express it how I felt . . . I needed more of those activities: (drama, symbolic work) because it was easier to explain, it was easier to understand, it was easier to *show*, rather than talking and being upset.

Psychodrama encourages people to show, rather than tell, how they felt. Action empowers.

Tom: It's much better when it's enacted: you have to use your imagination when someone's talking to you but when they're actually *showing* you it becomes more realistic.

For someone to be able to show or tell of their experiences there must be an audience: in the first instance this is the therapist, later there may be a group audience. (The word 'audience' derives from the Latin 'audire', to hear.) In considering individual and group therapy therefore we must first consider what participants in the research found helpful or not helpful in the behaviours of the therapist.

Therapist skills and qualities

What people have found helpful above all in me, as a therapist, has been my capacity to listen without judging and, as one person put it, my ability not only to listen but also to *hear* what people are saying. Other qualities that they have appreciated are my ability to be dependable, respectful, trustworthy, supportive, positive, warm, safe, playful. Therapist skills they have appreciated have been my facilitation of group process, holding the boundaries of time and space, being both professional and yet relaxed/calm/informal, my ability to share my own experiences, be creative, to motivate, not pushing yet confronting in a supportive way. It was my ability to relate, to establish a warm, friendly relationship that formed the basis of all therapeutic work. In research into what people with serious mental illness wanted in individual therapy, 'Friendliness was the quality most desired in a therapist' (Coursey *et al.*, 1995: 283).

Tom: I like his presence as a personality: he's particularly friendly. He's always reassuring . . . other groups in the past I left it because I was getting a bit paranoid . . . in this group I felt all right . . . he's a very polite man. He's not overpowering, he's very easy to get along with.

Jill: We've been building up trust, it does take me a while to get to know folk . . . He's very friendly, puts you at ease . . . I liked him very much as a person as well. I found him very easy to talk to. He's a very colourful character. He's very open. If something's happened to him that's related to what (had happened to you) . . . he'll talk about that with you, not too personal but he has . . . like when he broke his leg how he felt . . . it's made you more equal: more's (like) going to see a friend and having a good chat than you know . . . I found him very professional as well . . . (with John) It's more level, you're more 1 to 1, it's more of a person to person, than a professional to a client. He doesn't look down on you . . .

I have tried to strike a balance between being supportive, accepting and sometimes confronting, while not pushing people beyond what they are ready to do or face.

Sheila: He's got a relaxing voice, he doesn't raise his voice, he calmly tells you . . . If he did have to challenge you he wouldn't come across as an angry person.

Two people wanted me to be more audible/visible:

Cheryll: You don't talk enough – you are the tree – I like that but I've got to come out of that. You're a faceless presence.

Jill: He doesn't push you, sometimes I think he'd better do . . . Sometimes I think he lets me get away with wittering . . . he lets me talk about general things

. . . (I need) a bit more guidance . . . sometimes I feel I'm repeating myself . . . If he gave me his opinion a bit more . . . on how things have gone or what I've said, his opinion . . . I'd like that, not whether he approves or disapproves, sometimes he seems too level. I'd like him a bit more involved. To participate a bit more: 'Let's try this . . . I'd like us to do this . . . I think we might try this to help with that problem we talked about last time.' I'd see him a bit more of an ally than someone to sound off on. I can talk to him a bit more and trust him. He's still a bit detached, (I want him to be more of) an ally in the fight against the demons!

Following this feedback I did change the way I was working: I had been over-cautious, intending to ensure I was not overpowering: **Jill** hereby asked for more when perhaps she was ready for a challenge. **Anton** however said that it would be unhelpful if the therapist was: Pushing things, making them rush. The balance between motivating and yet not pressurising, between waiting for the person to be ready and giving permission, even modelling playfulness, has not been easy to achieve: I have been a prompter, waiting in the wings, for just that fulcrum moment to offer the useful stimulus to enable the person to take the next step (Jennings, 1990; Cox and Theilgaard, 1994).

At her final follow-up interview **Jenny** said it had been helpful that:

(a) There were no pressure. (b) You didn't let big gaps happen . . . where . . . we just sat there and nothing said or did anything . . . 'cause . . . I can do that and just trap off . . . (and that as a therapist I offered) (c) Listening and (d) some of the guidance . . . of how to cope or what to do . . . without being pressured.

The skills of the group facilitator

The skills of the group facilitator can enable a positive group process. The participants' opinions of my group facilitation skills included the following:

Sheila told me: it was very positive the group: it got you through the bad times as well as the good times. I think we worked well. That's down to you. You had a lot to do with it . . .

Later, speaking to a research assistant, she said:

John's got a happy attitude. He's not singling us out. We're all asked to give our own opinions. None of us are criticised. There's no backbiting. There's a lot of positive vibes. I think we've got fairly close . . . If we are having a bad time he'll probably say to someone else what do you think, what's your opinion on it? And you find out what other people are thinking about you: they're not saying it outside or behind your back, they're actually confronting you with it. (This is inclusion rather than exclusion, tending towards cohesion and universality.) *Because he involved us all, and didn't just concentrate on one person: no matter what we were working at we were always involved individually . . . If we weren't grasping what the group was doing that particular time he explained it to us: which I think was important as well because otherwise you'd have been feeling, well what do I do next?*

Harry confirms **Sheila**'s last point: *He'd explain what he was about to do before going through the session which is brilliant I think.*

Explaining what was happening or what I proposed to do, giving information and helping them understand, empowered people:

Tina: *John **encourages** us. If someone's trying to get in (to the conversation) he'll say 'Let's hear . . . (what they have to say)'. He is sort of in control, not of what's being said . . .*

I have given permission and supported people in the creative risk taking of therapy. One way of encouraging has been by me modelling playfulness and role taking in the drama:

Pat: (It was helpful that we were) *exploring different ways of talking to people and generally being able to let your hair down and mess about. You participated: that made it fun.*

What was helpful in individual therapy?

In psychosis I have suggested there is a loss of self (see Chapter 3). Through therapy people can rediscover themselves, become more authentic and expand their sense of self. The therapeutic relationship enabled **Pat** to be more genuine and give up denial as a survival strategy. At her 27th individual session she said: *I've stopped confabulating since I came to see you.*

At her 32nd individual session **Gloria** said: *I'm starting to come into my own self.* The sessions had helped her focus, gain self-respect and a greater sense of control in her life, regain herself in both a cultural and psychological sense. She was able to assert her rights, let go of past attitudes, losses and feelings, communicate more with others and renew her creative activities.

Cheryll (Chapter 8) and **Harry** (Chapter 11) both confirmed that through therapy they gained a greater sense of their authentic self and consequently, increased confidence and well-being.

Individual versus group therapy

Participants were asked, 'Did you find the individual work more or less helpful/ unhelpful, the same or different from group work?'

Ben: Individual work was more direct. Group work helped me to learn to listen to others.

Anton said it was easier to concentrate in individual therapy (one hour): the longer group time (two hours) and the number of people made it difficult for him to concentrate. It may be better to run such a group for an hour and a half.

Sheila said of her individual assessment sessions: I've enjoyed my chats with John over the past weeks and he has helped me a great deal . . . (after first group session:) I feel so relaxed to know that I can be involved if I want to be because we all listen to each other . . . everyone there are caring and I'm glad to be part of this group. (This comment suggests the benefit of being listened to increases with a group compared to individual work as there are more people listening. How was the group?) It was very helpful. I normally find it quite hard to be in a group but because we all worked together and we got on quite well the harmony was there, if someone got upset we were able to comfort them and understand what they were going through. (The individual work) was really helpful. He made me feel as though **I was important**. (Such attention strengthens the ego and raises self-esteem.) I liked everything he did: he made you feel special in a lot of ways when you were feeling down.

Of the group **Dave** said he enjoyed being in a group of oddballs – marvellous characters, enjoyed the humour and relationships . . . There is a lot to be said positively for group therapy (even though it can be publicly painful) which I didn't realise at first when I was fixed with the idea only 1 to 1 sessions were helpful.

The relationship with the therapist achieved in pre-group individual work helped to sustain people through the first weeks of the group when they were settling into new relationships: these relationships can be safely facilitated by the therapist.

Pat (Were you interested in group work after you had been in individual therapy?): Yes because I'd found the (individual) sessions . . . helpful . . . I found it more helpful coming to see you on your own but at the same time it was important . . . to work as a group . . . People become de-socialised . . .

Of 349 individual sessions 56 were lost through non-attendance (293 sessions were actually attended).

Of 340 group sessions 103 were lost through non-attendance (237 were actually attended).

This shows that people were more likely to attend individual therapy. I suggest this may be due to the therapeutic alliance being stronger in individual therapy.

Group therapy

Group therapy enables people to relate and draw support, enrichment and enjoyment from each other. The principal ways this is done in dramatherapy and psychodrama are through playful encounter, drama, talk and listening. As people continue to attend a group, to express themselves, communicate, share disclosures, they benefit by becoming less isolated, discovering they have things in common. They value the social opportunity. Members looked forward to the group and felt motivated:

Theo: It helped to mix with others. It got me out every Monday to socialise.

Leah: Today I was looking forward to the group because I was lonely all week at home.

Sheila: Mostly I'm 'up', especially on a Monday because I'm so looking forward to going to the group. I find Monday afternoons I just can't wait for three o'clock . . . I just enjoyed it. I found it hard sometimes having to go to the group but when I got there I enjoyed myself even if it was hard going and probably afterwards there was a lot of thought in it. I think because I had something to look forward to during the week as well to the next Monday that spurred me on a lot as well.

Yalom (1985: 3) has written of the benefits of group therapy including universality, group cohesion, catharsis, the corrective recapitulation of the family group, learning social behaviours, practising altruism and the instillation of hope. In groups people have an experience of inclusion as opposed to exclusion, rejection or abandonment. From these shared experiences interpersonal confidence and social skills develop. They learn coping strategies from each other.

Universality

By 'universality' Yalom (1985: 7) meant that in group therapy people discover they are not alone with their difficulties, that they share experiences. Given the role of isolation in the generation and exacerbation of voices (see Chapter 2) this is a significant therapeutic factor. This leads to group cohesion and the development of interpersonal trust and confidence. As the men in the first research group sang:

> We're all in the same boat: We all have fears . . .

Jimmy valued the group as an opportunity: To meet other people, share what it's like to be schizophrenic, talk about problems . . . to achieve something, to understand, to know that other people can relate to me and talk to me . . .

Pat, who valued her prior experience of individual dramatherapy, said that the group is different in as much that there are other people who've had the same kind of experiences and you realise you're not alone.

Sheila: We shared things with each other that we hadn't shared with anyone else and we discussed things that we wouldn't normally do: I think that was really helpful as well because we trusted each other . . . I've learned a lot over the weeks since the group started and come to terms with some of my problems because I now know others feel the same . . . each one of us is helping the other . . . I'm feeling better in myself now: I know there are people that have the same problem as me. I'm not a special person that's been picked out for other people to pick on.

Tina (What in particular have you found helpful?): Talking with the other people, just sharing your experiences of your illness . . . It's good to talk to other people who hear voices and to hear their stories. It's the first time I've spoken to someone else who hears voices. It makes me feel that I'm not on my own. They have the same problems as I have. People poorlier than I am. They're all nice people.

Group cohesion and positive attachment

Sharing experiences develops group cohesion. **Tom** said that the therapist

gets people to 'bare their souls' if you like, tell their story. You find yourself wanting to let people know about yourself. It's interesting to hear other people's predicament . . . when we're talking about the voices some people's differ, some are almost the same . . . In the group you can say anything really . . . it was a very jovial atmosphere . . . you could let people know what you were into . . . strike up relationships, friendships . . . in Drop-In you don't always get to talk about, you tend not to talk about things: I think it's in (therapy) groups you talk about your personal life.

Jimmy: We're becoming much more together in the group . . . it's nice to have understood each other . . . we've got a friendly familiar feeling for each other.

Many had experiences of abusive relationships, when they were bullied, when the other was domineering, and the relationship had a lack of boundaries. In therapy these experiences can be shared and such sharing be a source of group cohesion. Cohesion is the result of people *connecting* with each other: becoming *attached* is the opposite of dissociation and loneliness.

Sheila: Even though we're all separate people we all seem to have something connected to each other . . . either hearing voices or being picked on . . . and I think, 'Oh I can connect with that person' . . . I was eager to meet up with Leah and Tom again and yourself. There's something in life that I was actually **attached to** and that I were enjoying . . . I **belonged** somewhere and I was mixing which I wasn't normally doing.

Sheila's positive attachment provided the basis for personal growth and change. People value *belonging*, establishing trusting relationships with others and achieve a positive attachment to each other.

> The process of group cohesion (or multiple attachment) undoubtedly mirrors the one-to-one therapeutic attachment relationship which, in turn, reflects our earliest attachment with caregivers. Learning occurs during that creative connection in the space between people. New brain patterns are laid down and these connect with body memories . . . these new learning experiences can replace earlier 'triggers' from body memories and so can prevent episodes of dissociation.
>
> (A. Bannister, personal communication, 16 March 2003)

Positive attachment experiences in therapy during which people have an opportunity to learn new ways of being and socialising therefore can lead to a diminution of voices (see pp. 232–5). Connecting with others (associating) can also result in connecting with feelings and other aspects of the self (instead of dissociating). Conversely there can also be some reaction to the end of therapy: the loss of which seemed to result in an increase in voices, possibly due to the increase in isolation (see Leudar and Thomas, 2000, 122).

Theo (at follow-up three months later) reported hearing more voices. He felt lonely, excitable, anxious, heard screams in bed. He felt suicidal. This matched his experience in the group: after five weeks in the group he said he was hearing fewer voices. Then after the seventh week he missed five sessions. He returned to the group saying that the voices had been worse recently: loneliness makes them worse. When I bottle things up the voices get worse.

When there is a break in therapy this feeling of isolation can return:

Tom: When we had that two weeks off when I couldn't talk . . . (he felt the loss of the group, missed the relationships and felt worse.) I had this bad dream and I woke up in the middle of the night and then this whispering down my ear . . . I was petrified, really scared and I thought 'Oh no, it's two weeks until the next session, I won't be able to tell anybody about it' and that really did get me down that did 'cause I missed going to the group itself . . . It was more like it was scarey, 'cause it had died down a bit over the few weeks, it had not gone away but right down, it had stopped for a few weeks and then I thought 'Oh No it's come back. It's going to start all over again.'

Diane reported that after therapy: The voices have got worse . . . The end of therapy increased her sense of isolation due to lack of support from her mother, therapist, social worker and support worker. Such an exacerbation of voices at the end of therapy is also reported by Carlyn who, after two years of therapy at the Red House Psychotherapy Unit, Manchester, complained her voices got worse as a consequence of the loss of support (Carlyn, 1997: 6). Achieving *attachment* means experiencing *loss*, missing the group or therapy after it's over: the relationships hold people. **Roger** after the first group said that on the last day he felt he was leaving friendship behind: *We'd made a **bond** with each other, friendship and understanding of each other's problems.* He benefited later from attending a second group. Others are more able to break out of their isolation after a period of therapy:

Dave (after therapy): *I'm not on my own, not unique, I can express myself better. I feel more self-respect. I have a sense of humour.* He became more involved in creative and social activities beyond the mental health services.

Trust and confidence

People discover they can trust others through the relationships in group therapy.

   Roger spoke of *making friends . . . It's helping me . . . it were hard for me to trust people . . . because with my ex-wife cheating on me and especially with my best friend . . .*

   As trust developed, so interpersonal confidence developed.

Dave: (In a drama session) *I was a mediator between Anton and Dillon: it felt good because of (the) personal relationship between Anton and Dillon: it was in my power to make things better . . . Where else could I have open discussion/shared experiences with people . . . and develop confidence in myself and other people . . .*

Leah: *I have been able to trust people and they trust me . . . I've been able to talk more to people than I thought I would.*

In group therapy the self is in relation to several others. This can be experienced as potentially threatening, especially by people who are paranoid, anxious or lacking in interpersonal confidence.

Anton: (What was unhelpful?) *Comments from other people: Roger seemed to have it in for me. Dillon wasn't helpful sometimes: we were all ill and sometimes things weren't helpful.*

Dramatherapy, in working through distance and structure, can manage intra-group hostility and provide safe opportunities for catharsis of such feelings. **Roger** was able to express his anger safely and thus achieve some distance from his potential violence, which he and others felt threatened by: *I'm more relaxed coming here: I don't react to threats with hostility but **step aside**.*

   As well as universality and cohesion the group also allowed people to benefit by realising their differences, their individuality.

Theo: It's made me realise there's people worse off than me: I realised it's not the end of the world: we're all the same but I'm not as bad as some others.

Theo considered the benefits of group work were:

- social
- relief from tension: being able to express himself, his frustrations and aggression
- discovering his acting ability and expanding his role repertoire
- assertiveness training
- insight into the sources of his voices in earlier experiences
- being able to voice: speak out his voices (saying 'Fuck off' without feeling bad)
- fun, laughter.

Catharsis

Dave and **Leah** confirm some of **Theo**'s points.

Dave: I'm actually feeling stronger and more confident by expressing my feelings and insecurities . . . I've accepted voices, there's not a lot can be done about it. I'm not on my own, not unique, I can express myself better.

Leah: I was impressed finally 'cause I almost stopped hearing voices . . . I really enjoyed the group . . . we had fun, excitement and happy memories. The group was good to my thoughts. The good thing was we talked about anything . . . I had expressed myself in the group about nightmares, hearing voices, aggressive behaviour and more . . .

What helped **Leah** was the opportunity to talk freely in the group, express feelings, share experiences, problems, finding others had similar experiences, not being alone, helping others, confidentiality.

Self-esteem

The achievement of coming to the group resulted in increased self-esteem.

Roger (After the second group: have you changed?): Yes. A lot. I'm getting out a lot more . . . I've got a lot more respect for (myself).

Feedback from other group members can raise self-esteem.

Pat: They said they would miss me and I said 'Why?' 'Because you're good fun to be around,' and I thought usually I'm moaning and groaning . . .

Pat had been criticised by her mother-in-law, husband and professionals about her behaviour as a mother. Her peer group relations validated her as an individual woman rather than identifying her solely with the role of mother.

Watkins (1998: 219) pointed out that 'Disturbing voices sometimes begin to disappear spontaneously as a person's self-esteem improves.'

Self-esteem is also raised by helping others in the group: Yalom lists the opportunity to be altruistic, to help others, as therapeutic:

Sheila: (How was the group?) It was very helpful. I normally find it quite hard to be in a group but because we all worked together and we got on quite well the harmony was there, if someone got upset we were able to comfort them and understand what they were going through.

In group therapy the therapeutic relationships are spread between members: they become auxiliaries to each other and research has shown that people benefit more from each other than they necessarily benefit from interventions by the therapist (Yalom, 1985).

The therapy of relationships: interpersonal learning

Dramatherapy enabled **Jimmy** to develop the ability to mix with people, rather than feel as if I was isolating myself and not feeling so fragile that I couldn't do a thing . . . I observed how, through the structured activities of dramatherapy, he moved into greater relatedness as the sessions continued. It's positive: it's helping me because it's helping me understand my own mind. It helps me to be able to express myself in a way that I couldn't do in other social situations.

From the group experience people learned coping skills and positive attitudes:

Tina: I used to feel it was a good morning spent . . . doing something, learning to cope, learning how other people cope.

Group therapy provides a corrective recapitulation of the family group (Yalom, 1985). It therefore offers people who have had dysfunctional socialisation another opportunity to learn more effective ways of relating to others. Family dysfunction, the lack of communication with and between mother and father, abuse, the breakdown of relationships, the impact of loss, all have a role in the onset of voices. Several reported that their parents divorced when they were young: **Simon** (aged 3); **Tina** (aged 4); **Roger** (aged 11). **Anton** spoke of the impact on him as a child of his mother's depressions, his father's hostility/criticism and of their arguments.

Roger: It goes back to when I was a child my Dad used to hit us a lot . . . he'd would come home from the . . . club legless. If there were no food on the table he'd hit my mother, my sisters and myself. It carried on till I were 11. And then at one time he tried to hit my Mam with an axe . . . I hope I'm not turning into another part of my Dad . . . the voice I hear, 'Self-destruct' is from my father.

After working in the dramatherapy group, on her grief and ambivalence resultant from her mother's death, **Sheila** said:

I've thought less negative thoughts about my mum as well since I've been going to the group. I'm talking to her again. I know she can't hear me. But I'm not getting upset as much as I was before which I think is good.

Psychodrama enabled **Roger** and **Sheila** (see Chapter 12) to change their relationship with their dead parent (of the opposite gender) from fear and distress to calmer acceptance.

Many had been subject to criticism, nagging, bullying, racism and being picked on: **Theo**, **Dave**, **Roger** and **Anton** (who were heterosexual) had all been subject to homophobic taunts which raised anxieties about their sexuality. The voices reproduce this negativity: the person has introjected it into the self, with resultant low self-esteem. She/he may become a scapegoat. **Dave** had been paranoid since the age of 13–14 when he was bullied at school and his mother had left home. His voices were all critical comments, insults: adolescent bullying voices replaying ad nauseam the bullying of his youth, destroying his self-esteem. His father had also been violent to him.

Simon's mother was mentally ill after his birth. She said to him as a child, 'I'll put "the Hoodoo" on you.' Later he wondered if he was possessed by demons:

On occasions my mother seems to be capable of being very irritating indeed and very frustrating. I don't know why. Sometimes I feel I have to be defensive to my own mother: feeling of being stalked . . . I feel I was being got at from lots of sides . . .

Therapy enabled **Roger**, **Sheila**, **Simon**, **Tina** and **Pat** to talk more and assert themselves with members of their family. During therapy **Pat** became more understanding of her husband's difficulties and their relationship improved.

The instillation of hope

Sheila: Since I've been in the group I'm looking at life differently. I've felt very positive this week.

From expressing suicidal feelings during the early sessions of his first group, **Roger** became progressively more hopeful. At the end of his second group he had been able to establish a new, loving relationship and said: dramatherapy has *brought myself out of my shell . . . Dramatherapy has helped me survive.* If I wouldn't have joined the dramatherapy group maybe I wouldn't be here. (This opinion echoes that of **Cheryll**: see Chapter 8.)

From the above I offer the following summary.

The benefits of dramatherapy and psychodrama

Social

The emergence from isolation is therapeutic and leads to a reduction of voices. Social skills can be learned and practised. People can be encouraged to become more assertive, to voice feelings and opinions. These activities lead to an improvement in a person's relationship with themselves and in their relationships with others.

Relief from tension

Since stress exacerbates voices, the person can benefit from relieving tension through relaxation, being able to express self, feelings, frustrations or aggression. Being creative raises self-esteem, and expands people's role repertoires, freeing them from debilitating constraints. Laughter resulting from having fun relaxes people.

Insight and integration

Therapy can enable people to gain insight into the sources of voices in earlier experiences. Working through these enables the person to own their voices and previously split off feelings, and thus achieve some resolution or integration of the intrapsychic difficulties that were the origin of the voices. Creative activity facilitates the integration of unconscious material, strengthens the ego, and promotes personal development.

Rehearsing a future

Recovery must be a possible future (Coleman, 1999): the instillation of hope is in itself therapeutic (Yalom, 1985). But hope cannot just be given to people: they must discover hope for the future through their own practical efforts and experiences. Dramatherapy and psychodrama offer the possibility of rehearsing situations and practising behaviours to achieve competence and confidence.

Distance and empowerment

Essential to safe and effective work are the therapeutic relationships (with the therapist and other group members) and the degree of distance the person needs at any one time so as not to be overwhelmed and further disempowered. The method can empower through choices and decisions being made by the people who hear voices. Their creative expression of will and responsibility for what is co-created is empowering. In dramatherapy and psychodrama people can experience being in control or letting go of control.

Prevention of suicide and self-harm

There is some evidence in my study that therapy reduces self-harm and suicidal behaviour as a result of the opportunity to express feelings and receive support. Therapeutic relationships hold people back from the brink.

Therapy and voices

What then was the impact of these creative action methods in therapy on the intensity and frequency of voice hearing? In the final follow-up interview people were asked: Has your attitude to your voices changed? Eight people answered, Yes. One person answered a mixed Yes and No. Three people answered, No.

Simon pointed out that it is possible to have different attitudes to different voices:
> Well there isn't a single attitude, because I hear different people. My attitude to them? Not a great deal. No.

The majority however reported they were less troubled by the voices.

Jenny: I'm not as scared any more.

Several people were more able to dismiss the voices:

Sheila: I try not to take much notice of them now. (Since I've been in the group) I can understand now they (voices) are not real, which I couldn't before . . . I've put my fingers up to the voices and said, 'Bugger you,' and said, 'I don't care what you say any more.' I kept repeating it to myself, 'I'm not bothered what you say any more.' Just walk round the flat doing it. I'm not as frightened in the flat as I was before.

Tina: I don't feel as desperate about them: I used to think what a terrible thing, mental illness. It doesn't bother me that I hear voices.

Some people gained greater understanding and a sense of the meaning of their voices.

Dillon: When I hear a comment (voice) I'm able to unpack its meaning more: that's helpful: it makes me understand how easy it is to get misunderstanding . . .

Gloria already had her own ideas about voices at the start of therapy: she believed they emerged from her unconscious mind with messages to help her and her conscious mind then had the task of processing them: I found them (the voices) threatening at first, now I can ascertain what messages are coming through, what's causing them and so understand them . . . (Dramatherapy) helped me understand why I was having problems.

For some people, therapy reduced their voice hearing. At the final interview people were asked: Are you hearing more voices or fewer voices or about the same than when we started work together? Seven people said they heard fewer voices; six heard the same amount; three found their voices less disturbing/aggressive; one person said they were more aggressive. **Roger**, after the closure of his first group, and **Diane** after the end of her individual therapy heard more voices: an emotional reaction to the loss of therapy and a recurrence of isolation. During therapy both of them had a reduction of voice hearing. By the fifth session of the first group **Roger** said he was hearing fewer voices due to attendance at the group. After the first group was over he said that the voices had been slowly dwindling away but that when the group had finished they'd come back with a vengeance. His care worker had noticed he was becoming more confident. **Roger** put this down to his experiences in the group: I'm more in control of the voices. After the second group he said he was more able to say 'No' to ideas, he was more confident and could block out voices.

Ten people said they heard fewer voices *during* their therapy. **Gloria** said that after twelve sessions of individual therapy she was hearing fewer voices and they were becoming supportive. At the end of her therapy she said: I seldom hear voices now.

Pat: There are fewer voices anyway . . . (Have the voices changed?) I don't hear as many. A lot of it is down to that (dramatherapy) because I didn't understand before.

Jenny (Mr is the name of her voice): The voice is a bit less . . . Mr sounds whiney. Mr can come big time but not as often . . . Mr doesn't have as much impact. I don't know why . . . I have got stronger with Mr . . . Mr sounds weaker and a bit silly sometimes . . .

Talking with others may weaken frequency/intensity of the voice hearing because the person's isolation is reduced.

Dave: I'm not sure personally if your groups alleviate voices directly; but it's positive to be in them and if voices are stress related then by alleviating this stress as happens in the group, then it's very useful . . .

In the final follow-up interview participants were asked: Have your voices changed? Seven said, Yes; four, No.

Theo said that the voices had *gone softer, not shouting, nice, kinder. The aggressive voice has gone. A mumbled voice – nonsense, easier to dismiss . . .*

Dave: *The same but not as disturbing as they were. I feel more confident.*

At the final follow-up interview people were asked: Has your ability to cope with the voices improved, lessened or remained the same? Ten people said their ability to cope had improved, three that it was at the same level and two said their ability to cope had got worse.

Jimmy: *It's something I have to live with: it's me who's producing the voices in the first place. So as long as I'm here the voices are going to stay.*

I had not set out with a treatment goal of reducing voices.

Treatment should not be aimed directly at curing or eliminating the experience [of voice hearing] itself but by helping the coping process.

(Romme, 1998: 53)

The aim of therapy is not to get rid of parts of the self, though resolution through expression and integration may result in a reduction of voices. Some of our work has indeed led to a diminution of the intensity of the voices. The empowerment of the person was more a treatment goal than symptom relief as the symptom is also part of the person and not necessarily to be removed but rather to be accepted and integrated. The attempt to remove aspects of the person that have been stigmatised in the past, such as being left handed or gay, would not now be seen as appropriate therapeutic goals. Some improvement in a person's ability to cope with voices may be signalled by their internalising/owning of the voices:

Tina: *Since I saw John I've begun to accept the voices are in my head, are mine.*

The projection of the voices out of the self into the environment (where many of them came from originally) may help the person to reject such noxious psychic material but reinforces his/her powerlessness.

Theo: *When I walk past vans the F word ended, occasionally I hear screaming – it's in my mind: I look back and there's no one there.*

Through a psychodrama (see Chapter 12) **Theo** was able to say the F word himself and this seemed to empower him: he owned the aggression in the word rather than projecting it into the environment.

Several people had learned other coping strategies:

Anton: *I agree with them and brush them off:* (I say, in reply to command hallucinations) '*I've done it* (or) *you do it*' (I'm) *more relaxed.*

Tom described how he put the psychodrama reported in Chapter 12 into practice:

> *If I heard the voices and I suddenly got up and switched the TV on that would be totally normal . . . That'd drown the voices out I reckon. If the voices are particularly prominent in the night it helps to have something normal to counteract, cancel them out . . . usually if I'm hearing voices I turn the light on, get in bed, listen to the radio: that usually helps me . . .* (Is that a way of helping yourself you've learned in the group?) *Well I picked up on it in the group: the thing I like about the group is the way you can help other people . . . or you can find out, they've got different* (ways of coping).

At final follow-up participants were asked: Have you changed? Nine said Yes. Two answered Not sure. One said No.

Tom (You wanted to understand yourself better.): *I think I do. I don't think of myself as someone special: I think of myself as a normal person now who happens to hear voices . . . I've matured. In some ways I can brush them* (voices) *aside.*

The results suggest that dramatherapy and psychodrama, for the majority of participants, promoted intrapsychic and interpersonal change.

From the above it is possible to assert that dramatherapy and psychodrama tended to reduce voices and their impact; to change the voices so that those that remained were less aggressive and threatening; to improve people's coping ability, enabling personal change and a change of attitude towards the voices in the direction of people feeling more in control. This may also be due to the interaction of these creative therapies with several other factors including medication and increased social relationships.

What was generally thought to be not helpful?

Of thirteen respondents to this question six could not think of anything unhelpful; of the other seven, two named interpersonal difficulties in the group as not helpful, two said the emotional aftermath of therapy was sometimes difficult and one said there was not enough support outside therapy. One said lack of consistent attendance at the group was unhelpful. The research assistants and I found it difficult to draw out participants' negative experiences: this may be due to some idealisation or that simply that the experience was generally positive. In analysing what was not helpful I have, in accordance with the emergent theory of distance (see Chapter 7) and to aid understanding, divided the responses into issues of *underdistance* and *overdistance*: these concepts are fundamentally linked to the relationship of *self* and *other*, that is, what degree of closeness or distance to the other can a vulnerable person tolerate? Safe and effective therapy in this theoretical frame will modulate the degree of distance a client needs at any particular time. Thus what was regarded as unhelpful can be analysed under the following headings:

- *Underdistance*
  The emotional aftermath of therapy; emotional material resurfacing; conflict. A feeling of 'too much', possibly overwhelming.
- *Overdistance*
  A lack of time/continuity; lack of depth; lack of closure. A feeling of 'too little/not enough'.

Underdistance

One woman withdrew from the second group because she felt overwhelmed: she used the audience chairs in two sessions but these did not provide sufficient distance for her. Shared intimacy can hold fears for people who have withdrawn from contact with others for fear of the danger of such contact.

Anton: Discussing things with other voice hearers is helpful but sometimes not helpful getting deeper into (a) voice: this might not be helpful. **Anton** is saying, in effect, he needed more distance from a voice.

Also feared and found to be difficult, if not unhelpful, was conflict in the group.

Simon: Felt a bit of difficulty with Jimmy at one stage but it didn't last very long. We didn't seem to hit it off too well. I don't know if it was a communication problem or a different clash of personalities or what. He seemed to get annoyed about something. I'm not so sure that some of it was particularly helpful.

Tina: To be quite frank there was only one thing I didn't like . . . I didn't like Jimmy's aggression . . . it didn't put me off coming . . . I thought he was like a spoiled brat. He wanted all the attention . . . It used to get me a bit worked up . . . (I got cross with) him. I did say once. But I don't think it was constructive . . . I think it's his illness and I sympathise with him. But I didn't like it.

The emotional aftermath of sessions may be experienced as not helpful:

Gloria: Opening up some of the old wounds. It seemed to unleash a lot of pain without having a cushion there for me to fall on. It later allowed me to systematically heal that wound . . . Some of the role play had an adverse effect rather than clarifying. Instead of coming out feeling I'd resolved something I came out feeling halfway through an issue – perhaps it was more deeply embedded: it took a number of sessions to dismiss, something had resurfaced . . . Some issues are still deeply embedded.

Jenny: One time at the beginning we did role play it were very hard I did a lot and when I went I never left it, I brought it home with me again. I got upset and angry with John. He should have known that I were going home with it and he didn't help me to get rid. So I wasn't going to go again because I didn't want that . . . I am going to come away with some feelings but not intense, not coming away without knowing how to cope with them, how to deal with them, how do I: I can't put myself back together and everything feels floating and in bits and that stayed like that for a while so I felt on my guard for a while. I don't know how to handle it when I come home. He were good at getting it out but no good at telling how to put it back. Perhaps finish a bit sooner and talk about what we'd done, and leave a bit more time at the end to stick myself together, pick up the pieces. He could give a bit of guidance on what to do. It's happened a couple of times; then I can't let myself get that far now where I'm in that position: I don't think it's a good thing . . . To let go sometimes and not be able to put it back together is just as bad as carrying it around.

Following this feedback I changed the way I was working, ensuring the last fifteen minutes were a time for re-integration, de-roling, reflection, closure, preparation to leave the session: in effect creating some distance from the material that had resurfaced during the session so that she could successfully contain it.

Overdistance

The lack of sufficient time in therapy was found to be unhelpful: the research was of an arbitrary length: twenty weeks for a group and forty-four individual sessions.

Harry: More time would be useful in therapy. A year only an hour a week it left me . . . a bit more time would be better.

Jenny: We should have talked about past things . . . (J.C.: We haven't had the time) or the courage . . . It takes a lot to get to know somebody: on both sides, it's not a one way thing it's a two way. With deep down things it takes a lot of digging up: sometimes you think they're best left buried. But you know they're there . . .

This is an argument against the fashion for brief therapy. Clients who have complex problems and difficulty forming an attachment may need longer in therapy for it to be effective. This is further evidenced in group therapy when people have difficulty attending and the consequent lack of continuity of membership damages the group:

Dave: It's not so good when people miss groups; it throws the bonding/empathy/ shared experiences and trust off balance for the following week. Having said that it's working as therapy in the smaller groups.

Simon: People not attending and it being such a small group: it did cause a bit of a difficulty in maintaining the continuity . . .

Tom: It was just a shame when people had times when they were off. I would have found it better if everyone could have been there at the same time . . . When we started the group . . . there were six including me . . . with it whittling down there's less people so there's more chance to talk . . .

Dave and **Tom** here both valued the smaller group: fewer members meant more space that was safer for those remaining. It seems smaller groups are less likely to be emotionally overwhelming.

Conclusion

The majority of opinions expressed by the participants who took part in this limited research study show that the creative action methods of dramatherapy and psychodrama can be helpful to people who hear voices. As a result, it is possible to state that dramatherapy and psychodrama promote intrapsychic and interpersonal change.

I have provided evidence that during therapy there was a reduction in the frequency, intensity, negativity of voices and an increase in self-esteem, coping ability, social skills. The reduction of isolation and stigmatisation that group therapy provides was seen as especially valuable. Appropriate use of action methods can then lead to the release of tension and the promotion of relaxation: the safe channelling of aggression and anger results in a reduction in aggressive voices. The study revealed that the fun inherent in these methods was especially valued and had many perceived therapeutic benefits. Furthermore during therapy there was evidence of a greater internalisation of the voices: participants owned what was previously seen as entirely outside of themselves with a consequent increase in insight, integration and ability to cope. The use of metaphor, dramatic distance and working in miniature were seen by participants as empowering them and consequently the therapeutic method did not overwhelm them.

From these research results it is possible to develop guidelines for good practice: the subject of the final chapter.

Chapter 14

Guidelines for good practice

I have attempted in this book to provide a theoretical framework, examples of practice and research results, to make a case for the effective practice of dramatherapy and psychodrama with people who hear voices or have psychotic experiences. This work is complex, difficult and can be, indeed often is, frightening and disturbing for the therapist. In this final chapter I therefore offer guidelines for good practice to provide a foundation for the work, focusing first on the therapist and then on the work with the clients.

The therapist's own madness

> We are all partly psychotic all of the time and all of us display psychotic parts of our personalities part of the time.
>
> (Young, 1995: 48)

Therapists must be aware of their own psychotic material so that this is not projected onto the client, e.g. their own tendency to act out omnipotent fantasies of being able to 'cure', rescue, save people who have been abandoned in the past and who struggle to survive; their own hostility and wish to deny unattractive aspects of the self; their own feelings of hatred, murderousness, madness. The therapist will take such material to supervision and where necessary to their own therapy. The therapist must be aware of what their own 'voices' might be saying. Furthermore Rosenfeld (1987: 8) warned that 'unskilled psychotherapy of the psychoses is a danger to the therapist's personality because it inevitably stimulates his feelings of omnipotence and helplessness' (quoted in Ellwood, 1995: 14). It is essential therefore that therapists wishing to work in this area do sufficient work in their own therapy on their own madness: this can then become a source of empathy and insight and ensure that therapists are not overwhelmed when their own psychotic parts are stimulated in the work with clients.

Coping with anxiety

During this work with clients, therapists will feel anxious. They need to be able to process anxiety: to practise their own physical relaxation, keep breathing and nurture their own self-respect.

Coping with and learning from the countertransference

Because of the overwhelming power of the feelings the voice hearer originally was unable to feel (and so split off or projected out of themselves) the therapist may be the first vessel available to contain these feelings. Melanie Klein argued that psychotic people 'form an immediate intense transference. This is because the subject, unable to distinguish between inner and outer worlds, attempts to shed the terrified unwanted parts of self into the therapist' (cited in Thomas, 1997: 68). The countertransference in working with psychotic people may therefore be overwhelming. The therapist must be prepared to feel confused, sick, terrified, lost, angry, hateful, disgusted, despairing etc. without either collapsing as if they were incompetent (i.e. be overwhelmed themselves) or attacking/criticising/rejecting the person who hears voices. By being congruent about their feelings the therapist can model emotional expression: feelings then can be voiced and the client perceive and relate to the therapist as a real person. The timing of such congruence must however be considered with the client's needs and capacity to tolerate such openness in mind. The therapist's negative feelings must not be expressed in ways that the client might experience as persecutory or punishing. The therapist must take such hostile feelings to supervision.

Professional relationships

This therapeutic work may take place in a psychiatric culture that can be overtly or covertly anti-therapy: professional jealousies, different philosophies, anxieties and responsibilities may make the work difficult and at times impossible. The therapist must be prepared to negotiate with other professionals and seek their support for the work. Indeed I would recommend co-therapy so that the therapist is not isolated in the work and groups can continue to meet when one therapist is ill or on holiday.

The psychodrama team

Zerka Moreno (1978: 163) advised that the psychodramatist should practise with professional auxiliary egos to take roles. Psychodrama with psychotic clients should be 'a team approach'. Thus the therapist is more able to achieve a better overview of the patient's needs and be able to determine the appropriate therapeutic intervention. This also may reduce the possibility of client and therapist being overwhelmed by transferences as these are 'broken up into multiple parts and carried by auxiliary egos.'

The therapeutic relationship

The difficulties of this work include establishing and sustaining the therapeutic relationship, especially with people who are paranoid. The therapeutic relationship can take time to become established and in true Morenean fashion this may mean the therapist will have to go to the person's home if they are too frightened to come out. An auxiliary ego/support worker may contribute to this process by bringing the client to therapy and accompanying them home. Prouty's pre-therapy (1990) offers a method of working with people whose ability to relate is severely impaired, to enable them to develop a therapeutic relationship. I recommend that therapy be once a week as this ensures the therapeutic relationship does not become too intense: the results of intensive psychoanalytic psychotherapy, several times a week, were found to be anti-therapeutic for this client group (see Chapter 1).

Positive support

The vulnerable ego is supported and strengthened by unconditional positive regard, non-judgemental acceptance and warmth from the therapist. This attitude will result in praise from the therapist to encourage and reinforce positive achievement and change. The client's self-esteem is raised through his or her own spontaneous, creative activity in therapy, the therapist's affirmations and by the group's praise.

Accepting the client's perspective and needs

The therapist must respect the defences of the person and proceed gradually, accepting their frame of reference and helping them work through delusions and hallucinations. Conscious insight may empower a person and therefore be helpful. If however it is imposed on the person by the interpretation of the therapist this may be unhelpful and unnecessary: dramatherapy can facilitate changes in behaviour without insight into unconscious processes. The appropriate treatment goal may shift from the integration of aspects of the personality, to acceptance of the multiplicity of the personality, to interpersonal play, to relaxation, to social skills training, to assertiveness training, to grieving and back again according to the person's needs at the time of treatment. In this I am influenced by Rogers' person-centred approach.

Working with the whole person

The therapist must provide a safe, accepting, supportive, nurturing environment within which no part of the self is rejected or split off: the person's voices, delusions, feelings, thoughts and fantasies are all accepted. The therapist gives permission for the unacceptable parts of the self to appear and be negotiated with: thus it becomes possible, if not to integrate split-off parts, at least to establish a relationship with them (at sufficient distance), such that the person feels less threatened and more in control, with choices rather than ultimatums. The therapy must be concerned with the whole person, not just the voices, but not ignoring the voices. Every person who struggles with a psychotic process has healthy parts and abilities: the whole person is not sick or disabled (see Mollon, 1996: 9–10). Manfred Bleuler (1978: 636) wrote: 'much of the inner life of the schizophrenic remains human, natural and healthy.' Creative therapy can work with both the distressed parts and the functioning healthy parts to enable growth. The whole self is acknowledged, learning from those aspects that are wise and strange: the mystery of the self is not reduced to pathology.

Feelings

Any feeling is accepted: an emotional re-education takes place whereby feelings can be felt, named, processed. The therapist

> is responsive, supportive and empathic in the face of painful emotions. Patients are enabled to develop psychological complexity only if they are shown, via [the therapeutic relationship] . . . a more complete and hence complex picture of themselves which supplies the hitherto denied or dismissed painful emotions or dominating unconscious dynamic themes in relation to themselves and others.
>
> (Dolan, 1996: 79)

Hostility, aggression, anger and frustration are allowed expression, even facilitated by the therapist, in safe ways. Split-off hostility, aggression and negativity need to be owned and/or returned to whom they originally belonged. Combined with humour this catharsis can release tension and provide integration of previously split-off feelings. Dramatherapy and psychodrama provide safe ways for feelings to be expressed.

Voices and delusions

Voices are listened to and meanings sought for what they are saying. Delusions can likewise be listened to and processed for their meanings. I have proposed that voices and delusions are metaphoric and contain meaning (see Chapter 3).

Boundaries

Clear boundaries of time, body, space are established in practice. Dramatherapy and psychodrama provide containing structures that clarify boundaries.

Structure

Given the difficulties voice hearers have concentrating (they may be distracted by voices or have difficulty focusing when habitually confused) the therapist provides structure and stimuli that aid concentration and focus. Structure reduces anxiety by providing a boundaried container. Creative structures, to be therapeutic, must be neither rigid nor empty, but provide a supportive, stimulating space for free play and autonomy (see Eigen, 1993: 347–348).

Dramatherapy and psychodrama provide structure and a safe, free place to play: the vulnerable self/ego can enjoy both the nurture of the therapist's positive regard and the encouragement to play. Play/drama enables the vulnerable ego to recapitulate developmental stages and grow stronger (see Cattanach, 1994: 28–40). Play allows the child part of the self to be present in the therapy (see Mollon, 1996: 11–12). Dramatherapy provides an environment 'with distinct boundaries and structure to ensure that the insecure personality will not be engulfed' (Johnson, 1981: 50, 60).

Sessions should not end in climactic emotional work but come to closure in calm reflection (which Slade (1995: 9) called 'de-climax'). De-roling from the drama enables the person/group be grounded in the here and now social reality. Reflection on experience promotes clear thinking. Before they leave the session people can be buoyed by some humour and positive appreciation, praise from the therapist or warmth from fellow group members expressed through handshakes, hugs or other closing activities.

The use of containing objects

In therapy objects such as buttons, toy chairs, animals and Babushkas can be used to hold projections in the space between therapist and client. Toy theatre can also be a container. Working in miniature with objects can empower people and keep material contained at a safe distance.

Metaphor

Dramatherapists can work without interpreting metaphoric material and so may be more able to work with delusions and voices than other therapists. The metaphor contains material at a safe distance. Interpreting the material would in effect prematurely collapse the distance provided by the metaphor. When the client is ready s/he will make the links and interpret their own material: the metaphor will carry across meaning at first unconsciously and later, when the person is stronger, consciously. The therapist must be willing to work without knowing the meaning, trusting the metaphoric process. Keeping an open mind and being able to hold different realities as coexisting is quite a trick: being able to both stay in a metaphor/delusion and keep track of here and now reality and the therapeutic process. The therapist needs to be both grounded and playful.

Distance

Voice hearers may have overdistanced themselves from overwhelming feelings. Dramatherapy enables people to play with distance: to find the aesthetic or middle distance, where feelings can be felt, observed and processed without overwhelming the person.

The audience

An audience space, two rows of chairs, is created in the group room where group members can withdraw from the activity and just watch. This enables people to stay in the room when overstretched by the activity, knowing they can temporarily withdraw. The group are told that sitting in a front row seat means they are willing to be drawn back in whereas sitting in the back row means they want to be allowed to sit quietly until ready to re-emerge. From this place the observer ego is still engaged and the person need not flee or dissociate. The therapist may visit anyone sitting in the back row or wait for them to re-emerge (see Chapter 10).

In individual psychodrama/dramatherapy the therapist must ensure they do not become over identified with any role or suffer role confusion (Casson, 1997a). Johnson (1992) suggested a playing space and a separate observing space so that the therapist may leave a role temporarily and witness the scene as an audience, before re-entering a role enactment (see also Mitchell, 1996: 73). The client can use such an audience space during an improvisation to distance themselves and observe. This also reduces the likelihood of a client dissociating to escape overwhelming material (Landy, 1996: 17).

The observer ego

Dramatherapy and psychodrama methods (such as the mirror and working at a distance) can engage and strengthen the observer ego, enabling the person to reflect on their experience rather than be overwhelmed by it.

Relaxation

Dramatherapy and psychodrama attend to the body. Relaxation and ways of reducing or managing stress can be explored, practised or learnt.

Breathing

Breathing is noticed, attended to, encouraged, practised: this experience of self-control counters tension, anxiety and panic and promotes relaxation.

The voice

The person's own voice, the voice of the vulnerable ego, is reinforced and supported by empathic affirmation, through talking, writing, singing and voice work.

Power and control

The person is empowered by the process: to choose, to change, to decide the direction of a therapy session or stop any activity. Clients need to find that the locus of control is substantially in their own hands, not only in those of the therapist or the voices. The process must empower. This can be done by the therapist offering clients a choice of several, different activities and the right to refuse any of the choices offered.

> Psychotherapy is a process of empowerment.
>
> (Wilkins, 1997: 51)

One difficulty is finding the most appropriate creative method: people who are paranoid are also more likely to be rigid and less able to be creative (Chadwick, 1997): progress may be slow and the therapist must be creative in finding small, safe steps a person can take. The client may give metaphoric clues to, or suggestions of, ways of working but the therapist must check whether the client wants to work in that way before proceeding so that the person owns the process. Sometimes a client will need permission and a little encouragement, which is not the same as being told what to do: 'You can experiment, give it a go and then if you want to stop, we can.'

Through such empowerment the person is able to own more of their experience and so feel in control. A therapy where the therapist is the expert, in control, can reproduce the experience of the person who has been controlled and disempowered by another in the past. The therapist must not abdicate their power and responsibility in an attempt to give power to the client who is not ready: they might simply then be overwhelmed again by such responsibility. The therapy must offer the opportunity for play: for control to be played with between the parties, to be shared and passed back and forth between the two (and shared with others in group therapy). The therapist becomes a playmate.

The right to say 'No' and 'Stop'

Dramatherapists and psychodramatists must enable clients to say 'No' to any technique or 'Stop' to any activity and to regard such refusals as therapeutic steps forward to be praised/supported. The methods can empower the client. Those techniques that do so are especially important in this work.

Role play

> Roles do not emerge from the self, but the self may emerge from roles.
>
> (Moreno, 1993: 47)

This suggests that role playing may enable the person to re-create themselves. Many psychotic people suffer role poverty: loss of roles in life. They benefit from the opportunity in drama to satisfy act hungers and play, in surplus reality, roles that the outer world does not give them opportunity to inhabit. (See Harrow (1952) for evidence that role taking leads to personality development in people diagnosed with psychotic illnesses, see also Chapter 5.)

Role reversal

Role reversing with a voice brings the person closer to the feeling contained in the voice. This can be empowering: as when a person is able to own their split-off aggression, but it can also be overwhelming, as the original (overwhelming and therefore split-off) feeling is accessed. Such role reversals therefore should be *brief*: a 'homeopathy' of role reversal can enable the client to tolerate small amounts of the feeling. Clients may feel 'worse' after such role reversals, as grief, anger and other feelings are released. For this reason such role reversals should not be done just before the end of the session. In a group, playing the role of another person's voice enables a voice hearer to explore at one remove (a safe distance) an element in their own voice hearing while also enabling the other person to develop their observer ego, gain insight, support and confront their voice.

Traumas

Traumas are acknowledged when they emerge into consciousness; with care and, at the client's pace, they are processed as far as the client chooses. The process will not be linear but spirallic with the client sometimes moving away from the painful experience: the therapist must respect the need for distance from over-whelming experiences. Therapy must not retraumatise.

Critics

Internal critics are examined and responded to: processing the criticism to establish what is true and valid as opposed to oppressive, invalid and out of date.

Individual/group therapy

Individual therapy may reinforce isolation and needs to be balanced by a programme of care that offers social activities. Therapy cannot substitute for good housing, creative support, voluntary or paid work, recreation (sport, physical activity), education, but must work with such a package of care. Individual therapy can be a preparation for group therapy.

Therapy groups for people who hear voices and have psychotic experiences are best small: it seems that a group of six is an optimal size but given dropouts it may be wise to start with eight people. People may need support to get to a group: maximising attendance is therapeutic not only for the individual but also for other members of the group. Group therapy may be followed by a period of individual therapy to follow-up issues that emerged in the group, at greater depth.

Time

Therapy with people who hear voices is not likely to be brief: while they can benefit from courses of relaxation, social skills and assertiveness training there will often be a need for long-term supportive counselling and/or creative psychotherapy. Planned breaks in the therapy can provide space to reflect, integrate, review but these may also be difficult if they result in a return to isolation. Group sessions will last between forty-five minutes and two hours, depending on the setting and the clients' needs. The greater the difficulty of the clients in concentrating and relating, the shorter the group.

Time past, present and future

Dramatherapy and psychodrama philosophy and practice emphasise the here and now; there is also the opportunity to rehearse the future: the methods do not promote regression. Past scenes may be revisited in both therapies but this is to gather strength and repair: rehearsal is to empower the person in future, not to repeat the past. *In working with people who have overwhelmingly traumatic pasts, therapy is better focused in the here and now* (see Coursey, 1995: 289, 297; Stanton *et al.*, 1984).

Closure

At closure the person should be offered support or enabled to find a self-help network: to end therapy and return the person to isolation is not helpful. Therefore a therapeutic task in the final period is to help the person focus on what they need for the future and enable them, and the services supporting them, to put such social supports into place before the close of therapy. People can move on from creative therapy to creative activities in the community.

Gentle courage

Dramatherapists have proceeded gently, cautiously. Moreno's heroic vision of the possibilities of psychodramatising hallucinations and delusions can inspire and deserves further exploration. We need both: caution and modesty emboldened by courage and spontaneity within a safe, structured, well-supported therapeutic environment.

It is my sincere hope that this volume (*whelm*: see Appendix 3) enables the development of safe and effective practice with people who hear voices and have psychotic experiences: that it empowers therapists and clients to work together towards recovery.

Afterword

A journey through an innovative book is a journey through a new landscape: pieces of topography, that perhaps have been seen before, are gathered together in new constellations and relationships, thus creating new ways of understanding. A journey through ourselves is also a new way of understanding, listening to our own voices and making manifest the dialogues with our inner as well as our outer voices. Who does not hear voices? It is only when the voices disable us and threaten to take us over, that we need the support of therapists like John Casson, in order to achieve some degree of balance.

He has created this new landscape with his thorough and comprehensive research of people who hear voices, carried out over six years. Very importantly he includes feedback from the people with whom he conducted his research, which focuses on the types of intervention that participants found most helpful or least helpful for their particular unwell being. This honest approach to participant feedback should be widespread in clinical practice. It brings a reality to what can often become rarefied conjecture concerning our 'professional' observations. Whatever 'measurement' we use in our research, it cannot replace the direct experience of group members. At the end of the day, if we want to know what is effective, 'ask the consumer'! It takes some humility on our part.

John Casson has also integrated a complex web of historical data, which embraces psychological and physical medicine, medical anthropology, theatre and drama, and the emergence of the artistic and action-based therapies. He includes theatre research in relation to psychoanalysis, and brings in key theatre figures such as Antonin Artaud and Goethe. Artaud's understanding of 'madness' through his own lifelong experience is a crucial contribution to theatre and its application in theatre and dramatherapy. Artaud *lived* his madness to its absolute extreme and suffered many years of deprivation, beatings, dousings and electric shocks during his almost nine years of incarceration in several different asylums. Yet his clarity of writing seems to override his behaviours as he manages his experience through the written and theatrical word:

> I say what I have seen and what I believe; and whoever says that I have not seen what I have seen, I will tear off his head.[1]

I was interned at Le Havre on my return from Ireland (from where de Valera's government had me deported on the orders of the Intelligence Service, which found me too revolutionary, that's to say too specifically Irish), I was, as I said, interned at Le Havre for having defended myself on the ship the Washington against an act of aggression which I suffered from a steward and a chief mechanic whom I accused of having been bribed by the police to make me disappear. That act of aggression having failed because the chief mechanic and the steward, who had cunningly entered my cabin with a monkey wrench, left again mad with fright, *I was myself accused of hallucinating* [my emphasis] according to the procedure of all police forces, English or French, which consists of putting in a strait-jacket and throwing into a mental hospital all those whom they have not killed or poisoned.[2]

John Casson reminds us that, historically, people who hear voices were often revered as mystics and prophets and he lists the extraordinary number of well-known people who have heard voices right up until the present day. He also reminds us that shamanistic practice relies on the receiving of wisdom through voices, which can be for prediction or for direct healing. However, the contemporary medical model categorises and dismisses the voices as hallucinations and aberrations. The voices are suppressed by medicine or ridicule, or people learn not to talk about them in order to progress through their treatment towards freedom.

> **Naomi:** Yes, doctor, you are right – there is no baby – I am being very good – I am not being silly anymore. I must not be silly. (in a whisper) But there is a baby, I know there is a baby. Where is she? What did they do to her?
>
> I know what the staff want to hear from me, if I am going to ease up on the medication and no more ECT. No talk of babies or they'll say I'm getting worse.[3]

This book weaves together the threads from psychiatry, theatre, shamanism, dramatherapy and psychodrama and allows us to understand the central position of theatre in this applied work. Theatre not only as tragedy but also, very importantly, as comedy is essential to the process of healing. How often we forget the therapeutic effect of laughter and fun. The staff of a long-stay psychiatric hospital, where I am currently working in Romania, spoke of the pleasure of seeing patients able to laugh again, after intensive theatre and dramatherapy work. We created their holiday for them, since they were unable to leave the hospital. We explained that we were bringing a holiday to them; and this did not preclude in depth dramatherapy with people, several of whom hear voices, through embodiment-projection-role. We included work with the Russian nesting dolls.

I believe that John Casson has written for the future. He presents a model of practice both for research and clinical application and rehabilitation. He dares to allow the people in his groups and one-to-one work, to find their own authentic voice and speak of their experiences without fear of ridicule and punishment. They also find their own voice of experience of their treatment programme without feeling they have to please doctors and therapists.

Trainers in all the artistic and performative therapies, especially those who are training dramatherapists or psychodramatists, should place this book on the essential reading list. Students will be reassured that they can undertake placements within psychiatry and really understand why they are applying dramatherapy. It is also an important book for psychological medicine of all orientations.

I hope this book will help us all to take a more humane attitude towards the many hearers of voices. Especially as we are living in an age of instant answers, 'reality entertainment', and fast-lane living, this book reminds us to be more reflective and to remember the fun and poetry in our lives.

Dr Sue Emmy Jennings
Consultant Dramatherapist and Author
Glastonbury UK and Zarnesti Romania

References

1 Artaud, A. *Collected Works V11: Heliogabalus and The New Revelation of Being, Letters*. Gallimard: Paris, 1976.
2 *Collected Works X1*: letters written at Rodez 1945–46 Gallimard: Paris, 1976.
3 Jennings, S. (2001) *Silver Apples of the Moon: an unquiet journey*. Original play on women and madness.

Voices interview

This interview is based on Romme (1994), a version of which appears in Romme and Escher (2000).

1   Do you hear voices?
2   What voices do you hear? (comment on their tone, volume, nature, age, gender)

- voice 1:
- voice 2:
- voice 3:

(a)   Do you know who they are/to whom they belong?
(b)   Have they names?
(c)   Where do they come from?
(d)   When did you first hear the voices?
(e)   How do you understand them? (e.g. What theory or explanation for the voices do you have?)
(f)   When do you usually hear voices?
(g)   Are there other times you hear voices? Such as:
(h)   What do they usually say?

3   How often do you hear voices?
4   Are you hearing voices now?
5   What are the voices saying now?
6   What do you feel about your voices?
7   What do your voices have to say about me asking about them?
8   What do your voices have to say about you taking part in this research?
9   What do you find helpful in coping with the voices?
10   What do you find unhelpful in coping with the voices?
11   Do you ever do things the voices tell you to? Such as:
12   Have the voices ever told you to harm yourself?
13   What happened then? (What did you do/how did you cope?)

14 Have the voices ever told you to harm someone else? What did you do/how did you cope with that?

15 Do you ever talk with your voices?

16 Do you have other experiences like this such as seeing images that others cannot see?

Appendix 2

The etymology of 'whelm'

Further research in the etymology of the word whelm led to the following interesting discoveries.

> whelm (hwelm): 1. intr: to overturn, capsize.
> 2. v. trans To turn (a hollow vessel) upside down or over or upon something so as to cover it. (Simpson and Weiner, 1989)

> hwealf: an arched or vaulted ceiling. (Bosworth, 1882)

In one ancient source the sky is likened to such a containing bowl or vaulted arch covering the earth.

The essential idea here is turning and covering.

As v is sometimes interchangeable with w (volv = wolw) I wondered then if there was a link between the word *whelm* and the word *volume*. The root of the latter is volvo/volvere: Latin for *turn* or *roll*.

> volume: volumen: coil, wreath, *roll*
> 1 a roll of parchment
> 2 a book
> (Simpson and Weiner, 1989)

> volvere: to roll, wind, turn round, twist round.
> volumen: anything rolled.
> volva (vulva) 1 any *covering*, husk, *shell* (which is a container)
> 2 the womb (which is a container) (Simpson, 1968)

(Note: **Cheryll** said that dramatherapy brings you out of your *shell*. An implicit image here is of *re-birth*. A *whelk* is a shell, a marine gastropod mollusc that clings, *attached* to the rocks to survive the overwhelming waves. It is a convex dome, a 'turned over' shell. A *whelp* is a young, *new born* animal. The word *shell* also contains the idea of covering, containing and the root *hel* within it, see below.)

Whelm also contains the idea of *rolling*: M.E. wheluen, whelven: hwelfen: 'He hwelfde at þare sepulchre-dure enne grete ston.' = He rolled (or turned) a great stone at the door of the sepulchre (Skeat, 1910). I then further hypothesised a connection between the words whelm and wheel.

Thus I realised there was a connection between the origin of the words *volume*, *whelm*, *roll* and *role*. A role was originally a roll of parchment or hide on which the script for the actor was written. My suggestion then in Chapter 7 that a role can be a whelm or container for the flow of emotion is entirely accurate. Can this be healing?

I then made a connection with the origins of the word heal: hele or hel.

Hel (which is contained within the word w*hel*m) originates from an Ayran root: **kel** as in the Latin celare: to hide, as in *conceal* and *occult*. It therefore retains the idea of cover. Hell is the place of the dead, covered by the earth: an abyss where they are overwhelmed, lost/hidden. A *helmet* covers (and so protects) the head.

hele: to hide, keep secret, cover: to keep silent. (Shipley, 1957)

Originally then a healer was one who covered up, concealed: there is even a suggestion that a healer was one who deceived. This is initially a surprising derivation as we perhaps like to think of healers as transparently honest: people of integrity. To heal a wound (a whelk, wheal, weal) however it may be best to cover it with a bandage or poultice. As wounds heal they are covered by a scab. A shaman might well dissemble, use tricks, masks, hide equipment or techniques. The placibo effect might heal despite the deceitful trick of the sugar pill. The word 'cover' returns as an idea of healing in the word *recovery*. The healer might keep silent to preserve the confidentiality of the client, keeping secret the source of the distress and so protecting the vulnerable person. A whelm also covers and protects. In the practice of dramatherapy the use of metaphors provides sufficient distance and a cover for the traumatic material which might otherwise overwhelm the client. The method thus protects the vulnerable. The w*hel*m is *hel*pful: indeed the words *health*, *help* and *well* are all connected. The water metaphor also is implicit in the word well: which contains health giving water that may be channelled through a whelm.

Purchasing the Five Story Self Structure

The Five Story Self Structure is being further developed as a method for group work. It has been used in group therapy and a co-operative game of free association and storytelling, Quintessence, has been developed (patent applied for). It has also been used in team building. The Five Story Self Structure is now available for purchase, with instructions, from:

Dr John Casson, Inscape Creative Psychotherapy and Counselling Service, Room 5, St Chads' Offices, Uppermill, Saddleworth, Oldham, OL3 6AP, UK or enquire through email: joncassun@beeb.net

www.quintessence5story.net

Comparative costings: hospital, medication and therapy

It is useful to be able, in these cost-conscious times, to compare the costs of different methods of treatment. I have therefore researched this to counter the myth that therapy is an expensive luxury.

Hospital

For the year 2001–2002

One day in-patient psychiatric bed cost	£191.21
Seven days:	£1,338.47
Thirty days:	£5,736.30
Three months:	£17,208.90

Figures taken from the Annual Financial Returns of NHS Trusts, 2001–2002.

Medication

In considering the cost of medications I am presenting the highest, middle and lowest costs of a range of medications: there are many gradations of dose and cost between these.

Atypical anti-psychotic medication per person per year: £3,758
(Risperidone 16mg daily)

£1,423
(Risperidone 6mg daily)

£523
(Zotepine 75mg daily)

Typical anti-psychotic medication per person per year: £529
(Sulpiride 1600 mg daily)

£226
(Holperidol 30 mg daily)

£37
(Chlorpromazine 75 mg daily)

Figures provided by the Pharmaceutical Adviser to Oldham Primary Care Trust based upon MIMS, March 2003 and Drug Tariff: these are for costs of medication dispensed in Primary Care.

Dramatherapy and psychodrama

In costing these I have added half-an-hour to individual therapy for preparation and note-taking afterwards costing an individual session at one and a half hours; for group therapy I have likewise costed a two-hour group session as three hours, including one hour for preparation and note-taking afterwards. I have chosen the highest grade of the senior 1 dramatherapy scale to ensure that these costings are not underestimates.

Senior I dramatherapist

Point 05 on the PV 13 scale: £26,055 from April 2002 (36 hours a week.)

Superannuation	£1,824
National insurance	£1,973
Total cost of dramatherapist	£29,852

One hour individual session:	£23.92
One year (forty-five sessions):	£1,076.39

Group session £47.84 (divided by six clients):	£7.97 per client
Twenty sessions £956.79 (divided by six clients):	£159.46 per client

Psychodrama psychotherapist

Point 31 on psychotherapist scale: £26,293 – from April 2002 (36 hours a week.)

Superannuation	£1,841
National insurance	£1,995
Total cost of psychodramatist	£30,129

One hour individual session: £24.14
One year (forty-five sessions):   £1,086.30

Group session £48.28 (divided by six clients):   £8.05 per client
Twenty sessions £965.67 (divided by six clients):   £160.95 per client

The Morenean method of psychodramatising suicidal ideation

Suicide is psychodramatically enacted but not without proper precautions taken, both during the action itself and afterwards; the patient is carefully monitored throughout this phase. One of the basic approaches here, after having enacted the suicide, is facing the consequences of this act by posing the question: Who will be most affected by your death? The answer provides the key for the next scene; the patient is warmed up to the role of that most affected other and put in role reversal; it may be a child, a lover, a mate, a parent, etc. An auxiliary ego is placed in the role of the patient. In the reversed role position, the patient is confronted with his or her own behaviour as well as with the issues cast up by the suicide and the interpersonal turmoil which the suicide engenders.

When the patient is unable to answer the question, or denies that anyone will be affected, a thorough exploration of the social atom is required. We have found that suicidal patients often have a phantom social atom, a 'death social atom' which includes loved persons who have died or are dying, thus pulling the patient into the death whirlpool. These are then the persons whose roles have to be taken by the patient in order to clarify the effects of the suicidal act. Once this purging has taken place the 'social atom of life' has to be explored in order to find suitable replacements there, the rekindling of contacts with potentially helpful agents in life itself. The pull towards death must be neutralised by a productive engagement in life.

(Z. Moreno and J. D. Moreno, 1984: 30–31)

My own view is that the actual act of suicide should not be rehearsed but the motivation for the act and the consequences, as above, should be explored and worked through.

References

Allen, J. (1994) 'An Exploration: does dramatherapy help clients with schizophrenia?' *Journal of the British Association for Dramatherapists*, vol 16, pp. 12–22.

Andersen-Warren, M. (1992) 'The Revenger's Tragedy: from spectators to participants', *Journal of the British Association for Dramatherapists*, vol. 14, pp. 4–8.

Andersen-Warren, M. (1996) 'Therapeutic Theatre', in S. Mitchell (ed.) *Dramatherapy Clinical Studies*, London, Jessica Kingsley.

Andersen-Warren, M. and Grainger, R. (2000) *Practical Approaches to Dramatherapy*, London, Jessica Kingsley.

Armstrong, F. (1996) The Unique Voice that Lives Inside Us All, in J. Pearson (ed.) *Discovering the Self through Drama and Movement: The Sesame Approach*, London, Jessica Kingsley.

Armstrong-Perlman, E. M. (1995) 'Psychosis: The Sacrifice that Fails?' in J. Ellwood (ed.) *Psychosis: Understanding and Treatment*, London, Jessica Kingsley.

Artaud, A. (1958) *The Theatre and its Double*, New York, Grove Press.

Ayckbourn, A. (1989) *Woman in Mind*, London, Faber and Faber.

Baars, B. J. (1997) *In the Theatre of Consciousness: The Workspace of the Mind*, New York, Oxford University Press.

Baarrs, M. (1996) 'Making the Present Come Alive', in J. Pearson (ed.) *Discovering the Self through Drama and Movement: The Sesame Approach*, London, Jessica Kingsley.

Bannister, A. (1997) *The Healing Drama: Psychodrama and Dramatherapy with Abused Children*, London, Free Association Press.

Bannister, A. (2000) 'Prisoners of the Family: Psychodrama with Abused Children', in P. F. Kellermann and M. K. Hudgins (eds) *Psychodrama with Trauma Survivors: Acting Out your Pain*, London, Jessica Kingsley.

Bannister, A. (2002) 'The Effects of Creative Therapies with Children who have been Sexually Abused', *Journal of the British Association of Dramatherapists*, vol. 25, no. 1, pp. 3–9.

Bannister, A. (2003) *Creative Therapies with Traumatised Children*, London and Philadelphia, PA, Jessica Kingsley.

Barrie, J. M. (1998) *Dear Brutus*, London, Samuel French (first published 1923, London, Hodder and Stoughton).

Beckett, S. (1954) *Waiting for Godot*, New York, Grove Press.

Bellack, A. S., Turner, S. M., Hersen, M. and Luber, R. F. (1984) 'An Examination of the Efficacy of Social Skills Training for Chronic Schizophrenic Patients', *Hospital and Community Psychiatry*, vol. 35, pp. 1023–1028.

Benedetti, G. (1983) *Todeslandschaften der Sele* (The soul's death landscapes), Gottingen, Verlag fur Medizinisch Psychologie.

Bentall, R. P. (ed.) (1990) *Reconstructing Schizophrenia*, London, Routledge.

Bielanska, A., Cechnicki, A. and Budzyna-Davidowski, P. (1991) 'Drama Therapy as a Means of Rehabilitation for Schizophrenic Patients', *American Journal of Psychotherapy*, vol. 45, no. 4, pp. 566–575.

Birdfield, T. (1994) 'Structuring the Group Dramatherapeutic Process for the Schizoid Individual: Experiences of a Closed Group', Postgraduate Diploma Project (unpublished), University of Exeter.

Birdfield, T. (1998–1999) 'The Healing Drama and Psychosis 1 and 2', *Journal of the British Association of Dramatherapists*, vol. 20, no. 3, pp. 20–27.

Blatner, A. and Blatner, A. (1988) *Foundations of Psychodrama: History, Theory and Practice*, New York: Springer.

Bleuler, M. (1978) 'The Long-term Course of Schizophrenic Psychoses', in L. C. Wynne, R. I. Cromwell and S. Matthysse (eds) *The Nature of Schizophrenia*, New York, Wiley.

Bloom, S. (1997) *Creating Sanctuary: Towards the Evolution of Sane Societies*, London, Routledge.

Bokun, B. (1986) *Humour Therapy*, London, Vita Books.

Bolton, G. (1979) 'Some Issues Involved in the Use of Role-Play with Psychiatric Patients', *Journal of the British Association of Dramatherapists*, vol. 2, no. 4, pp. 11–13.

Bosga, D. (1993) 'Parapsychology and Hearing Voices', in M. Romme and S. Escher (eds) *Accepting Voices*, London, MIND Publications.

Bosworth, J. (1882) *An Anglo-Saxon Dictionary*, Oxford, Clarendon Press.

Bouchard, S., Vallieres, A., Roy, M., *et al.* (1996) 'Cognitive Restructuring in the Treatment of Psychotic Symptoms in Schizophrenia: A Critical Analysis', *Behaviour Therapy*, vol. 27, pp. 257–277.

Boyle, M. (1990) *Schizophrenia: A Scientific Delusion?* London, Routledge.

Brecht, S. (1969) *Revolution at the Brooklyn Academy of Music, The Drama Review*, ed. R. Schechner, vol. 13, no. 3 (T43), New York University.

Breggin, P. (1993) *Toxic Psychiatry*, London, HarperCollins.

Bremner, J. D., Krystal, J. H., Charney, D. S. and Southwick, S. M. (1996) 'Neural Mechanisms in Dissociative Amnesia for Childhood Abuse: Relevance to the Current Controversy surrounding "False Memory Syndrome"', *American Journal of Psychiatry*, July, 153, p. 7 (Suppl. 71).

Browne, R. (1843) Crichton Royal Institution Case Books (Case 193) vol. 3.

Browne, W. A. F. (1837) *What Asylums Were, Are, and Ought to Be*, Edinburgh, Adam and Charles Black.

Brun, B., Pedersen, E. W. and Runberg, M. (1993) *Symbols of the Soul, Therapy and Guidance through Fairy Tales*, London, Jessica Kingsley.

Burke, A. (1984) Racism and Psychiatric Distress Among West Indians in Britain, *International Journal of Social Psychiatry*, vol. 30, pp. 50–68.

Byron, G. G. (Lord) (1970) *Poetical Works*, ed. F. Page, J. Jump (new edition), Oxford, Oxford University Press.

Carlyn, K. (1997) 'After the Red House', *Voices Magazine*, issue 18, pp. 6–7.

Carney, F. (1952) *The Righteous are Bold*, Dublin, James Duffy.

Carriere, J-C. (1988) *The Mahabharata*, London, Methuen.

Casson, J. (1979) 'Shamanistic Elements of Oriental Theatre with Special Reference to the Traditional Forms of Drama in Sri Lanka', unpublished MA thesis, University of Birmingham.

Casson, J. (1984) 'The Therapeutic Dramatic Community Ceremonies of Sri Lanka', *Journal of the British Association for Dramatherapists*, vol. 7, no. 2, pp. 11–18.

Casson, J. (1986) 'Starting Life as a Dramatherapist', *Journal of the British Association for Dramatherapists*, vol. 9, no. 2, pp. 25–32.

Casson, J. (1990) 'Dramatherapy into Psychodrama: An Account of a Therapy Group for Women Survivors of Sexual Abuse (with Pam Corti)', *Journal of the British Psychodrama Association*, vol. 5, no. 2, pp. 37–53.

Casson, J. (1994) 'The Therapeutic Elements of Drama', *Newsletter of the British Association for Dramatherapists*, Spring, pp. 10–11.

Casson, J. (1995) 'The Therapeutic Value of Performance', *Newsletter of the British Association for Dramatherapists*, Summer, pp. 10–13.

Casson, J. (1997–1998) 'Shamanism, Dramatherapy and Psychodrama', *Cahoots Magazine*, 62, pp. 52–56; 63, pp. 55–56; 64, pp. 56–60; 65, pp. 49–56.

Casson, J. (1997a) 'Psychodrama in Individual Psychotherapy', *Journal of the British Psychodrama Association*, vol. 12, nos 1 and 2, pp. 5–20.

Casson, J. (1997b) 'Dramatherapy History in Headlines: Who did What, When, Where?', *Journal of the British Association for Dramatherapists*, vol. 19, no. 2, pp. 10–13.

Casson, J. (1997c) 'The Therapeusis of the Audience', in S. Jennings (ed.) *Dramatherapy Theory and Practice 3*, London, Routledge.

Casson, J. (1998a) 'The Stage: The Theatre of Psychodrama', in P. Holmes and M. Karp (eds) *The Handbook of Psychodrama*, London, Routledge.

Casson, J. (1998b) 'The Hall of Mirrors: the Mirror Technique in Dramatherapy, Psychodrama and Playback Theatre', *Journal of the British Psychodrama Association*, vol. 13, nos 1 and 2, pp. 2–21.

Casson, J. (1998c) 'Right/Left Brain and Dramatherapy', *Journal of the British Association for Dramatherapists*, vol. 20, no. 1, pp. 12–15.

Casson, J. (1999a) 'Evreinoff and Moreno: Monodrama and Psychodrama, Parallel Developments or Hidden Influences?', *Journal of the British Psychodrama Association*, vol. 14, nos 1 and 2, pp. 20–30.

Casson, J. (1999b) 'Dramatherapy, Psychodrama and Dreamwork', *Journal of British Association for Dramatherapists*, vol. 21, no. 1, pp. 15–18.

Casson, J. (2000a) 'Maxwell Jones: Dramatherapy and Psychodrama, 1942–9', *Journal of the British Association of Dramatherapists*, vol. 22, no. 2, pp. 18–21.

Casson, J. (2000b) 'Dramatherapy, Psychodrama and Dance Movement Therapy', (article reprinted from 1995), *Journal of the British Psychodrama Association*, vol 15, no. 2, pp. 41–65.

Casson, J. (2001a) 'J. W. von Goethe and J. C. Reil: Theatre Therapy One Hundred Years before Moreno', *British Journal of Psychodrama and Sociodrama*, vol. 16, no. 2, pp. 118–127.

Casson, J. (2001b) 'The Social, Role and Cultural Atoms', *British Journal of Psychodrama and Sociodrama*, vol 16, no. 2, pp. 15–22.

Casson, J. (2002) 'Dramatherapy and Psychodrama as Psychotherapeutic Interventions with People Who Hear Voices (auditory hallucinations)', unpublished PhD thesis, Manchester Metropolitan University.

Cattanach, A. (1994) 'The Developmental Model of Dramatherapy', in S. Jennings,

A. Cattanach, S. Mitchell, A. Chesner and B. Meldrum (eds) *The Handbook of Dramatherapy*, London, Routledge.

Chadwick, P. K. (1992) *Borderline: A Psychological Study of Paranoia and Delusional Thinking*, London, Routledge.

Chadwick, P. K. (1997) *Schizophrenia: The Positive Perspective*, London, Routledge.

Chadwick, P., Birchwood, M. and Trower, P. (1996) *Cognitive Therapy for Delusions, Voices and Paranoia*, Chichester, Wiley.

Chu, J. A. and Dill, D. L. (1990) 'Dissociative Symptoms in Relation to Childhood Physical and Sexual Abuse', *American Journal of Psychiatry*, 161 (suppl. 18), pp. 145–153.

Clayton, M. (1994) 'Role Theory and its Application in Clinical Practice', in P. Holmes, M. Karp, and M. Watson (eds) *Psychodrama since Moreno*, London, Routledge.

Coleman, R. (1998) Opinions given to John Casson during research interview: unpublished research document.

Coleman, R. (1999) *Recovery an Alien Concept*, Gloucester, Handsell.

Coleman, R. (2001) Statement in article on the Inaugural Meeting of Scottish Hearing Voices Network, *Voices Magazine*, Summer issue.

Cook, C. (1917) *The Play Way*, London, Heinemann.

Cosgrove S. (1982) 'The Living Newspaper, History, Production and Form', unpublished dissertation, Hull University.

Coursey, R. D., Keller, R. E. and Farrell, E. W. (1995) 'Individual Psychotherapy with Persons with Serious Mental Illness: The Clients' Perspective', *Schizophrenia Bulletin*, vol. 21, no. 2, pp. 283–301.

Cox, M. (1978a) *Coding the Therapeutic Process*, Oxford, Pergamon Press.

Cox, M. (1978b) *Structuring the Therapeutic Process: Compromise with Chaos*, Oxford, Pergamon Press.

Cox, M. (1992) *Shakespeare Comes to Broadmoor: The Performance of Tragedy in a Secure Psychiatric Hospital*, London, Jessica Kingsley.

Cox, M. and Theilgaard, A. (1987) *Mutative Metaphors in Psychotherapy: The Aeolian Mode*, London, Tavistock.

Cox, M. and Theilgaard, A. (1994) *Shakespeare as Prompter*, London, Jessica Kingsley.

Crichton Royal Institution (1844) *Fifth Annual Report of the Hospital*, Dumfries, Crichton Royal Institution.

Crichton Royal Institution (1850) *Eleventh Annual Report of the Hospital*, Dumfries, Crichton Royal Institution.

Csikszentmihalyi, M. (1990) *Flow: The Psychology of Optimal Experience*, New York, Harper and Row.

Deane, W. N. and Hanks, V. A. (1967) 'Helping Chronic Schizophrenic Patients to Experience their True Feelings by Means of Psychodrama', *Group Psychotherapy*, vol. 20, nos 1–2, pp. 43–52.

Dennett, D. C. (1991) *Consciousness Explained*, London, Allen Lane.

Department of Health (DoH) (1999) *National Service Framework for Mental Health, Modern Standards and Service Models*, London, DoH.

Dickinson, E. (1975) *The Complete Poems*, edited by T. H. Johnson, London, Faber and Faber.

Diener, G. and Moreno, J. L. (1972) *Goethe and Psychodrama*, Psychodrama and Group Psychotherapy Monograph no. 48, New York, Beacon House (also published 1971 in *Group Psychotherapy and Psychodrama*, vol. 24, no. 1–2).

Dolan, B. (1996) *Perspectives on Henderson Hospital*, Sutton, Surrey, Henderson Hospital.

Dowie, C. (1987) *Adult Child/Dead Child*, Rushden, Northants, Reed Book Services.

Drake, R. E. and Sederer, L. I. (1986) 'The Adverse Effects of Intensive Treatment of Chronic Schizophrenia', *Comprehensive Psychiatry*, vol. 27, no. 4 (July/August), pp. 313–326.

Drury, N. (1989) *The Elements of Shamanism*, London, Elements Books.

Eaton, W. W., Romanoski, A., Anthony, J. C. and Nestadt, G. (1991) 'Screening for Psychosis in the General Population with a Self-report Interview', *Journal of Nervous and Mental Disease*, vol. 179, pp. 689–693.

Edwards, R. (1993) 'The Magic Truth Mirror', *Journal of the British Association for Dramatherapists*, vol. 15, no. 2, pp. 8–12.

Eigen, M. (1993) *The Psychotic Core*, Northvale, NJ, Jason Aronson.

Eliade, M. (1989) *Shamanism: Archaic Techniques of Ecstasy*, London (Penguin) Arkana.

Ellenberger, H. F. (1994) *The Discovery of the Unconscious*, London, Fontana.

Ellwood, J. (1995) *Psychosis: Understanding and Treatment*, London, Jessica Kingsley.

Emunah, R. (1994) *Acting for Real*, New York, Brunner/Mazel.

Engel, G. L. (1977) 'The Need for a New Medical Model: A Challenge for Biomedicine', *Science*, vol. 196, no. 4286, pp. 129–136.

Escher, S., Romme, M. and Buiks, A. (1998) 'Small Talk: Voice Hearing in Children', *Open Mind: The Mental Health Magazine*, no. 29 (July/August), pp. 12–14.

Eshowski, M. (1993) 'Practising Shamanism in a Community Mental Health Centre', *Shamanism*, vol. 5, no. 4 and vol. 6, no. 1 (double issue).

Esquirol, J. D. E. (1832) 'Sur les illusions des sens chez les aliénes', *Archives Générales de Médicine*, vol 2, pp. 5–23.

Estall, P. and Read, A. (1981) 'Dramatherapy and Psychodrama in a Psychiatric Day Hospital', *Journal of the British Association of Dramatherapy*, vol. 4, no.3, pp. 8–11.

Evreinoff, N. (1927) *The Theatre in Life*, New York, Brentano's.

Fairweather, G. W., Simon, R., Gebhard, M. E. *et al.* (1960) 'Relative Effects of Psychotherapeutic Programs: A multicriteria comparison of four programs for three different patient groups', *Psychological Monographs General and Applied*, vol. 74, pp. 1–26.

Ferenczi, S. (1920) 'The Further Development of an Active Therapy in Psycho-Analysis', an address delivered at the Sixth International Congress of Psycho-Analysis, translated by J. I. Suttie and compiled by J. Rickman (1980) *Further Contributions to the Theory and Technique of Psycho-Analysis*, London, Maresfield Reprints.

Fisher, S. and Greenberg, R. (1989) *The Limits of Biological Treatments for Psychological Distress*, Hillside, NJ, Lawrence Erlbaum.

Fontaine, P. (1999) *Psychodrama Training: A European View*, Leuven, Belgium, Federation of European Psychodrama Training Organisations.

Forrester, J. (1980) *Language and the Origins of Psychoanalysis*, London, Macmillan.

Fox, J. (1987) *The Essential Moreno*, New York, Springer.

Frederick, J. and Cotanch, P. (1995) 'Self-Help Techniques for Auditory Hallucinations in Schizophrenia', *Issues in Mental Health Nursing*, vol 16, no. 3 (May–June), pp. 213–224.

Freud, S. (1911) 'Psycho-analytical notes on an autobiographical account of a case of paranoia (dementia paranoides)', *Standard Edition*, vol.11, London: Hogarth.

Freud, S. (1924) 'The Loss of Reality in Neurosis and Psychosis', reprinted in A. Richards (ed.) Penguin Freud Library, vol. 10, London, Penguin.

Freud, S. (1926) 'Inhibitions, Symptoms and Anxiety', *Standard Edition*, vol. 17, London: Hogarth.

Freud, S. and Breuer, J. (1973) *Studies on Hysteria*, Penguin Freud Library, vol. 3, London, Penguin.

Fyfe, W. H. (1967) *Aristotle's Art of Poetry*, Oxford: Clarendon Press.

Gersie, A. (1987) 'Dramatherapy and Play', in S. Jennings (ed.) *Dramatherapy: Theory and Practice for Teachers and Clinicians*, London, Croom Helm.

Gersie, A. (1990) *Storymaking in Education and Therapy*, London, Jessica Kingsley.

Gersie, A. (1997) *Reflections on Therapeutic Storymaking*, London, Jessica Kingsley.

Goethe, J. W. von (1973) *Lila, a Play with Song and Poetry in Four Acts*, translated by O. Danielsson, published privately by O. Danielsson.

Goethe, J. W. von (1989) *Wilhelm Meister's Apprenticeship*, translated by E. A. Blackall and V. Lange, New York, Suhrkamp.

Goldberg, D. and Huxley, P. (1992) *Common Mental Disorders: A Bio-Social Model*, London, Routledge.

Goldman, E. E. and Morrison, D. S. (1984) *Psychodrama: Experience and Process*, Dubuque, IA, Kendall/Hunt.

Goldschmied, E. (1987) 'Creative Play with Babies', in S. Jennings (ed.) *Creative Therapy*, Banbury, Dramatherapy Consultants in Association with Kemble Press.

Goldstein, M. (1991) 'Psychosocial (Nonpharmacologic) Treatments for Schizophrenia', *Review of Psychiatry*, vol. 10, pp. 116–135.

Goleman, D. (1996) *Emotional Intelligence*, London, Bloomsbury Paperbacks.

Grainger, R. (1990) *Drama and Healing*, London, Jessica Kingsley.

Grainger, R. (1992) 'Dramatherapy and Thought Disorder', in S. Jennings S. (ed.), *Dramatherapy Theory and Practice 2*, London, Routledge.

Grainger, R. (1995) *The Glass of Heaven: The Faith of the Dramatherapist*, London, Jessica Kingsley.

Greenberg, I. A. (ed.) (1975) *Psychodrama Theory and Therapy*, London, Souvenir Press.

Greenfield, S. (2002) *The Private Life of the Brain*, London, Penguin.

Grimmelshausen, H. J. C. von (1999) *Simplicissimus*, a new translation by Mike Mitchell, Sawtry, Cambs, Dedalus.

Grinspoon, L., Ewalt, J. R. and Shader, R. I. (1972) *Schizophrenia: Pharmacotherapy and Psychotherapy*, Baltimore, MD, Williams and Wilkins.

Grof, S. (1986) 'Introduction', *Revision*, vol. 8, no. 2, pp. 3–4.

Grotowski, J. (1968) *Towards a Poor Theatre*, New York, Simon and Shuster.

Gruber, L. N., Mangat, B., Balinder, S. and Abou-Taleb, H. (1984) 'Laterality of Auditory Hallucinations in Psychiatric Patients', *American Journal of Psychiatry*, vol. 141, pp. 586–588.

Haddock, G. (1995) 'Stress and Hearing Voices', *Hearing Voices Magazine*, issue 16, p. 6.

Haddock, G. and Bentall, R. P. (1993) 'Focusing', section in Chapter 10, in M. Romme and S. Escher (eds) *Accepting Voices*, London, MIND Publications.

Haddock, G. and Slade, P. (1996) *Cognitive-Behavioural Interventions with Psychotic Disorders*, London, Routledge.

Hage, P. (2003) 'Losing our voices', *Voices Magazine*, Spring.

Haggard, E. A. (1964) 'Isolation and Personality', in P. Worchel and D. Byrne (eds) *Personality Change*, London, Wiley.

Harms, E. (1957) 'Modern Psychotherapy – 150 Years Ago', *Journal of Mental Science*, vol. 103, pp. 804–809.

Harms, E. (1960) 'Johann Christian Reil', *American Journal of Psychiatry*, vol. 116, pp. 1037–1039.

Harris, J. B. (1997) 'Working with Psychosis', unpublished training handout.

Harrison, G., Amin, S., Singh, S. P., Croudace, T. and Jones, P. (1999) 'An Increased Incidence of Psychiatric Disorders Repeatedly Reported among African-Caribbeans in the UK', *British Journal of Psychiatry*, vol. 175, pp. 127–134.

Harrow, G. (1952) 'Psychodrama Group Therapy: Its Effects upon the Role Behaviour of Schizophrenic Patients, Group Psychotherapy', *Journal of Sociopathology and Sociatry*, vol. 5, nos 1, 2 and 3, pp. 316–320.

Healy, D. (1993) *Psychiatric Drugs Explained*, London, Mosby Year Book Europe.

Hillman, J. (1983) *Archetypal Psychology: A Brief Account*, Dallas, TX: Spring.

Hogarty, G., Anderson, C. M., Reiss, D. J. *et al.* (1986) 'Family Education, Social Skills Training and Maintenance Chemotherapy in the Aftercare of Schizophrenia', *Archives of General Psychiatry*, vol. 45, pp. 633–642.

Hogman, G. and Sandamas, G. (2000) *A Question of Choice* (Survey by NSF, Mind, MDF), London, National Schizophrenia Fellowship.

Honig, A. (1992) 'Psychotherapy with Command Hallucinations in Chronic Schizophrenia: the use of action techniques within a surrogate family setting', *Journal of the British Psychodrama Association*, vol. 7, no. 2, pp. 19–37.

Hudgins, M., Druker, K. and Metcalf, K. (2000) 'The Containing Double', *British Journal of Psychodrama and Sociodrama*, vol. 15, no. 1, pp. 58–77.

Hunter, R. and Macalpine, I. (1964) *Three Hundred Years of Psychiatry*, London, Oxford University Press.

Iljine, V. (1909) 'Improvising Theatre Play in the Treatment of Mood Disorders', paper published in Russian, Kiev, quoted by H. Petzold (1973) *Gestalttherapie und Psychodrama*, Nicol, Kassel.

Iljine, V. (1910) 'Patients Play Theatre: a way of healing body and mind', paper published in Russian, quoted by H. Petzold (1973) *Gestalttherapie und Psychodrama*, Nicol, Kassel.

James, A. (2001) *Raising our Voices: An Account of the Hearing Voices Movement*, Gloucester, Handsell.

James, W. (1890/1950) *The Principles of Psychology, vol 1*, New York: Dover (original work published 1890).

Janet, P. (1889) *L'Automatisme psychologique: Essay de psychologie experimentale sur les formes inferieures de l'activite humaine*, Paris, Felix Alcan. Reprinted 1973, Paris, Société Pierre Janet/Payot.

Jaynes, J. (1990) *The Origin of Consciousness in the Breakdown of the Bicameral Mind*, London, Penguin.

Jenkyns, M. (1996) *The Play's the Thing*, London, Routledge.

Jennings, S. (1990) *Dramatherapy with Families, Groups and Individuals: Waiting in the Wings*, London, Jessica Kingsley.

Jennings, S. (1992) 'The Nature and Scope of Dramatherapy', in M. Cox (ed.) *Shakespeare Comes To Broadmoor*, London, Jessica Kingsley.

Jennings, S. (1996) 'Brief Dramatherapy: The Healing Power of the Dramatised Here and Now', in A. Gersie (ed.) *Dramatic Approaches to Brief Therapy*, London, Jessica Kingsley.

Jennings, S. (ed.) (1997) *Dramatherapy Theory and Practice 3*, London, Routledge.

Jennings, S. (1998) *Introduction to Dramatherapy: Theatre and Healing. Ariadne's Ball of Thread*, London, Jessica Kingsley.

Jennings, S. and Minde, A. (1995) *Art Therapy and Dramatherapy: Masks of the Soul*, London, Jessica Kingsley.

Jennings, S., Cattanach, A., Mitchell, S., Chesner, A. and Meldrum, B. (1994) *The Handbook of Dramatherapy*, London, Routledge.

Johnson, D. (1981) 'The Schizophrenic Condition', in G. Schattner and R. Courtney (eds) *Drama in Therapy 2*, New York, Drama Books Specialists.

Johnson, D. R. (1984) 'Representation of the Internal World in Catatonic Schizophrenia', *Psychiatry*, vol. 47, no. 4, pp. 299–314.

Johnson, D. R. (1992) 'The Dramatherapist in Role', in S. Jennings (ed.), *Dramatherapy Theory and Practice 2*, London, Routledge.

Jones, P. (1996) *Drama as Therapy, Theatre as Living*, London, Routledge.

Jung, C. G. (1972) *Man and his Symbols*, London, Aldus.

Jung, C. G. (1974) *Dreams*, translated by R. F. C. Hull, London, Routledge and Kegan Paul.

Kagan, J. (1994) *Galen's Prophecy*, New York, Basic Books.

Karon, B. and VandenBos, G. (1981) *The Psychotherapy of Schizophrenia: The Treatment of Choice*, New York, Jason Aronson.

Kellermann, P. F. and Hudgins, M. K. (2000) *Psychodrama with Trauma Survivors: Acting Out your Pain*, London, Jessica Kingsley.

Kelly, G. A. (1955) *The Psychology of Personal Constructs*, vols I and II, New York, Norton.

Killick, K. (1995) 'Working with Psychotic Processes in Art Therapy', in J. Ellwood (ed.) *Psychosis: Understanding and Treatment*, London, Jessica Kingsley.

Killick, K. and Schaverien, J. (1997) *Art, Psychotherapy and Psychosis*, London, Routledge.

Kipper, D. A. (1986) *Psychotherapy through Clinical Role Playing*, New York, Brunner/Mazel.

Kushner, T. (1992a) *Angels in America, a Play, Part One: Millennium Approaches*, London, Nick Hern.

Kushner, T. (1992b) *Angels in America, a Play, Part Two: Perestroika*, London, Nick Hern.

Lacan, J. (1997) *Ecrits: A Selection*, translated by A. Sheridan, London, Routledge.

Lahad, M. (1992) 'Story-making in Assessment Method for Coping with Stress: six-piece story-making and BASIC Ph', in S. Jennings (ed.) *Dramatherapy Theory and Practice 2*, London, Routledge.

Laing, R. D. (1960) *The Divided Self*, London, Penguin.

Landy, R. (1986) *Drama Therapy Concepts and Practices*, Springfield, IL: Charles Thomas.

Landy, R. (1993) *Persona and Performance: The Meaning of Role in Drama, Therapy, and Everyday Life*, London, Jessica Kingsley.

Landy, R. (1996) *Essays in Drama Therapy: The Double Life*, London, Jessica Kingsley.

Langley, D. (1983) *Dramatherapy and Psychiatry*, London, Croom Helm.

Leudar, I. and Thomas, P. (2000) *Voices of Reason, Voices of Insanity*, London, Routledge.

Levinson, H. (1966) 'Auditory Hallucinations in a Case of Hysteria', *British Journal of Psychiatry*, vol. 112, pp. 19–26.

Lewis, P. (1993) *Creative Transformation: The Healing Power of the Arts*, Wilmette, IL, Chiron.

Liddell, H. G. and Scott, R. (1996) *Greek–English Lexicon*, Oxford, Clarendon Press.

Lindkvist, M. (1998) *Bring White Beads When You Call on the Healer*, New Orleans, LA: Rivendell House.

Lindqvist, M. (1994) 'Religion and the Spirit', in P. Holmes, M. Karp and M. Watson (eds) *Psychodrama since Moreno*, London, Routledge.

Littlewood, R. and Lipsedge, M. (1982) *The Aliens and the Alienists: Ethnic Minorities and Psychiatry*, Harmondsworth, Penguin.

Lloyd-Jones, H. (trans.) (1979) *Aeschylus: Oresteia, Eumenides*, London, Gerald Duckworth.

Logan, J. C. (1971) 'Use of Psychodrama and Sociodrama in Reducing Negro Aggression', *Group Psychotherapy and Psychodrama*, vol. 24, pp. 138–149.

Lowenfeld, M. (1935) *Play in Childhood*, London, Gollancz.

McDougall, J. (1986) *Theatres of the Mind*, London, Free Association Press.

McDougall, J. (1989) *Theatres of the Body*, London, Free Association Press.

McGee, T. F., Starr, A., Powers, J., Racusen, F. and Thornton, A. (1965) 'Conjunctive Use of Psychodrama and Group Psychotherapy in a Group Living Program with Schizophrenic Patients', *Group Psychotherapy, American Society of Group Psychotherapy and Psychodrama*, vol. 18, no. 3, pp. 127–135.

McLuskie, M. (1983) 'Dramatherapy in a Psychiatric Hospital', *Journal of the British Association of Dramatherapists*, vol. 6, no. 2, pp. 20–25.

Marineau, R. F. (1989) *Jacob Levy Moreno 1889–1974*, London, Tavistock.

Marshall, R. (1995) 'Schizophrenia: a constructive analogy or a convenient construct?', in J. Ellwood (ed.) *Psychosis: Understanding and Treatment*, London, Jessica Kingsley.

Martensson, L. (1998) *Deprived of Humanity: The Case against Neuroleptic Drugs*, Geneva, The Voiceless (Movement Les Sans-Voix) and Association Ecrivans, Poetes and Cie.

Martin, S. A. (1996) 'I Voice Therefore I Know I Am', *The Arts in Psychotherapy*, vol. 23, no. 3, pp. 261–268.

Martindale, B. V., Bateman, A., Crowe, M. and Margison, F. (2000) *Psychological Approaches and their Effectiveness*, London, Gaskell.

Masson, J. (1989) *Against Therapy*, London, Collins.

Masson, J. (1992) *The Assault on Truth: Freud and Child Sexual Abuse*, London, Fontana.

Mead, G. H. (1934) *Mind, Self and Society*, Chicago, University of Chicago Press.

Meehl, P. E. (1962) 'Schizotaxia, Schizotypia, Schizophrenia', *American Psychologist*, vol. 17, pp. 827–838.

Mehl, L. E. (1988) 'Modern Shamanism: integration of biomedical with traditional world views', in G. Doore (ed.) *Shaman's Path*, Boston, MA, Shambhala.

Mental Health Foundation (MHF) (1997) *Knowing our own Minds*, London, MHF.

Miller, D. (1972) 'Psychodramatic Ways of Coping with Potentially Dangerous Situations in Psychotic and Non-Psychotic Populations', *Group Psychotherapy and Psychodrama*, vol. 25, pp. 57–68.

Miller, M. P. (2000) On *Anatomy of a Madman*, BBC Radio 3, 8 February.

Minkowski, E. (1970) *Schizophrenia, Lived Time*, Evanston, IL: Northwestern University Press.

Mitchell, R. (1987) 'Dramatherapy in In-Patient Psychiatric Settings', in S. Jennings (ed.) *Dramatherapy: Theory and Practice for Teachers and Clinicians*, London, Croom Helm.

Mitchell, S. (1994) 'The Theatre of Self Expression: a "therapeutic theatre" model of dramatherapy', in S. Jennings *et al.*, *The Handbook of Dramatherapy*, London, Routledge.

Mitchell, S. (1996) *Dramatherapy, Clinical Studies*, London, Jessica Kingsley.

Mollon, P. (1996) *Multiple Selves, Multiple Voices: Working with Trauma, Violation and Dissociation*, Chichester, Wiley.

Moreno, J. L. (1939) 'Psychodramatic Shock Therapy', *Sociometry, a Journal of Inter-personal Relations*, vol. 2, no. 1, Psychodrama Monographs no. 5, New York, Beacon House.

Moreno, J. L. (1945a) *A Case of Paranoia Treated through Psychodrama*, Psychodrama Monographs no. 13, New York, Beacon House.

Moreno, J. L. (1945b) *Psychodramatic Treatment of Psychoses*, Psychodrama Monographs no. 15 (first published 1940 in *Sociometry, a Journal of Inter-Personal Relations*, vol. 3), New York, Beacon House.

Moreno, J. L. (1952) *Group Psychotherapy, Psychodrama and Sociometry 4*, New York, Beacon House.

Moreno, J. L. (1965) *The Voice of J. L. Moreno*, interviewed by James Sacks, audiotape, copyright Marcia Karp, New York.

Moreno, J. L. (1971) *The Words of the Father*, New York, Beacon House.

Moreno, J. L. (1983) *The Theatre of Spontaneity*, Ambler, PA, Beacon House.

Moreno, J. L. (1985) *The Principles of Spontaneity: Psychodrama*, 4th edition, vol. 1, Ambler, PA, Beacon House.

Moreno, J. L. (1993) *Who Shall Survive?* Student Edition, Roanoke, VI: American Society of Group Psychotherapy and Psychodrama, Royal Publishing Co.

Moreno, J. L. and Moreno, Z. T. (1970) *Origins of Encounter and Encounter Groups*, Psychodrama and Group Psychotherapy Monographs no. 45, New York, Beacon House.

Moreno, J. L. and Moreno, Z. T. (1975) *Psychodrama Third volume: Action Therapy and Principles of Practice*, New York, Beacon House.

Moreno, Z. T. (1966) *Psychodramatic Rules, Techniques and Adjunctive Methods*, Psychodrama and Group Psychotherapy Monographs no. 41, New York, Beacon House.

Moreno, Z. T. (1978) 'The Function of the Auxiliary Ego in Psychodrama with special reference to Psychotic Patients', *Group Psychotherapy, Psychodrama and Sociometry* (official organ of the American Society of Group Psychotherapy and Psychodrama), vol. 31, pp. 163–166.

Moreno, Z. T. and Moreno, J. D. (1984) 'The Psychodramatic Model of Madness', *Journal of the British Psychodrama Association*, vol. 1, no. 1, pp. 24–34.

Moreno, Z. T., Blomkvist, L. D. and Rutzel, T. (2000) *Psychodrama, Surplus Reality and the Art of Healing*, London, Routledge.

Murphy, G. (1937) 'The Mind is a Stage: adjusting mental problems in a spontaneity theatre', *Forum*, vol. 97, pp. 277–280.

National Institute for Clinical Excellence (NICE) (2003) 'Schizophrenia: core interventions in the treatment and management of schizophrenia in primary and secondary care (NICE guidelines)', taken from the website:. http://www.nice.org.uk/Docref.asp?d=42460.

Nayani, T. H. and David, A. S. (1996) 'The Auditory Hallucination: a phenomenological survey', *Psychological Medicine*, vol. 26, pp. 177–189.

Nettle, D. (2001) *Strong Imagination: Madness, Creativity and Human Nature*, Oxford, Oxford University Press.

Newham, P. (1993) *The Singing Cure*, London, Rider.

Nitsun, M., Stapleton, J. H. and Bender, M. P. (1974) 'Movement and Drama Therapy with Long-stay Schizophrenics', *British Journal of Medical Psychology*, vol. 47, pp. 101–119.

Onions, C. T. (1988) *The Shorter Oxford English Dictionary*, vols I and II, London, Guild Publishing.

Parker, I., Georgaca, E., Harper, D., McLauglin, T. and Stowell-Smith, M. (1995) *Deconstructing Psychopathology*, London, Sage.

Parrish, M. (1959) 'The Effect of Short Term Psychodrama on Chronic Schizophrenic Patients', *Group Psychotherapy, Journal of Sociopathology and Sociatry*, vol. 12, no.1, pp. 15–26.

Pearson, J. (ed.) (1996) *Discovering the Self through Drama and Movement: The Sesame Approach*, London, Jessica Kingsley.

Perry, J. (1974) *The Far Side of Madness*, Englewood Cliffs, NJ, Prentice Hall.

Perry, J. (1986) 'Spiritual emergence and renewal'. *Revision*, vol. 8, no. 2, pp. 33–38.

Perry, J. (1987) *The Self in Psychotic Process*, Dallas, TX, Spring.

Pettiti, G. (1989) 'The Use of Video as an Externalising Object in Drama Therapy', *Journal of the British Association for Dramatherapists*, vol 12, no. 1, pp. 3–9.

Petzold, H. (1973) *Gestalttherapie und Psychodrama*, Nicol, Kassel.

Pinel, P. (1801) *Traite medico-philosophique sur l'alientation mentale*, 2nd edition, Paris, Brosson.

Pirandello, L. (1994) *Six Characters in Search of an Author*, London, Methuen.

Pisk, L. (1990) *The Actor and his Body*, London, Harrap.

Powley, D. (1981–1982) 'Images of Power (on the medium of video)', *Journal of the British Association for Dramatherapists*, vol. 5, nos 3 and 4, Winter/Spring.

Prouty, G. (1986) 'The Pre-Symbolic Structure and Therapeutic Transformation of Hallucinations', in M. Wolpin, J. Storr and L. Kreuger (eds) *Imagery*, vol. 4, New York, Plenum.

Prouty, G. (1990) 'Pre-Therapy: a theoretical volution in the person-centred/experiential psychotherapy of schizophrenia and retardation', in G. Lietaer, J. Rombauts and R. Van Balen (eds) *Client Centred and Experiential Therapy in the Nineties*, Leuven, Leuven University Press.

Prouty, G. (2000) 'Pre-Therapy and the Pre-Expressive Self', in T. Merry (ed.) *Person Centred Practice: The BAPCA Reader*, Ross-on-Wye, PCCS Books (previously published in *Person-Centred Practice*, vol. 6, no. 2, pp. 80–88).

Radmall, B. (1995) 'The Use of Role Play in Dramatherapy', *Journal of the British Association of Dramatherapists*, vol 17, nos 1 and 2, pp. 13–26.

Rauch, S. L., Van Der Kolk, B. A., Fisher, R. E., *et al.* (1996) 'A Symptom Provocation Study of Post-traumatic Stress Disorder using Positron Emission Tomography and Script Driven Imagery', *Archives of General Psychiatry*, vol. 53, pp. 380–387.

Read, J. (1997) 'Child Abuse and Psychosis: A Literature Review and Implications for Professional Practice', *Professional Psychology: Research and Practice*, vol. 28, No. 5, pp. 448–456.

Reich, W. (1980) *Character Analysis*, New York, Farrar, Straus and Giroux.

Reil, J. C. (1803) *Rhapsodien uber die Anwendung der psychischen Cur-Methoden auf Geisteszerruttungen*, Halle, Curt.

Roberts, G. and Holmes, J. (1999) *Healing Stories, Narrative in Psychiatry and Psychotherapy*, Oxford, Oxford University Press.

Rogers, C. (1959) 'A Theory of Therapy, Personality and Interpersonal Relationships as Developed in the Client Centred Framework', in S. Koch (ed.) *Psychology: A Study of Science*, New York, McGraw-Hill.

Romme, M. (1994) Unpublished research questionnaire for assessing people who hear voices, given to me by Prof. Romme.

Romme, M. (1998) *Understanding Voices: Coping with Auditory Hallucinations and Confusing Realities*, Runcorn, Cheshire, Handsell.

Romme, M. (2001) 'Breaking Down Social Taboos', *VOICES Magazine* (Hearing Voices Network, Manchester) Spring, pp. 7–8.

Romme, M. and Escher, S. (1993) *Accepting Voices*, London, MIND Publications.

Romme, M. and Escher, S. (1996) 'Empowering People Who Hear Voices', in G. Haddock and P. Slade (eds) *Cognitive-Behaviour Interventions with Psychotic Disorders*, London, Routledge.

Romme, M. and Escher, S. (2000) *Making Sense of Voices*, London, MIND Publications.

Rosenfeld, H. (1987) *Impasse and Interpretation*, London, Tavistock.

Rosenzweig, S. and Shakow, D. (1937) 'Play Technique in Schizophrenia and Other Psychoses', *American Journal of Orthopsychiatry*, vol. 7, pp. 32–47.

Roth, A. and Fonagy, P. (1996) *What Works for Whom? A Critical Review of Psychotherapy Research*, New York, Guilford Press.

Rowan, J. (1991) *Subpersonalities: The People Inside Us*, London, Routledge.

Rowan, J. (1993) *Discover Your Subpersonalities*, London, Routledge.

Ryle, G. (1990) *The Concept of the Mind*, London, Penguin.

Sachs, O. (1991) *A Leg to Stand On*, London, Picador.

Sarbin, T. (1954) 'Role Theory', in G. Lindzey (ed.) *Handbook of Social Psychology*, vol. 1, Cambridge, MA, Addison-Wesley.

Sayler, O. M. (1922) *The Russian Theatre*, New York, Brentano's.

Schattner, G. and Courtney, R. (eds) (1981) *Drama in Therapy 2*, New York, Drama Books Specialists.

Scheff, T. J. (1979) *Catharsis in Healing, Ritual and Drama*, London, University of California Press.

Schutzenberger, A. (1998) *The Ancestor Syndrome*, London, Routledge.

Scoble, S (1978) 'Dramatherapy with Psychotic Adults', *Journal of the British Association for Dramatherapists*, vol. 1, no. 4, pp. 13–16.

Scull, A. (1979) *Museums of Madness*, London, Penguin.

Scull, A. (ed.) (1991) *The Asylum as Utopia, W. A. F. Browne and the mid-19th Century Consolidation of Psychiatry*, London, Routledge.

Seth-Smith, F. (1997) 'Four Views of the Image', in K. Killick and J. Schaverien (eds) *Art, Psychotherapy and Psychosis*, London, Routledge.

Shepherd, M. (ed.) (1982) *Psychiatrists on Psychiatry*, Cambridge, Cambridge University Press.

Shin, L. M., McNally, R. J., Kosslyn, S. M., *et al.* (1997) 'A Positron Emission Tomography Study of Symptom Provocation in PTSD', *Annals of the New York Academy of Sciences*, vol. 821, pp. 521–523.

Shipley, J. (1957) *Dictionary of Early English*, London, Peter Owen.

Shorter, E. (1997) *History of Psychiatry*, New York, John Wiley.

Simpson, D. P. (1968) *Cassells Latin–English, English–Latin Dictionary*, London, Cassells.

Simpson, J. A. and Weiner, E. S. C. (1989) *Oxford English Dictionary*, Oxford, Clarendon Press.

Sims, A. (1991) *Symptoms in the Mind*, London, Baillière Tindall.

Skeat, W. W. (1910) *An Etymological Dictionary of the English Language*, Oxford, Clarendon Press.

Slade, P. (1980) *Child Drama* (first edition 1954), London, Hodder and Stoughton.

Slade, P. (1995) *Child Play: Its Importance for Human Development*, London, Jessica Kingsley.

Slade, P. and Bentall, R. (1988) *Sensory Deception: Towards a Scientific Analysis of Hallucinations*, London, Croom Helm.

Snow, S. (1996) 'Focusing on Mythic Imagery in Brief Dramatherapy with Psychotic Individuals', in A. Gersie (ed.) *Dramatic Approaches to Brief Therapy*, London, Jessica Kingsley.

Sophocles (1994) *Antigone, Oedipus the King, Electra*, translated by H. D. F. Kitto, Oxford, Oxford University Press.

Spence, J. D. (1985) *The Memory Palace of Matteo Ricci*, London, Penguin.

Spencer, E. (1910) *The Works of Edmund Spencer*, edited by R. Morris, Globe Edition, London, Macmillan.

Spolin, V. (1996) *Improvisation for the Theatre*, Evanston, IL, Northwestern University Press.

Stanton, A. H., Gunderson, J. G., Knapp, P. H., Frank, A. F., Vannicelli, M. L., Schitzer, R. and Rosenthal, R. (1984) 'Effects of Psychotherapy on Schizophrenic Patients: 1: design and implementation of a controlled study', *Schizophrenia Bulletin 10*, pp. 520–563.

Stone, H. and Winkelman, S. (1987) *Embracing our Selves*, San Raphael, CA, New World Library.

Stone, M. (1998) *Healing the Mind*, London, Pimlico.

Thomas, P. (1997) *The Dialectics of Schizophrenia*, London, Free Association Books.

Thompson, E. (1998) *The Actors are Come Hither: A Tribute to Elsie Green*, Philip Walton Partners, Coggers, Leatherhead Road, Oxshott, Surrey, KT22 0ET.

Tien, A. Y. (1991) 'Distribution of Hallucinations in the Population', *Social Psychiatry and Psychiatric Epidemiology*, vol 26, pp. 287–292.

Truax, C. B. (1963) 'Effective Ingredients in Psychotherapy: an approach to unravelling the patient–therapist interaction', *Journal of Counselling Psychology*, vol. 10, pp. 256–263.

Tselikas, E. and Burmeister, J. (1997) 'The Drum, the Mouse and the Boy in the Glass Palace: brief dramatherapy with a client with chronic catatonic schizophrenia', in S. Jennings (ed.) *Dramatherapy Theory and Practice 3*, London, Routledge.

Tsuang, M. T. and Faraone, S. V. (2002) 'Diagnostic Concepts and the Prevention of Schizophrenia', *Canadian Journal of Psychiatry*, vol. 47, no. 7.

van der Wijk, J-B. (1996) 'Brief Dramatherapy with Adolescents', in A. Gersie (ed.) *Dramatic Approaches to Brief Therapy*, London, Jessica Kingsley.

Voices magazine (2002) Hearing Voices Network, 91 Oldham Street, Manchester M4 1LW, Winter issue.

Wallace, C. J. and Liberman, R. P. (1985) 'Social Skills Training for Patients with Schizophrenia: a controlled clinical trial', *Psychiatric Research*, vol. 15, pp. 243–248.

Warmsley, T. (1984) 'Teaching Psychiatry: Scientific Myth', *Bulletin of Royal College of Psychiatrists*, vol. 8, no. 6, pp. 109–110.

Warner, S. (2000) *Understanding Child Sexual Abuse: Making the Tactics Visible*, Gloucester, Handsell.

Watkins, J. (1998) *Hearing Voices: A Common Human Experience*, Melbourne, Australia, Hill of Content.

Wells, H. G. (1911) *Floor Games*, London, Frank Palmer (1931, London, Dent)
http://digital.library.upenn.edu/webbin/gutbook/author?name=Wells%2C%20H.%20G.
http://ibiblio.org/gutenberg/etext03/flrgm10.txt

Wilkins, P. (1997) 'Psychodrama and Research', *British Journal of Psychodrama and Sociodrama*, vol. 12, nos 1 and 2, pp. 44–61.

Winn, L. (1994) *Post Traumatic Stress Disorder and Dramatherapy*, London, Jessica Kingsley.

Winnicott, W. D. (1991) *Playing and Reality*, London, Routledge.

Worchel, P. and Byrne, D. (1964) *Personality Change*, London, Wiley.

Wynne, L. C., Cromwell, R. L. and Matthysse, S. *et al.* (1978) *The Nature of Schizophrenia: New Approaches to Research and Treatment*, New York, Wiley.

Yalom, I. D. (1983) *Inpatient Group Psychotherapy*, New York, Basic Books.

Yalom, I. D. (1985) *The Theory and Practice of Group Psychotherapy*, New York, Basic Books.

Yates, F. R. (1966) *The Art of Memory*, London, Routledge and Kegan Paul.

Young, R. M. (1995) 'The Ubiquity of Psychotic Anxieties', in J. Ellwood (ed.) *Psychosis: Understanding and Treatment*, London, Jessica Kingsley.

Author index

Subject index